THE ROLE OF OXYGEN RADICALS
IN CARDIOVASCULAR DISEASES

THE ROLE OF OXYGEN RADICALS IN CARDIOVASCULAR DISEASES

A Conference in the European Concerted Action on Breakdown in Human Adaptation – Cardiovascular Diseases, held in Asolo, Italy, 2-5 December 1986

edited by

A. L'Abbate
Institute of Clinical Physiology, CNR, Pisa, Italy

and

F. Ursini
Institute of Biochemistry, Padova, Italy

KLUWER ACADEMIC PUBLISHERS
DORDRECHT / BOSTON / LONDON

for the Commission of the European Communities

Library of Congress Cataloging in Publication Data

The Role of oxygen radicals in cardiovascular diseases.

Based on a meeting held in Asolo, Italy on Dec. 2-5, 1986.
"Published for the Commission of the European Communities, Directorate-General Telecommunications, Information Industries, and Innovation, Luxembourg"--T.p. verso.
1. Cardiovascular system--Pathogenesis--Congresses.
2. Active oxygen--Pathophysiology--Congresses.
I. L'Abbate, A. II. Ursini, F. III. Commission of the European Communities. Directorate-General for Telecommunications, Information Industries, and Innovation. [DNLM: 1. Cardiovascular Diseases--etiology--congresses. 2. Free Radicals--congresses.
3. Oxygen--adverse effects--congresses. WG 100 R745 1986]
RC669.R65 1988 616.1'07 88-13706

ISBN-13: 978-94-010-7716-3 e-ISBN-13: 978-94-009-2697-4

DOI: 10.1007/978-94-009-2697-4

Publication arrangements by
Commission of the European Communities
Directorate-General Telecommunications, Information Industries and Innovation, Scientific and Technical Communications Service, Luxembourg

Softcover reprint of the hardcover 1st edition 1988

Published by Kluwer Academic Publishers,
P.O. Box 17, 3300 AA Dordrecht, The Netherlands.

Kluwer Academic Publishers incorporates the publishing programmes of
D. Reidel, Martinus Nijhoff, Dr W. Junk and MTP Press.

Sold and distributed in the U.S.A. and Canada
by Kluwer Academic Publishers,
101 Philip Drive, Norwell, MA 02061, U.S.A.

In all other countries, sold and distributed
by Kluwer Academic Publishers Group,
P.O. Box 322, 3300 AH Dordrecht, The Netherlands.

CONTENTS

PREFACE

Growing experimental evidence is beeing produced in support of the thesis that lipid peroxidation is an important mediator of both vascular and myocardial tissue derangement. Although the role of the free-radical system in human cardiovascular pathology remains speculative, nevertheless the potential implications of such a system in both pharmacological therapy and prevention of major cardiovascular diseases, such as myocardial infarction, cardiomyopathy and arrhythmias, justify the increasing interest of clinical cardiologists in this research area.

Furthermore, present-day clinical cardiology permits to reproduce in man such experimental models as ischemia and reperfusion, e.g. during percutaneous transluminal angioplasty, and even to gain histological and histochemical access to byoptic myocardial tissue.

Upon above premises the idea of a multidisciplinary discussion meeting was conceived, aimed to confront clinical expectations with acquired basic information, and to discuss the validity of experimental models in the light of pathological and clinical findings in man.

To this purpose, a unique group of experts in the field of free-radicals, from all over the world, was asked to make the topic accessible to clinical cardiologists, with the primary aim of projecting results and ideas towards potential clinical research; this is, in fact, the object of the European Concerted Action "Breakdown in Human Adaptation - Cardiovascular Diseases", in the frame of which the meeting was held.

My personal impression is that this experience was profitable for both cardiologists and basic scientists. They are now aware of the risk of a dichotomy between experimental research and clinical reality, and of the need for a more strict collaboration, capable to better orient research towards health care.

Following the meeting, manuscripts were reviewed by the authors, taking into consideration arguments and results emerged during the wide and lively discussion. While on one hand this delayed the publication of the volume, on the other it ensured information updating.

Finally, I wish to thank Professor Fulvio Ursini for his great organizing and editing effort, as well as all the authors and discussants for their precious collaboration.

Antonio L'Abbate

LIST OF CONTRIBUTORS

Dr. Adolfo Alexandre
Istituto di Chimica Biologica
via F. Marzolo 3
I - 35131 Padova

Prof. Giorgio Baroldi
Istituto di Fisiologia Clinica, CNR
Divisione "A. De Gasperis"
Ospedale Niguarda-Cà Granda
Piazza Ospedale Maggiore 3
I - 20162 Milano

Prof. Alberto Bindoli
Istituto di Chimica Biologica
via F. Marzolo 3
I - 35131 Padova

Enrique Cadenas
Dept. of Pathology II
University Hospital
S-58185 Linkoping
Sweden

J.A. Kelvin Davies, Ph.D
University Southern California
Toxicology and Biochemistry
1985 Zonal Avenue
Los Angeles, California 90033
USA

Dr. Thomas L. Dormandy
Dept. Chemical Pathology
Whittington Hospital
St.Mary's Wing
Highgate Hill
London N19 5NF
United Kingdom

Prof. Lars Ernster
Dept. of Biochemistry
Arrhenius Laboratory
University of Stockholm
S - 10691 Stockholm
Sweden

Prof. L. Flohé
Grunenthal GMBH
Center of Research
Zieglerstrasse 6
D - 5100 Aachen, DEN
FRG

Bruce A. Freeman, Ph.D.
Dept. of Anesthesiology
Univ. of Alabama at Birmingham
Birmingham, AL 35294
U.S.A.

Prof. David J. Hearse
The Rayne Institute
St. Thomas' Hospital
London SE1
United Kingdom

Dr. Toshihisa Ishikawa
Institute of Physiological Chemistry I
University of Dusseldorf
Moorenstrasse 5
D 4000 Dusseldorf 1
West Germany

Prof. Jim Kehrer
Institute of Physiological Chemistry I
University of Dusseldorf
Moorenstrasse 5
D 4000 Dusseldorf 1
West Germany

Prof. J.F. Koster
Dept. of Biochemistry I
Medical Faculty
Erasmus University - Rotterdam
POBox 1738
3000 DR Rotterdam
The Netherlands

Dr. D.O. Levitsky
Laboratory of Membranes and Ion Transport
Institute of Experimental Cardiology
USSR Cardiology Research Center
3rd Cherepkovskaya Street 15A
Moscow 121552
USSR

Prof. G.P. Novelli
Istituto Anestesiologia
Policlinico di Careggi
I - 50139 Careggi-Firenze

Prof. Giuseppe Rotilio
Dipartimento di Biologia
II Università di Roma - Tor Vergata
via Orazio Raimondo
I - 00173 (La Romanina) Roma

Dr. Alex Sevanian
University Southern California
Inst. for Toxicology
J. Stauffer Pharmaceutical Sciences
Center
1985 Zonal Avenue
Los Angeles, California 90033
USA

Prof. Fulvio Ursini
Istituto di Chimica Biologica
via F. Marzolo 3
I - 35131 Padova

Dr. Kunio Yagi
Institute of Biochemistry
Yagi Memorial Park
Mitake Gifu 5055-01
Japan

OXYGEN TOXICITY: BIOCHEMICAL, PHYSIOLOGICAL AND PATHOLOGICAL ASPECTS

Lars Ernster
Department of Biochemistry, Arrhenius Laboratory, University of Stockholm, S-196 91 Stockholm, Sweden

By way of introduction to this Discussion Meeting on the Role of Oxygen Radicals in Cardiovascular Diseases it seems appropriate to review current information concerning the sources and consequences of oxygen-radical production in animal cells (Figure 1), their biochemical mechanisms, physiological and pathological implications, and possible biological and pharmacological preventive devices.

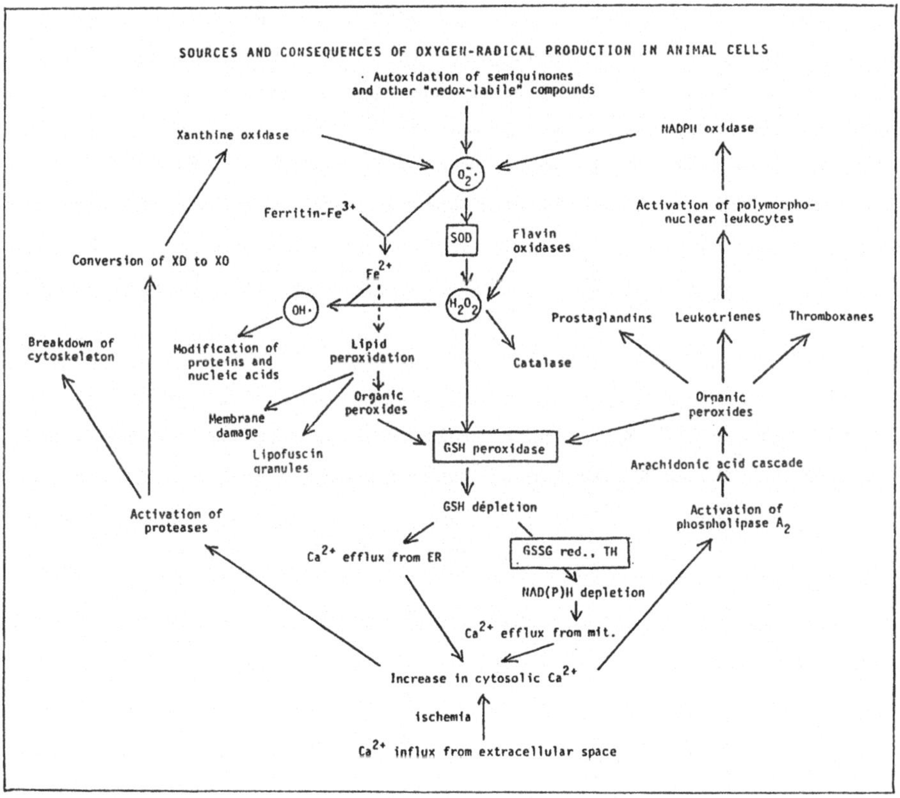

Figure 1

The following aspects may be relevant to the problems to be discussed at this Meeting:

1. Pathways of superoxide-radical ($O_2 \cdot^-$) formation by way of xanthine oxidase, NADPH oxidase, and autoxidation of semiquinones and other "redox-labile" compounds, including components of the mitochondrial respiratory chain. Prevention of quinone-induced $O_2 \cdot^-$ formation by DT diaphorase.

2. Mobilization of Fe^{2+} from ferritin-Fe^{3+} by $O_2 \cdot^-$, and initiation of lipid peroxidation with consequent membrane damage and accumulation of lipofucsin granules ("age pigments"). Mechanism of lipid peroxidation and its prevention by antioxidants.

3. Removal of $O_2 \cdot^-$ by way of superoxide dismutase (SOD), with the formation of H_2O_2. Fe-catalyzed hydroxyl-radical (OH·) formation and consequent modification of proteins and nucleic acids.

4. Removal of H_2O_2 and of organic peroxides by way of glutathione (GSH) peroxidase, with consequent depletion of cellular GSH and NAD(P)H via glutathione reductase (GSSG red.) and nicotinamide nucleotide transhydrogenase (TH), leading to a release of Ca^{2+} from the endoplasmic (ER) and mitochondria (mit.), and an increase in cytosolic Ca^{2+}.

5. Ca^{2+}-induced activation of cytosolic proteases, resulting in a breakdown of the cytoskeleton (with a consequent "blebbing" of the cell surface) and a conversion of xanthine dehydrogenase (XD) to xanthine oxidase (XO).

6. Ca^{2+}-induced activation of phospholipase A_2, with an increase in the level of free arachidonic acid and thus an activation of the "arachidonic acid cascade". Stimulation of leukocyte adhesion to endothelium by leukotrienes, causing activation of NADPH oxidase.

7. Factors involved in tissue injury caused by oxygen radicals, in particular that following ischemia and reperfusion, and possible preventive measures.

A recent paper discussing some of the above problems is found in the reference given below.

Reference

Ernster, L., 1986. Oxygen as an environmental poison. Chemica Scripta, 26: 525-534.

MORPHOLOGIC DIFFERENCES IN MYOCARDIAL NECROSIS AND ATHEROSCLEROTIC PLAQUE. WHAT IS THEIR PATHOGENETIC MEANING ?

G. Baroldi

Institute of Clinical Physiology CNR, Dpt of Milan, Centro De Gasperis "Niguarda" Hospital, Milan. Institute Biomedical Sciences, Dpt. Cardiovascular Pathology, Medical School, University of Milan, "Sacco" Hospital, Milan. Special research projects "Atherosclerosis" and National Cardiopulmonary Group of the National Research Council, Rome Italy.

Frequency and extension of different types of myocardial necrosis and variables of the coronary atherosclerotic plaque have been examined and statistically compared in 200 fatal acute infarct, 208 sudden unexpected death, 50 chronic ischemia cases and 97 healthy controls. In pratically all infarct cases the pathognomonic coagulation or infarct necrosis was associated with coagulative myocytolysis (contraction band necrosis) and in half of cases with colliquative myocytolysis. In sudden death and chronic ischemia coagulative myocytolysis prevailed. The three different morpho-functional types of myocardial cell death indicate that pathogenic mechanisms (adrenergic overstimulation or catecholamine depletion) other than ischemia may explain complications and cause of death in ischemic heart disease. In respect of plaque variables many significant divergencies were shown among the ischemic groups and between the latters and healthy controls. In particular lympho-plasmacellular reaction at the plaque level was significantly more frequent and extensive in ischemic patients (100 per cent in acute infarcts), all or most of the plaque being involved by this process. Topographical correlation with thrombosis, regional myocardial necrosis (both infarct and contraction band necrosis) and perivascular nervous structures was demonstrated. These findings suggest the working hypothesis that "active plaque" may corresponds to active phases of ischemic heart diseases by release of substances directly active on smooth muscle cells (spasm) and myocardial fibers (regional impairment of contractility), or by irritation or degeneration of the pericoronary nerves.

Is questionable if the classic pathogenic concept may explain onset, course, complications and death in the different patterns of ischemic heart disease (IHD). In this complex, not yet fully understood pathogenic mosaic one is tempted to conclude according to his own view with little consideration for findings from other specific fields. Radiologists look at and believe in cineangiographic imagings, biochemists in experimental models which mimic only a small, if any, part of the natural history of the disease, pathologists in dead structures, often unable to explain dynamics and sequential course of all events.

In the present controversial pathogenic contest two facts seem worthy of consideration in attempting to have an integrated view.

DIFFERENT TYPES OF MYOCARDIAL NECROSIS IN ISCHEMIC HEART DISEASE

Fatal acute infarct. In this condition the necrosis is pathognomonic. It consists in a monofocal lesion which ranges from less than 10 per cent to more than 50 per cent of the ventricular mass. The earliest (few seconds) functional change is the lost of contraction with paradoxical bulging. Attenuation of the muscle fibers and elongation of their nuclei are the first reliable structural modifications consequent to the mechanical effect on irreversibly relaxed myocells by the interventricular pressure. Subsequently within 6-8 hours an increasing centripetal infiltration of polymorphonuclear leukocytes occurs. The latter, particularly in large infarcts, becomes massive and disappears by lysis of these elements within one week. Already in the first day the intramural vessels undergo wall degeneration and secondary thrombosis. The repair process consists in centripetal detersion of the allosarcoplasmic structures by macrophages leading to empty sarcolemmal tubes undergoing collagenization.

An opposite pattern of myocell necrosis is visible at the periphery of the infarct where the blood supply is present and polymorphonuclear infiltration generates. A rim of myocardial cells interdigitating with the infarcted ones shows hypercontraction with subsequent irregular rupture of the myofibrils and anomalous cross band formation. In the majority of cases (about 90 per cent) an identical plurifocal lesion, often confluent, are seen in the adjacent normal myocardium and in other non infarcted cardiac regions. This type of necrosis does not show polymorphonuclear infiltration - only at the rim where it is evoked by the infarct necrosis - and vessel thrombosis. The repair process only is similar, with macrophagic cleaning which leads to characteristic "alveolar" foci of empty sarcolemmal tubes with subsequent fibrosis.
Finally in about half of the fatal infarct cases a third different damage can be seen in the subendocardial and perivascular myocardial layers, generally preserved by the infarct necrosis. The myocells show an increasing disappearance of myofibrils paralleled by edematous vacuolization resulting again in empty sarcolemmal tubes.(Baroldi _et al._, 1974, Siver _et al._, 1980).

Unexpected sudden coronary death - In selected cases

(dead within 10 minutes, out-of-hospital while acting their usual life-style, without history of IHD, not under medical care and without any medical intervention and resuscitation maneuvers) the frequency of histologically demonstrable infarct necrosis plus contraction bands was 17 per cent, necrosis with hypercontraction and anomalous bands 72 per cent, necrosis with myofibrillar colliquation 8 per cent (Baroldi et al., 1979).

Chronic ischemia - In patients who died following aorto-coronary by-pass graft the frequency of infarct was 72 per cent, coagulative myocytolysis 89 per cent and colliquative myocytolysis 54 per cent.

Healthy controls - Normal people who died instantaneously or in short periods (minutes) after an accident without any medical and resuscitation attempts the unique lesion found was contraction band necrosis. It was present in 19 per cent of the cases, being minimal in extension but in three cases with extensive plurifocal damage.

The diagnostic morpho-patological identification of any nosologic entity is based on specific structural changes. Identical or similar damage may result from several causes acting through the same pathogenic mechanism. In turn different functional-structural changes indicate different pathogenic mechanisms linked with different causes. In ischemic heart disease three different types of irreversible damage exist. The myocell may die:

1) in irreversible relaxation ("atonic death" or infarct necrosis or coagulation necrosis). The pathogenic mechanism is nutrient blood flow reduction while the cause(s) are still controversial (coronary thrombus, vasoconstriction/spasm, extravascular compression of the intramural branches, platelet aggregates etc).

2) in irreversible hypercontraction ("tetanic death" or coagulative myocytolysis or contraction band necrosis). This lesion can be found in numerous human (pheochromocytoma, malignant hyperthermia, transplanted heart etc.) and experimental (hemorrhagic shock, reflow, "Calcium paradox" etc.) conditions. In particular the lesion is specific for catecholamine cardiotoxicity. The typical myofibrillar rhexis with band formation is likely due to the mechanical rhythmic action of the normal contracting myocardium on rigid, hypercontracted elements. At present many data support the concept that Ca++ inflow following a direct toxic effect on the myocell is the pathogenic mechanism. Experimentally it has been shown that the quantity of damage is dose-depending irrespectively from ECG changes, blood flow, hemodynamics (similar qualitative and quantitative damage with both isoproterenol and norepinephrina despite dissimilar ECG, hemodynamic and biochemical profile). In this large series of experiments in dog in no one instance infarct necrosis was demonstrated (Todd _et al._, 1985a, 1985b).

3) In progressive failure ("failing death" or colliquative myocytolisis). This lesion is seen in any

condition with low output syndrome of different etiologies. The pathogenesis of this progressive lost in contraction-relaxation coupling is still unknown, even if catecholamine "depletion" seems to have a role. In six hearts with dilated cardiomyopathy (NYHA class III-IV) explanted from patients undergone heart transplant a severe reduction of noradrenaline and betareceptors in respect to normal has been found. It must be noted that no significant myocardial fibrosis was present. An egual noradrenaline reduction was observed in endomyocardial biopsy in patients with dilated cardiomyopathy with minor cardiac dysfunction (NYHA class II) (unpublished data).

Three types of damage which motivate to review (Baroldi, 1975) and more precisely define causes and pathogenesis in ischemic heart disease. In 200 fatal infarcts the size of infarct necrosis was less than 20 per cent. Too small to explain per se complications and death. Furthermore in no one instance was possible to document an expansion of the primitive infarct necrosis. The "border zone" seems more normal myocardium at risk of metabolic disorders rather than jeopardized by ischemia. Experiments support the view that regional lost of contraction increases compensatory contractility and blood flow of the normal myocardium likely via cardiac reflexes. Coagulative myocytolysis (contraction band necrosis) may indicate adrenergic overstimulation linked with malignant arrhythmia. In experimental permanent acute coronary occlusion in dog both contraction bands and ventricular fibrillation were prevented by a betablocker (Baroldi <u>et al.</u>, 1977) (propranolol). On the other hand colliquative myocytolysis is the histological hallmark of cardiac failure following infarct.

In sudden coronary death we know from monitorized patients by Holter that they die very shortly without ischemic ecgraphic changes. 81 per cent of resuscitated people by defibrillation do not show an infarct. Again overadrenergic regional stimulation linked with contraction bands may suggest the following two possibilities: one, more rare, an histologically undetectable (because of rapidity of death) large infarct triggers in predisposed patients the same mechanism as in documentated fatal infarcts; two (in most of these cases) a primitive adrenergic overstimulation may occurs.

<u>LYMPHO-PLASMACELLULAR INFILTRATES IN CORONARY ATHEROSCLEROTIC PLAQUE</u>

Morphologic variables (fibrosis, proteoglycan accumulation, atheroma, calcification, intimal vascularization, hemorrhage and lympho-plasmacellular infiltrates) of the atherosclerotic plaque have been quantified and compared with degree and length of lumen reduction, intimal and medial thickness in 3640 histological coronary sections. These were systematically sampled from eight selected segments of 358 ischemic hearts (100 fatal acute infarct, 208 sudden coronary death, 50 chronic ischemia) and 97 control hearts (normal people dying by accident). Statistical analysis showed significant divergencies in frequency and extension of the morphologic variables among the three groups of IHD and between the latters and controls, independently from degree of stenosis and intimal thickness (Baroldi et al., in press). In particular the lympho-plasmacellular reaction showed:

1. 100 per cent frequency in acute infarcts, 85 per cent in chronic ischemia, 85 per cent in sudden death and 64 per cent in controls. Frequency was paralleled by extension.

2. Its presence in all or most plaques found in each single ischemic patient in contrast to control cases (absent or only one plaque involved).

3. Excess in inflammatory elements in vessels supplying infarcted areas and areas with contraction band necrosis.

4. Correlation with occlusive and mural coronary thrombus.

5. Peculiar tropism for the adventitial nervous structures at the plaque level.

6. Relative high frequency (32 per cent) in plaque with mild lumen reduction (< 50 per cent) and minor intimal thickness (< 600 micr.) in relation to proteoglycan accumulation.

7. Absence in normal vessel wall.

The nature of this inflammatory process is still unknown. Some data support the hypothesis of an autoimmune process. However what seems important to establish is if this "active" inflammatory component of a chronic process (atherosclerotic plaque) may or not correspond to the active phase(s) of the disease; in keeping with alternating active-inactive phases as in any chronic process. Substances released from these elements may directly act on smooth muscle cells (spasm) and/or myocardial cells (regional impairment of contractility); or indirectly by irritation or degeneration of the pericoronary nervous structures.

Stenosing atherosclerosis and thrombosis are considered the main factors in the natural history of all IHD patterns. Several fact however contradict their direct cause-effect relation. The first episode of the disease may ensue independently from degree and number of severe stenosis. The latter can not predict course, complications and death. In about half of the general atherosclerotic population an identical stenotic damage exist without evidence of IHD. The size of the infarct is unrelated, as it should be, to the number of severe stenosis. Thrombosis occurs mainly at the level of severe stenosis already by-passed by collaterals and its occlusive effect - as shown experimentally (Kouri *et al.*, 1965) - seems inconsistent on blood flow distribution. The stenotic lesions pre-exist for months or years to the first symptom in apparently normal and active people with any type of stress.

All these facts point out that on the background of the atherosclerotic process some events other than stenosis or thrombosis may be responsible. Different types of myocardial necrosis and "active" atherosclerotic plaque may help us in better understanding this complex disease, its complications and cause of death.

References

Baroldi, G., 1975. Different types of myocardial necrosis in coronary heart disease: a pathophysiological review of their functional significance. Am. Heart J., 89: 742-752.

Baroldi, G., Silver, M.D., Lixfeld, W., McGregor, D.C., 1977. Irreversible myocardial damage resembling catecholamine necrosis secondary to acute coronary occlusion in dogs: its prevention by propanolol. J. Molec. Cell. Cardiol., 9: 687-691.

Baroldi, G., Falzi, G., Mariani, F., 1979. Sudden coronary death. A postmortem study in 208 selected cases compared to 97 "control" subjects. Am. Heart J., 98: 20-31.

Baroldi, G., 1983. Diseases of coronary arteries. In "Cardiovascular Pathology", Silver, M.D., ed., Churchill Livingstone Inc. New York, 317-391.

Baroldi, G., Silver, M.D., Mariani, F., Giuliano, G.. Variation of coronary atherosclerotic plaque morphology in relation to clinical patterns of ischemic heart disease and healthy controls. Am. J. Cardiov. Path. in press.

Khouri, E.M., Gregg, D.E. and Loweschn, H.S., 1968. Flow in the major branches of the left coronary artery during experimental coronary insufficiency in the unanesthetized dog. Circul. Res. 23: 99-106.

Silver, M.D., Baroldi, G., Mariani, F., 1980. The relationship between acute occlusive coronary thrombi and myocardial infarction studies in 100 consecutive patients. Circulation 61: 219-227.

Todd, G.L., Baroldi, G., Pieper, G.M., Clayton, F.C., Eliot, R.S., 1985. Experimental catecholamine-induced myocardial necrosis. I Morphology, quantification and regional distribution of acute contraction band lesions. J. Molec. Cell. Cardiol. 17: 317-338.

Todd, G.L., Baroldi, G., Pieper, G.M., Clayton, F.C., Eliot, R.S., 1985. Experimental catecholamine-induced myocardial necrosis.II Temporal development of isoproterenol-induced contraction band lesions correlated with ECG, hemodynamic and biochemical changes. J. Molec. Cell. Cardiol. 17: 647-656.

FREE RADICALS AND CIRCULATORY SHOCK

Gian Paolo Novelli
Institute of Anesthesiology and Intensive Care, University of Florence, Policlinico Careggi, 50134 Florence (Italy).

ABSTRACT

Circulatory shock is a severe pathologic state caused by several agents (trauma, sepsis, surgery, etc.) and characterized by diffuse tissue hypoperfusion and ischemic damage. The search for mediator/s of circulatory shock is relevant, as they are thought to be identical to those of all ischemia-related conditions.

Recent reports seem to indicate that leukotrienes and oxygen radicals can play a role as mediators of circulatory shock.

Data concerning the role of leukotrienes are conflicting and their complete effect is still unknown.

Experiments on the role of oxygen radicals in the physiopathology of circulatory shock have been performed using phenylbutyl-nitrone (PBN), a spin-trapper, as scavenger.

PBN was effective to prevent death after administration of lethal doses of endotoxin, after trauma or superior mesenteric artery occlusion in rats. PBN was also effective in preventing metabolic acidosis, hemoconcentration and membrane stiffness (as measured by spin-labels and ESR) after lethal trauma.

When injected 60 minutes after trauma, PBN was able to reverse traumatic shock.

The results of this study suggest that oxygen radicals play a key role in the physiopathology of circulatory shock and ischemia-related conditions.

INTRODUCTION

Circulatory shock is a syndrome of tissue hypoperfusion and of cellular hypoxia consequent to several stressors, i.e. to hypovolemia, trauma, sepsis, burn, surgery and myocardial insufficiency.

The prominent events in circulatory shock are related to ischemia or to ischemia/reperfusion: increase of capillary permeability, decrease of transmembrane potentials, increase of cell membrane permeability, decrease of energy utilization, etc. are therefore present.

The research in the field of the pathogenesis of circulatory shock is strictly linked to that in the field of the pathogenesis of ischemia and ischemia/reperfusion conditions.

The pathways involved in the passage from stress to ischemia, shock and, in case, death are not well recognized and the search for common mediator/s is in progress. This search could represent the basis for relevant therapeutic programs.

A putative mechanism was suggested many years ago by Fine and his coworkers

(1965) who stressed endotoxin of gram-negative bacteria as the common pathogenetic mediator of all shock states.

In recent years more and more mediators have been considered as the common basis for ischemia and circulatory shock. Among these, products of the metabolic pathway of eicosanoids and oxygen radicals are those of major interest.

The role of each of these two mechanisms is under investigation in many laboratories and attempts to prepare drugs effective in preventing the production of leukotriens or in scavenging the reactive species of oxygen are in course. Those drugs would have a large spectrum of use, including all conditions of tissue hypoperfusion and ischemia - both general and local - before the evolution toward circulatory shock and irreversible cellular damage.

Some products of the metabolic pathway of eicosanoids have been shown by Lefer (1985) to fulfil most of the criteria postulated for humoral mediators of ischemia and shock. Among these, thromboxane A2, leukotriene C4 and leukotriene D4, are all able to constrict arteries (mostly cutaneous, mesenteric and coronary), to induce adherence of white blood cells to be endothelium, therefore contributing to increased capillary permeability (Samuelsson and Hammarstrom, 1982).

Macrophages, monocytes and granulocytes are capable of generating leukotrienes during endotoxic shock and ischemia, (Piper et al, 1984; Bottoms et al., 1985) probably as a consequence of their "self killing" after activation.

However, the exact role of leukotrienes in these conditions is difficult to be determined, due to technical difficulties in their measurement in plasma and tissues. Endotoxin lethality has recently been reported to be prevented in mice by a leukotriene antagonist, by the inhibition of leukotriene biosynthesis or by the dual lipoxygenase and ciclooxygenase inhibitor BW 755C but not by inhibitors of ciclooxygenase alone (Hagmann et al., 1984). In other experiments the same dual inhibitor BW 755C prevented the increase in plasma prostanoids after endotoxin but failed to increase survival of rats (Mc Kechnie et al., 1985).

In other experiments, nefazatrom, an effective lipoxygenase inhibitor, is reported to protect against traumatic shock (Lefer and Messenger, 1982).
Since leukotriene C4 is converted to D4, which exerts more potent circulatory effects in the rat, Hock and Lefer (1985) investigated the selective D4 antagonist LY-171883 in traumatized rats.

Results are conflicting but consistent with the concept of an involvement of leukotrienes in the pathophysiology of circulatory shock and ischemia.

Unfortunately, leukotriene antagonist specificity is low and these substances are also active on the oxygen radical system (Lefer, 1985).

Therefore, in order to clarify the pathogenesis of shock and ischemia related conditions, the role of oxygen radicals was also investigated (Novelli and De Gaudio, 1983).

The involvement of oxygen radicals in the pathophysiology of ischemia and circulatory shock has received significant experimental support; endotoxin, hypoxia and ischemia/reperfusion are well accepted as causes of unbalance in the oxygen radicals system, due to both an increased production and a decreased inactivation.

Oxygen radicals overproduction, related to shock - inducing conditions seems to be due to:

a - the mitochondrial electron chain transport;

b - the xantine - oxidase activity; the role of xanthineoxidase in oxygen radical pathology is supported by experiments with allopurinol;

c - the arachidonic acid cascade activated by phospholipase, granulocytosis, etc., leading to the production of leukotrienes whose putative role of unique mediators of shock and ischemia has been previously discussed;

d - the granulocyte activation as response to complement activation and to various chemiotactic factors, including leukotrienes; aggregated granulocytes in the capillaries can induce oxygen radicals generation (Goldstein et al., 1975) as well as ischemia secondary to mechanical obstruction.

There are a lot of reports concerning the relationship between oxygen radicals and shock related events (i.e. lung damage, myocardial depression, diffuse intravascular coagulation, increased capillary permeability, etc.) but few papers are focused on the shock status as a whole.

A possible approach to the evaluation of the role of oxygen radicals in shock is the study of the scavenging systems, and the documentation of improvement of the syndrome by the activation of these systems and its worsening by their depression.

In brief:

a - administration to rats of physiological scavengers (reduced glutathione or alpha-tocopherol) prevents endotoxin and whole body trauma shock (Novelli and De Gaudio, 1983);

b - administration of a drug with scavenger property prevents whole body trauma shock (Lefer et al., 1981);

c - inhibition of scavenging enzymes (diethyl-di-thiocarbamate) increases lethality after endotoxin or whole body trauma (Novelli and De Gaudio, 1983);

d - administration of superoxide dismutase decreases mortality after burns (Saez et al., 1984);

e - administration of alpha-tocopherol, allopurinol, reduced glutathione and superoxide-dismutase lessens the metabolic and cardiovascular effects of prolonged administration of endotoxin in rats (McKechnie et al., 1986).

Moreover, in our laboratory we faced the problem of "capturing" oxygen radicals immediately after their generation (Novelli et al., 1984).

This goal was achieved using the spin-trapper phenyl-butyl-nitrone (PBN), which is one of the most prone trappers of superoxide and hydroxyl radicals (Rosen and Rauckman, 1984). Experiments were performed injecting PBN in vivo a) before shock producing maneuvers, b) when shock was in course.

MATERIALS AND METHODS

All the experiments were performed on male Wistar rats (200g).

Endotoxic shock was provoked by Escherichia Coli lipopolysaccharide (Difco O111: B4) 20 mg/Kg i.p.

SMAO shock was provoked by a rotating drum, submitting rats to 1200 revolutions after light anesthesia (pentobarbital 10 mg/Kg i.p.).

The spin-trapper PBN was administered in 1 ml of olive oil, as previously described (Novelli et al., 1986). Plain olive oil, 1 ml, was injected in control experiments.

Drugs or fluids were never administered.

To measure the evolution of shock the following parameters were used:

a - survival at 3, 6, 12 and 24 hours,

b - hematocrit value, measured in duplicate by a micromethod on arterial blood,

c - acid-base status measured by a micromethod (Instrumentation Laboratories, Milano) on arterial blood and reported as pH and base excess (BE),

d - the physico-chemical status of microsomal and mitochondrial membranes labelled with four different spin-labels (with the doxyl unity localized in position 5, 6, 12, 16) and ESR (Bruker 200D) as previously described (Novelli et al., 1986).

EXPERIMENTS

A preliminary trial was performed injecting the PBN (125 mg/Kg i.p.) to rats daily for six days.

The following series of experiments were performed:

1. experiments directed to evaluate whether PBN (150-100-50 mg/Kg i.p.) or its solvent alone prevented death after lethal doses of endotoxin, trauma or SMAO. The

spin-trapper was administered 5 minutes before shock-provoking procedures; no fluid therapy was given.

2. experiments directed to evaluate whether PBN (150 mg/Kg i.p.) or its solvent alone affected the appearance of traumatic shock as measured in experimental conditions as in (1) by pH, base excess, hematocrit. Blood sampling was performed before and immediately after trauma, and after 3 and 6 hours. Animals submitted to blood sampling were sacrificed.
3. experiment directed to assess if PBN (150 mg/Kg) or its solvent alone affected survival when administered at various intervals after trauma. The spin-trapper was given 30 or 60 minutes after the end of whole body trauma and no fluid therapy was given.
4. experiments directed to assess if PBN (150 mg/Kg i.p.) or its solvent alone affected pH, base excess and hematocrit in traumatized rats. Experimental conditions were as in (3) and blood sampling was as in (2).
5. experiments directed to evaluate if PBN (150 mg/Kg i.p.) or methylprednisolone (30 mg/kg i.p.) or plain olive oil prevented the physico-chemical damage of cell membranes consequent to traumatic shock. Experimental conditions were as in (1); animals were sacrificed immediately after trauma.

RESULTS

Preliminary trials showed no effect of repeated doses of PBN alone. Figure 1 summarizes the massime increase in survival after three types of lethal shock. The number of traumatic shock experiments is not uniform, due to the early death of some animals in the rotating drum.

Figure 2 shows the evolution of hemoconcentration and metabolic acidosis after trauma.

Figure 3 is indicative of the dramatic effect on survival of PBN, although administered after trauma.

Also in this case the number of experiments is not uniform among groups, due to early death of some animals during rotation.

Figure 4 confirms the existence of circulatory shock at the time of PBN injection and evidences its rapid effect.

In figure 5 the ESR spectra obtained from membranes of normal and shocked rats are reported. The spectra from membranes of rats submitted to trauma after PBN or methylprednisolone are identical to those of control rats, so indicating that both drugs protect cell membranes against peroxidative damage (fig. 6).

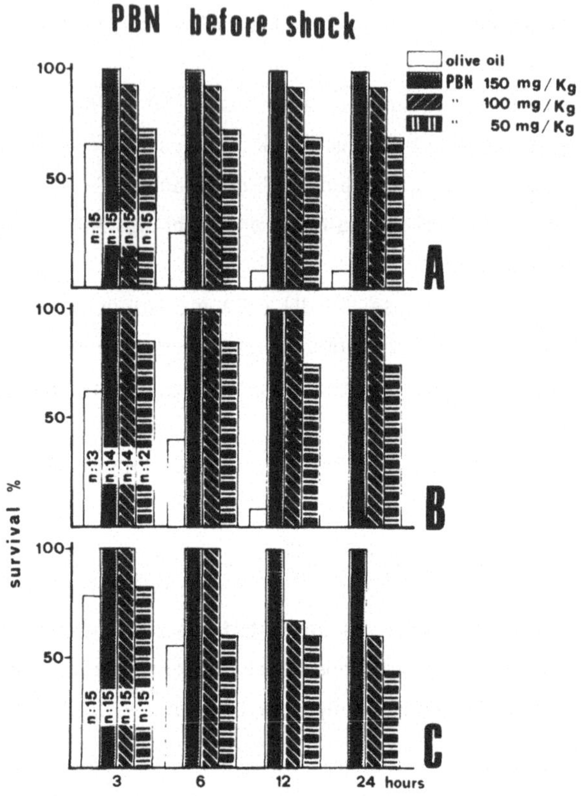

Fig. 1: % survival of rats submitted to lethal doses of endoxin (A), trauma (B) or SMAO (C) and pretreated with PBN or olive oil.
It must be noted that all control animals died within 24 hours.
Statistical differences are always highly significant except at 3 hours.

DISCUSSION

The experimental models of circulatory shock proposed in this study are relevant both as models of ischemia-reperfusion and with regard to the clinical syndrome.

The results confirm that PBN is able to prevent the lethal effects of trauma, endotoxin and SMAO, in absence of any other drug or fluid therapy.

The complete prevention of death obtained by PBN in the three models of circulatory shock seems to be attributed to its trapping action on oxygen radicals.

In fact, no other biological effects of PBN have been identified until present except for a scavenging action. Similar effects of PBN have been observed by McKechnie et al. (1986) who reported a significant improvement in survival and metabolic derangement of rats during intravenous infusion of endotoxin. Other reports concern the prevention afforted by PBN of the chemical damage of alveolar surfactant induced by endotoxin (Yanev et al., 1986).

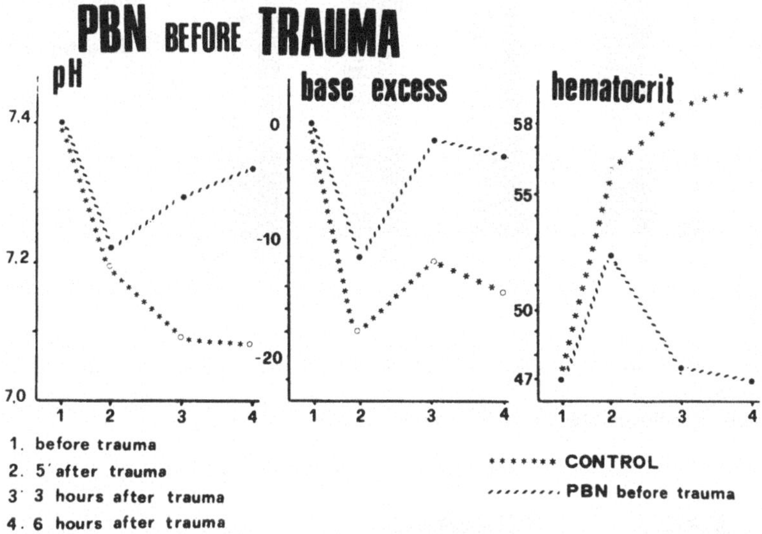

Fig. 2: Blood parameters in a typical experiment of trauma after PBN. Examined parameters were affected by trauma but rapidly returned toward normal values without any additional therapy in PBN treated rats.

Therefore, although the exact mode of action is still to be clarified, PBN is to be considered a scavenger.

The effect of PBN injected 30 or 60 minutes after the end of trauma (when circulatory shock was confirmed by metabolic acidosis and hemoconcentration) seems to be due to a more complex phenomenon than the simple trapping of oxygen radicals.

At that moment, in fact, the generation of oxygen radicals has already taken place and cellular damage is occurring. It can be hypothesized that PBN is active not only on oxygen radicals but also on other free radicals, thus interrupting the self perpetuating chains of lipoperoxidation.

In any case, the experiments of this study strongly support the role of oxygen radicals in circulatory shock, and suggest that in ischemia and shock the production of leukotrienes may be the consequence of the uncontrolled oxygen radical overproduction.

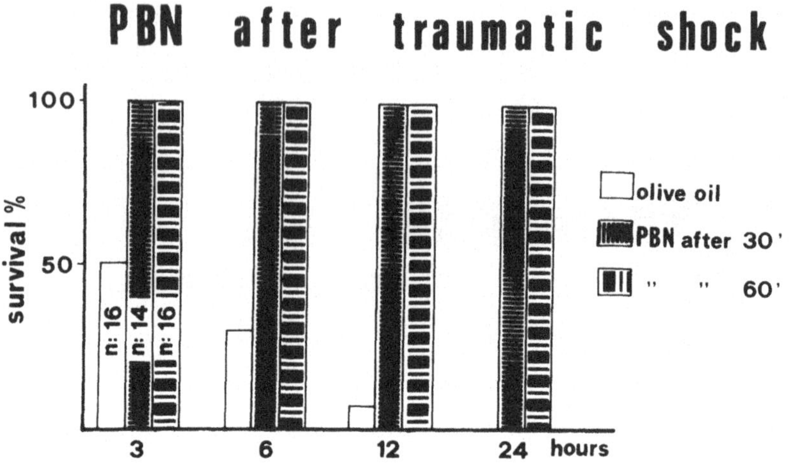

Fig. 3: % survival of rats submitted to a lethal dose of whole body trauma and pretreated by PBN or olive oil.
All the statistical differences were highly significant.

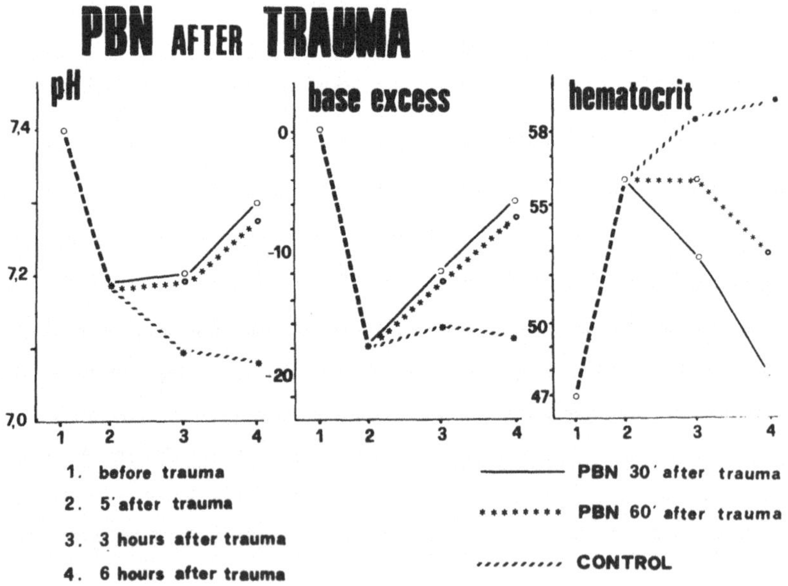

Fig. 4: blood parameters in typical experiments on shocked rats receiving PBN at two intervals after trauma.

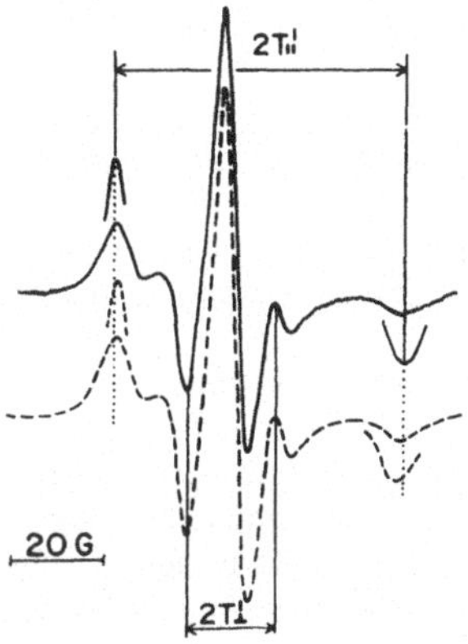

Fig. 5: Typical ESR spectrum of 5-SASL (localized near the surface) taken from membranes of liver mitochondria of rats submitted to traumatic shock (full line) and of control rats (dashed line). The same linear-shape was obtained for microsomial fraction. Calculation performed on the ESR spectrum indicates that in shocked rats there is a decrease of fluidity of the membranes near the surface with reduced molecular movements.

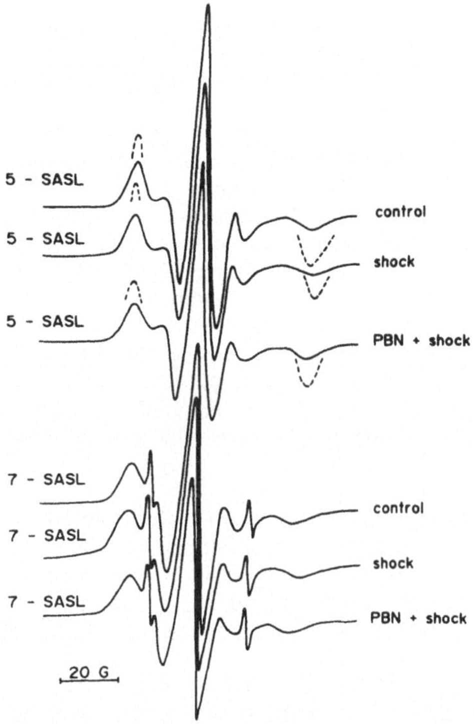

Fig. 6: ESR spectra of C-5 (5-SASL) and C-7 (7-SASL) from cell membranes of rats submitted to whole body trauma after PBN, methylprednisolone or plain olive oil. Only the spectra from untreated shocked rats are indicative of reduction of membrane fluidity.

REFERENCES

Bottoms, G.D., Johnson, M.A., Lamar, C.H., Fessler, J.F. and Turek, J.J., 1985. Endotoxin-induced eicosanoid production by equine vascular endothelial cells and neutrophils. Circ. Shock, 15: 155-162.

Fine, J., 1965. Current status of the problem of traumatic shock. Surg.Gynec.Obst., 120: 537.

Goldstein, I.M., Rood D., Kaplan, H.B. and Weissman, G., 1975. Complement and immunoglobulins stimulate superoxide production by human leukocytes independently of phagocytosis. J. Clin. Invest., 56: 1155-1158.

Hagmann, W., Denzlinger, C. and Keppler D., 1984. Role of peptide leukotrienes and their epatobiliary elimination in endotoxin action. Circ. Shock, 14: 223-235.

Hock, C.E. and Lefer, A.M., 1982. Protective effects of a new LTD 4 antagonist (LY-171883) in traumatic shock. Circ. Shock, 17: 263-272.

Lefer, A.M. and Messenger, M., 1982. Protective action of nefazatrom in traumatic shock. Arzneimittel. Forsch, 32: 1089-1091.
Lefer, A.M.n 1985. Eicosanoids as mediators of ischemia and shock. Fed. Proc.,44: 275-280.
McKechnie, K., Furman, B.L. and Parratt, J.R., 1985. Metabolic and cardiovascular effects of endotoxin infusion in conscious unrestrained rats: effects of methylprednisolone and BW755C. Circ. Shock, 15: 205-216.
McKechnie, K., Furman, B.L. and Parratt, J.R., 1986. Modification by oxygen free radical scavengers of the metabolic and cardiovascular effects ofendotoxin infusion in conscious rats. Circ. Shock, 19: 429-440.
Novelli, G.P. and De Gaudio, A.R., 1983. Oxygen free-radicals in shock states. In: D. Lewis and U. Haglund (Editors), Shock Research, Amsterdam, Elsvier, pp. 31-42.
Novelli, G.P., Bordi, L. and De Gaudio, A.R., 1984. Trapping of free-radicals prevents endotoxin shock. 1st Meeting of European Shock Society - Manchester, 8th Sept.
Novelli, G.P., Martini, G., Bordi, L., Consales, G., Porciani, S. and Becciolini, A., 1986a. Fluidity of mitochondrial and microsomal membranes in traumatic shock as studied by ESR. In: G.P. Novelli and F. Ursini (Editors), Oxygen free radicals in shock, Karger, Basel, pp. 46-52.
Novelli, G.P., Angiolini, P., Consales, G., Lippi, R. and Tani, R., 1986b. Anti-shock action of phenyl-t-butyl-nitrone, a spin trapper. In: G.P. Novelli and F. Ursini (Editors), Oxygen free radicals in shock, Karger, Basel, pp. 119-124.
Novelli, G.P., Angiolini, P., Tani, R., Consales, G. and Bordi, L., 1986c. Phenyl-t-butyl-nitrone is active against traumatic shock in rats. Free Rad. Comm.1: 321-327.
Piper, P.J., 1984. Formation and action of leukotrienes. Physiol. Rev., 64: 744-761.
Rosen, G.M. and Rauckman, A., 1984. Spin trapping of superoxide and hydroxylradicals. Methods in enzimology 105: 198-209.
Samuelsson, B. and Hammarstrom, S., 1982. Leukotrienes, a novel group of biologically active compounds. Vitam. Horm. 39: 1-30.
Yanev, A., Momchilova, A., Koumanov, K., Novelli, G.P. and Nicolov, N., 1986. N-t-butyl-phenylnitrone antioxidant effect on the alterations in phosphilipid composition of alveolar surfactant and lungs in endotoxin shock rats. In: G.P. Novelli and F. Ursini (Editors). Oxygen free radicals in shock, Karger, Basel, pp. 193-196.

REPERFUSION ARRHYTHMIAS: DO FREE RADICALS PLAY A ROLE?

David J Hearse

Cardiovascular Research
The Rayne Institute
St Thomas' Hospital
London SE1, U.K.

ABSTRACT

Oxygen-derived free radicals are produced in the myocardium under both normal and pathological conditions. These intermediates can be extremely toxic and are able to induce severe cellular injury including membrane lipid peroxidation. Evidence is presented that free radicals may play a role in the genesis of reperfusion-induced ventricular fibrillation and that anti-free radical interventions, acting as anti-oxidants, possess potent anti-arrhythmic properties.

INTRODUCTION

The objective of this article is to review recent studies, from the Cardiovascular Research Group in the Rayne Institute at St Thomas' Hospital, which have contributed to the testing of the hypothesis that free radicals may play a role in the genesis of reperfusion-induced ventricular arrhythmias.

ISCHEMIA- AND REPERFUSION-INDUCED ARRHYTHMIAS

A variety of arrhythmias occur as a consequence of myocardial ischemia and reperfusion. These include ventricular fibrillation, ventricular tachycardia and premature ventricular contractions. The underlying mechanisms and the pharmacological control of ischemia-induced arrhythmias are relatively well characterized (Parratt, 1982). In contrast, reperfusion-induced arrhythmias are less easily controlled and their mechanisms are less well understood. Interest in reperfusion-induced arrhythmias has recently been stimulated by the realization that they are a clinically encountered event.

CLINICAL RELEVANCE OF REPERFUSION-INDUCED ARRHYTHMIAS

As recently reviewed (Manning and Hearse, 1984, Hearse et al 1987) reperfusion-induced arrhythmias are observed under a number of clinical circumstances. These can be conveniently sub-divided on the basis of the duration of the preceding period of ischemia, which may range from seconds to weeks, or even longer. Reperfusion after seconds or minutes of ischemia can be associated with the relief of coronary artery spasm. Although the degree of ischemic injury sustained during the period of spasm may be relatively minor, the tissue is rendered sufficiently irritable to permit the precipitation of serious reperfusion-induced arrhythmias which may account for some cases of sudden cardiac death. On a longer time scale, and in a different setting, reperfusion of the whole heart after minutes or hours of ischemia occurs during cardiac surgery and again, serious arrhythmias, including ventricular fibrillation are frequently encountered. Reperfusion after hours of ischemia occurs with thrombolysis or angioplasty, which are recently introduced procedures for the disruption of coronary occlusions. Successful reflow is often marked by the occurrence of ventricular arrhythmias.

Since reperfusion-induced arrhythmias may represent a lethal event in otherwise viable tissue, there is a clear need to understand their mechanisms of origin and develop pharmacological means for their effective control.

FACTORS INFLUENCING THE VULNERABILITY OF THE HEART TO REPERFUSION-INDUCED ARRHYTHMIAS

THE DURATION OF THE PRECEDING PERIOD OF ISCHEMIA

This is perhaps the most important determinant of the vulnerability of the heart to reperfusion-induced arrhythmias. As previously reviewed (Manning and Hearse, 1984), there is a bell-shaped relationship between the incidence of reperfusion-induced arrhythmias and the duration of preceding ischemia. The example in Figure 1 shows this relationship for the isolated rat heart with regional ischemia.

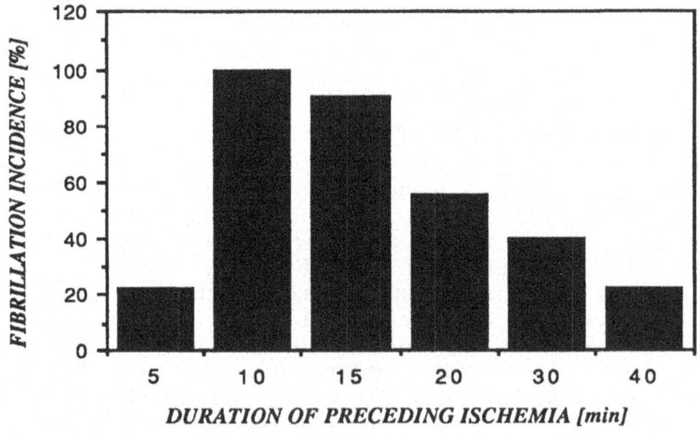

FIGURE 1: The relationship between the vulnerability of the heart to reperfusion-induced arrhythmias and the duration of preceding ischemia.

There is increasing vulnerability to reperfusion-induced ventricular fibrillation as the duration of ischemia increases from 0 to 10 min, at which time all hearts fibrillated upon reperfusion. With longer durations of ischemia there is a declining vulnerability such that after 30 or 40 min of ischemia reperfusion becomes electrophysiologically benign. Similarly shaped curves can be demonstrated for the rat heart in vivo, the guinea pig heart, the dog heart, and the rabbit heart. Different species and different preparations exhibit optima at different times, probably reflecting different rates of development of tissue injury and cell death. In this connection heterogeneity of injury in reversibly injured tissue has been proposed (Manning and Hearse, 1984) to be a very important factor in the genesis of serious arrhythmias.

ION DISTRIBUTION

Intracellular potassium loss together with extracellular potassium accumulation is thought to be an important factor in the genesis of both ischemia- and reperfusion-induced arrhythmias (Geddes, 1987). Other ionic perturbations such as magnesium loss and calcium overload, which probably reflect ischemia- and reperfusion-induced sarcolemmal injury, are also thought to be important determinants of electrical instability and tissue injury.

METABOLIC FACTORS

Patterns of substrate utilization, particularly the metabolism of fatty acids, has long been associated with the genesis of arrhythmias during ischemia (Kurien et al 1971). More recently lysophosphatide accumulation has also been linked with electrical instability in the ischemic and reperfused heart (Corr et al 1987). While abnormal fatty acid metabolism is generally associated with an increased vulnerability to arrhythmias, glucose utilization (and in particular glycolytic ATP production) has been proposed to protect cell membranes and reduce vulnerability of the heart to arrhythmias (Opie et al 1979).

RECEPTORS AND CYCLIC AMP

Activation of adrenergic receptors, increased tissue cyclic AMP content and the consequent increase in slow inward calcium current have long been associated with the induction of arrhythmias during ischemia. However, despite the undoubted arrhythmogenic effects of catecholamines, and the anti-arrhythmic effects of receptor blockade or catecholamine depletion, the cyclic AMP hypothesis has been challenged (Manning et al 1985). The possibility remains that catecholamines may, at least in part, exert their arrhythmogenic effects by non-receptor-mediated mechanisms e.g. free radical production arising from catecholamine oxidation (Bhagat et al 1980).

FREE RADICALS

Recently, two British groups, Woodward and Zakaria (1984) in Bath and Manning, Coltart and Hearse (1984) in London, have proposed the hypothesis that oxygen-derived free radicals, such as the superoxide and hydroxyl radical, generated during the early moments of reperfusion, may initiate membrane injury leading to the development of severe ventricular arrhythmias. During the last two years, considerable evidence has accumulated in support of this hypothesis, and in particular, the possibility that the xanthine oxidase pathway may represent an important source of cytotoxic free radicals. In the following sections some of these findings are overviewed.

SOURCE OF FREE RADICALS IN THE ISCHEMIC AND REPERFUSED MYOCARDIUM

Free radicals may emanate from a number of sources and cellular mechanisms, and their production occurs under both normal and pathological circumstances (Figure 2).

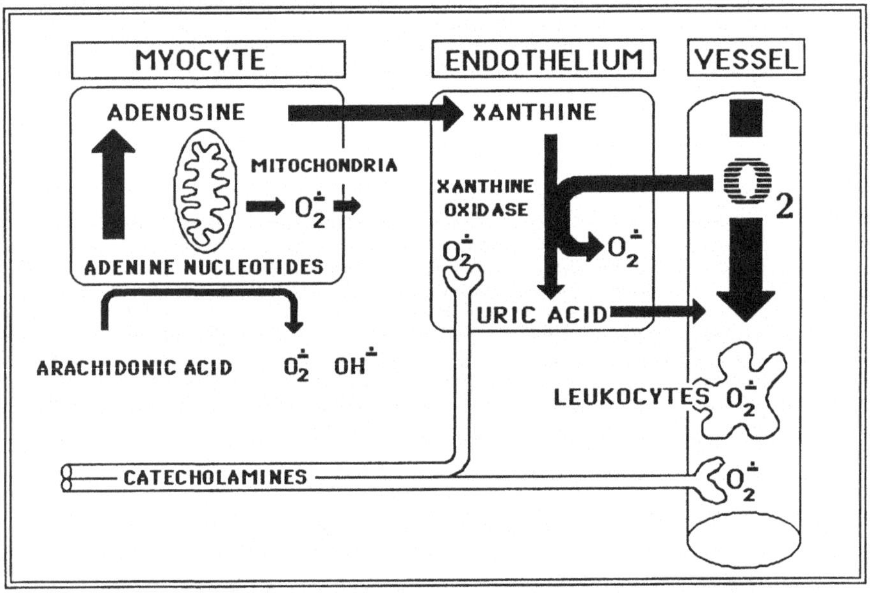

FIGURE 2: Free radical production by the xanthine oxidase and other pathways

The xanthine oxidase pathway (McCord, 1984), the arachidonic acid pathway (Halliwell and Gutteridge, 1985), invading leukocytes (Lucchesi et al 1984), catecholamine oxidation (Singal et al 1983) and mitochondrial activity (Turner and Bovaris, 1980) can all lead to the production of a variety of oxygen intermediates including superoxide, hydrogen peroxide and the hydroxyl radical.

Whatever their source, free radicals can be extremely cytotoxic and they are capable of causing major membrane injury by initiating lipid peroxidation or by altering the activity of membrane-bound enzyme systems which control ionic movement (Hess and Manson, 1984). The cell possesses highly efficient protective mechanisms, including anti-oxidants such as tocopherol and ascorbate or the enzymes superoxide dismutase and catalase, all of which are designed to prevent free radical-induced injury under normal conditions. However, it has been argued (McCord, 1984) that, under conditions of ischemia and reperfusion, these protective mechanisms may be overwhelmed and severe free radical-mediated injury may occur. McCord (1984) and Hess and colleagues (Hess and Manson, 1984) have developed the concept that ischemia can "prime" the myocardium for free radical-induced injury. In this regard, it has been shown that ischemia promotes the conversion of xanthine dehydrogenase to xanthine oxidase. This occurs at a time when hypoxanthine and xanthine, the substrates for xanthine oxidase, are accumulating in the cell as a consequence of the ischemia-induced degradation of adenine nucleotides. Ischemia also activates the arachidonic acid pathway and can cause the dissociation of the intramitochondrial electron transport system; both events can result in the production of superoxide. These factors, and others such as invading leukocytes and catecholamine degradation, create a scenario for free radical production and major tissue injury during ischemia and particularly during reperfusion.

IN VIVO STUDIES WITH XANTHINE OXIDASE

Investigating whether the activity of xanthine oxidase may influence tissue injury and the vulnerability of the heart to reperfusion-induced ventricular fibrillation, Manning et al (1984) used the anesthetised rat with coronary artery ligation (5 min) and reperfusion. They demonstrated (Figure 3) that allopurinol (20 mg/kg, 24 hours before study plus 20 mg/kg intravenously 15 minutes prior to study), an inhibitor of both xanthine oxidase and xanthine dehydrogenase, reduced the incidence of reperfusion-induced ventricular fibrillation from 67% (12/18) to 11% (2/18). In additional studies, Manning (1986), showed that folic acid solution (which contains the xanthine oxidase inhibitor pterinaldehyde) also reduced the incidence of reperfusion-induced ventricular fibrillation (67% to 17%) as did soybean trypsin inhibitor (which blocks the conversion of xanthine dehydrogenase to the superoxide-producing xanthine oxidase).

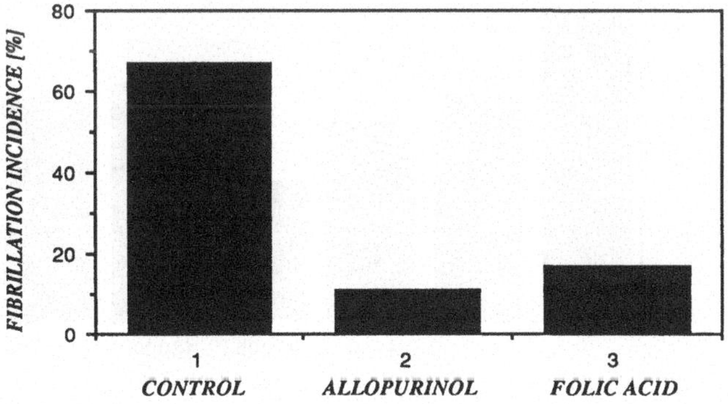

Figure 3: Xanthine oxidase inhibitors and reperfusion-induced ventricular fibrillation.

Manning was also able to show that the administration of superoxide dismutase (35000 IU/kg, intravenously 3 min before ischemia and again 2 min before reperfusion), catalase (400,000 IU/kg, intravenously 3 min before ischemia and again 2 min before reperfusion) or the combination of the two, were able to reduce the incidence of reperfusion-induced ventricular fibrillation.

IN VIVO STUDIES WITH ANTI-OXIDANT ENZYMES

Riva et al (1986) extended the in vivo studies to establish dose-response relationships for the anti- arrhythmic properties of superoxide dismutase and catalase against reperfusion-induced ventricular fibrillation (Figure 4). At their optimal doses, superoxide dismutase (27000 IU/kg) and catalase (42,000 IU/kg) reduced reperfusion-induced ventricular fibrillation from its control incidence of 73% to 33% and mortality fell from 47% to 7% and 13% respectively.

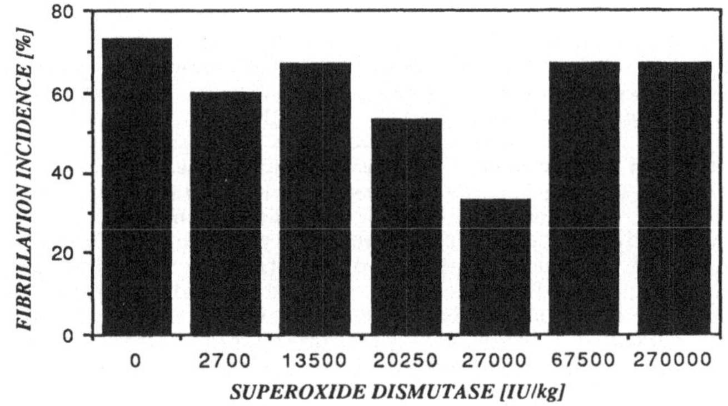

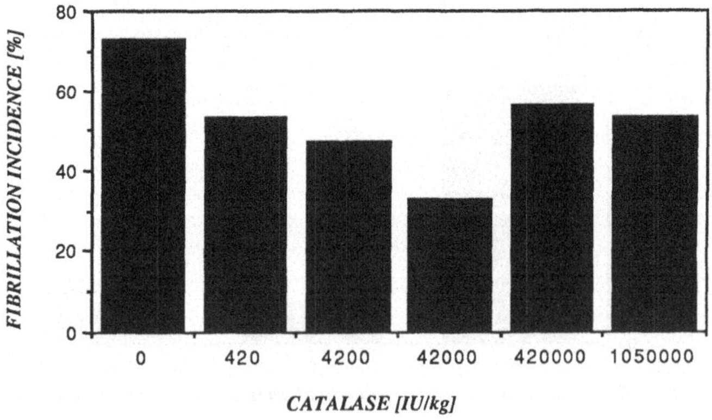

FIGURE 4: In vivo dose response characteristics for the anti-arrhythmic properties of superoxide dismutase and catalase

IN VITRO STUDIES

Bernier et al (1986) investigated whether six agents, that are known either to inhibit free radical formation or to scavenge free radicals once they are produced, can reduce the incidence of reperfusion-induced arrhythmias in the isolated rat heart with coronary artery ligation (10 min, the time for maximum vulnerability to reperfusion-induced ventricular fibrillation in vitro) and reperfusion. The results (Figure 5)

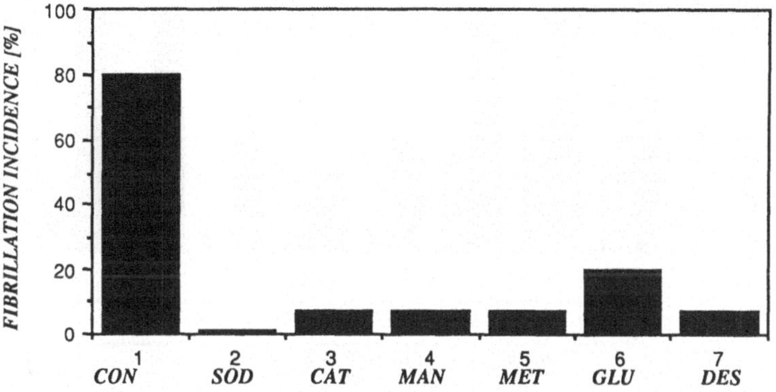

FIGURE 5: The anti-arrhythmic effect of a variety of free radical inhibitors or scavengers. CON = control, SOD = superoxide dismutase, CAT = catalase, MAN = mannitol, MET = methionine, GLU = glutathione, DES = desferrioxamine

demonstrate that superoxide dismutase (100,000 IU/liter), catalase (1,000,000 IU/liter), mannitol (50 mmoles/liter), methionine (10 mmoles/liter), glutathione (0.01 mmoles/liter) and desferrioxamine (0.15 mmoles/liter) reduced the incidence of reperfusion-induced ventricular fibrillation from 80% to 0%, 7%, 7%, 7%, 20% and 7% respectively. Bernier et al (1986) also carried out dose-response studies for each intervention and demonstrated a clear dose-dependency for each intervention.

In additional studies with free radical *generating* systems (xanthine oxidase plus hypoxanthine and also ferric chloride-ADP) Bernier et al (1986) were able to *increase* the vulnerability of hearts to reperfusion-induced arrhythmias. Furthermore, this increase could be ameliorated by superoxide dismutase, catalase, mannitol, methionine or desferrioxamine.

ALTERNATIVE NON-FREE RADICAL-MEDIATED MECHANISMS OF ACTION

Despite the wide and diverse group of interventions studied it must be concluded that although each has an ability to influence free radical production, alternative mechanisms of action may be involved. Thus, allopurinol may be acting via purine salvage, methionine and glutathione may exert some effects upon intermediary metabolism and mannitol may exert osmotic effects.

Bernier and Hearse (1986) have recently used glucose and mannitol in the isolated rat heart in an attempt to dissociate the metabolic, osmotic and free radical scavenging properties of hexose molecules. It was found that the non-metabolizable sugar mannitol exerted a dose-dependent anti-arrhythmic effect (Figure 6)

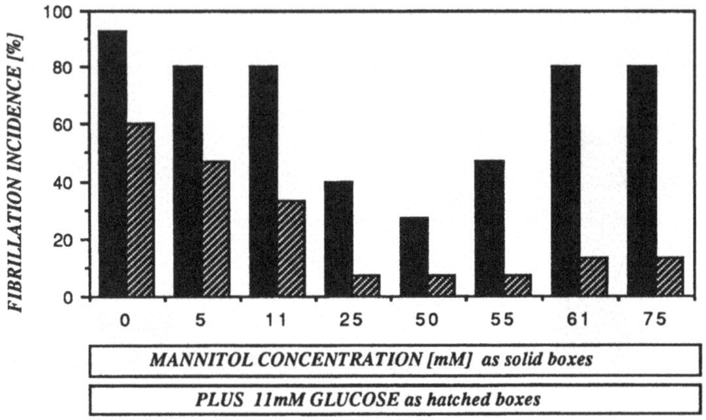

FIGURE 6: The dose-dependent anti-arrhythmic effect of mannitol in the presence and absence of glucose

which could be greatly potentiated by the addition of small quantities (11 mmoles/liter) of glucose. However, glucose alone exerted no significant anti-arrhythmic effect when used at 11 mmoles/liter. In seeking to assess the relative importance of osmotic properties, hearts were perfused with various combinations of mannitol plus glucose with an identical osmotic load. Striking differences were observed such that good protection (Figure 7)

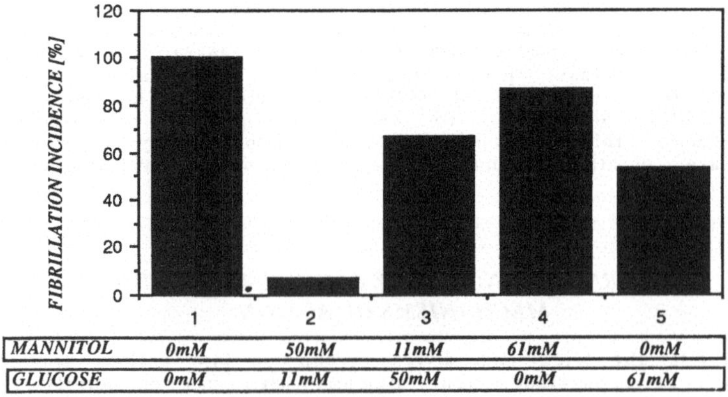

FIGURE 7: The relative anti-arrhythmic effect of different combinations of glucose and mannitol with an identical osmolarity

was only observed with high concentrations of mannitol (50 mmoles/liter) plus low concentrations of glucose (11 mmoles/liter) where reperfusion-induced ventricular fibrillation was reduced from its control value of 100% to 7%. In contrast, when high concentrations of glucose (50 mmoles/liter) were combined with low concentrations of mannitol (11 mmoles/liter) 67% of the hearts fibrillated. These and other studies have led Bernier and Hearse (1986) to dismiss osmotic effects and also question whether free radical scavenging is the major mechanism by which hexose molecules exert their potent anti-arrhythmic effects.

FREE RADICALS AND ARRHYTHMIAS: INDIRECT EVIDENCE WHICH MAY BE CIRCUMSTANTIAL

The association between the production of free radicals and the genesis of reperfusion-induced arrhythmias is *indirect* and as such may be *circumstantial*. As stressed earlier, alternative mechanisms may be involved. In order to prove a *direct* relationship it would be necessary to detect and quantify free radicals in the preparations under study. This is difficult due to the very short half life of the radicals which are thought to be involved. Recently Garlick and Hearse, in collaboration with Slater and Davies from Brunel University, have used electron spin resonance (ESR) in an attempt to detect and quantify free radical production in the isolated rat heart during reperfusion after a short period of ischemia (Garlick et al 1986). Rat hearts were perfused with the spin trap N-tert-butyl-alpha-phenylnitrone (PBN) at a concentration of 3 mmoles/liter. After 35 min of aerobic perfusion the hearts were rendered ischemic for 15 min and then they were reperfused either *aerobically* or *anoxically*. Sequential aliquots of coronary effluent were extracted into toluene and ESR spectra were recorded. Large signals were obtained during the first 4 min of aerobic reperfusion. Much smaller signals were obtained during anoxic reperfusion. Although the initial free radical species formed were probably superoxide and hydroxyl, the ESR signals were suggestive of a carbon-centred free radical adduct formed by secondary reactions with membrane lipids. Thus, evidence was obtained, within the time frame during which reperfusion-induced arrhythmias occur, that free radicals are formed and that membrane damage is likely to result. Free radical-induced membrane injury would, of course, be likely to render the heart more susceptible to reperfusion-induced arrhythmias.

FREE RADICAL SPIN TRAPS AND ARRHYTHMIAS

Since free radical spin traps act essentially as free radical scavengers, removing free radicals through the formation of relatively stable adducts, it could be hypothesized that spin trap agents should possess anti-arrhythmic properties. This has been tested by Hearse and Tosaki (1987a, 1987b) who demonstrated (Figure 8)

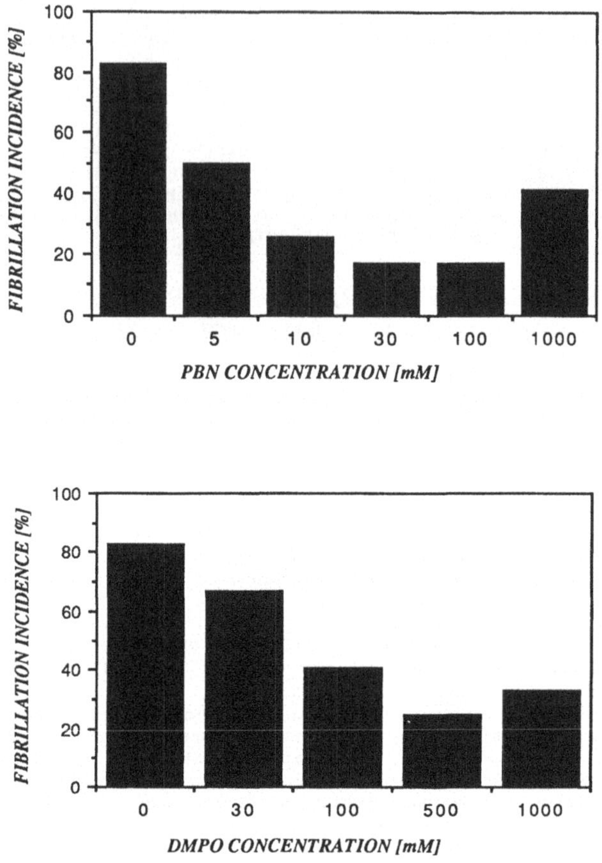

FIGURE 8: The anti-arrhythmic properties of PBN and DMPO

that both PBN and DMPO (5, 5-dimethyl-1- pyrroline N-oxide) were able to exert a dose-dependent anti-arrhythmic action against reperfusion-induced ventricular fibrillation in the isolated rat heart.

CONCLUDING COMMENTS

There is now a growing body of evidence that free radicals, generated during ischemia and reperfusion, may be an important factor in precipitating the occurrence of ventricular fibrillation. In a variety of preparations, both in vivo and in vitro, free radical scavengers, or inhibitors of free radical production, have been shown to dramatically reduce the vulnerability of the heart to reperfusion-induced ventricular fibrillation. Conversely free radical generating systems can increase the vulnerability to arrhythmias. It must be conceded that these findings are currently limited to the rat heart and that they are indirect and may be circumstantial. However, recent studies have provided a *direct* demonstration of a burst of free radical production at a time when arrhythmias would normally be expected to occur.

While free radicals may finally prove to be an important determinant of vulnerability to ventricular arrhythmias (and thus provide for the development of novel anti-arrhythmic agents) it must be stressed that many other triggers are likely to exist. It may well transpire that it is the pattern of interaction between these multiple triggers that determines whether an individual heart develops a potentially lethal disorder of cardiac rhythm.

REFERENCES

Bernier M, Hearse DJ. 1986. The anti-fibrillation effect of glucose in the isolated rat heart: is it an osmotic, metabolic or anti-freeradical-mediated mechanism? Circulation 74: (Suppl II) abstract 1359.

Bernier M, Hearse DJ, Manning AS. 1986. Reperfusion-induced arrhythmias and oxygen-derived free radicals. Studies with anti-free radical interventions and a free radical-generating system in the isolated perfused rat heart. Circulation Research 58: 331-340.

Bhagat BD, Rao PS, Dhalla NS. 1980. The role of catecholamines in the genesis of arrhythmias. Advances in Myocardiology 2: 117-121

Corr PB, Saffitz JE, Sobel BE. What is the contribution of altered lipid metabolism to arrhythmogenesis in the ischemic rat heart? In: Life Threatening Arrhythmias During Ischemia and Infarction. Eds. DJ Hearse, AS Manning, MJ Janse. Raven Press, New York, 1987.

Garlick PB, Davies MJ, Slater TS, Hearse DJ. 1986. Detection of free radical production in the reperfused rat heart using a spin trap agent and electron spin resonance. Circulation 74: (Suppl II) abstract 1393.

Geddes LS. What are the effects of potassium on the electrophysiology of acute ischemia? In: Life Threatening Arrhythmias during Ischemia and Infarction Eds. DJ Hearse, AS Manning, MJ Janse. Raven Press, New York, 1987.

Halliwell B, Gutteridge JMC. Free radicals in Biology and Medicine. Clarendon Press, Oxford 1985.

Hearse DJ, Manning AS, Janse MJ (Eds). Life-threatening arrhythmias during ischemia and infarction. Raven Press, New York, 1987.

Hearse DJ, Tosaki A. 1987a. Free radicals and reperfusion-induced arrhythmias: protection by spin trap agent PBN in the rat heart. Circulation Research 60: 375-383.

Hearse DJ, Tosaki A. 1987b. Reperfusion-induced arrhythmias and free radicals: studies in the rat heart with DMPO. Cardiovascular Pharmacology, In the press.

Hess ML, Manson NH. 1984. Molecular oxygen: friend or foe? Journal of Molecular and Cellular Cardiology 16: 969-985.

Kurien VA, Yates PA, Oliver MF. 1984. The role of free fatty acids in the production of ventricular arrhythmias after acute coronary artery occlusions. European Journal of Clinical Investigation. 1: 225-241.

Lucchesi BR, Romson JL, Jolly SR. Do leukocytes influence infarct size? In: Therapeutic Approaches to Myocardial Infarct Size Limitation. Eds. DJ Hearse, DM Yellon. Raven Press, New York, 1984.

McCord JM. Are free radicals a major culprit? In: Therapeutic Approaches to Myocardial Infarct Size Limitation. Eds. DJ Hearse, D M Yellon, Raven Press, New York 1984.

Manning AS. 1986. Reperfusion-induced arrhythmias: a possible role for xanthine oxidase-derived free radicals. Journal of Molecular and Cellular Cardiology 18: (Suppl 1) abstract 197.

Manning AS, Coltart DJ, Hearse DJ. Ischemia- and reperfusion-induced arrhythmias in the rat: effects of xanthine oxidase inhibition with allopurinol. Circulation Research, 55: 545-550.

Manning AS, Hearse DJ. 1984. Reperfusion-induced arrhythmias: mechanisms and prevention. Journal of Molecular and Cellular Cardiology 16: 497-518.

Manning AS, Kinoshita K, Buschmans E, Hearse DJ. 1985. The genesis of arrhythmias during myocardial ischemia: dissociation between changes in cyclic AMP and electrical instability in the rat. Circulation Research 57: 668-675.

Opie LH, Muller C, Nathan D, Daries P, Lubbe WF. Evidence for role of cyclic AMP as a second messenger of arrhythmogenic effects of beta stimulation. In: Advances in Cyclic Nucleotide Research Eds. P Hamet, H Sands, 12: 63-70, Raven Press, New York, 1980.

Opie LH, Nathan D, Lubbe WF. 1979. Biochemical aspects of arrhythmogenesis and ventricular fibrillation. American Journal of Cardiology. 43: 131-148.

Parratt JR (Ed). Early arrhythmias resulting from myocardial ischemia. MacMillan Press, London,1982.

Riva E, Hearse DJ, Manning AS. 1986. Free radical quenching and reperfusion-induced arrhythmias: dose-response studies for superoxide dismutase and catalase in the anesthetized rat. Journal of Molecular and Cellular Cardiology 18: (Suppl 2) abstract 65.

Singal PK, Beamish RE, Dhalla NS. 1983. Potential oxidative pathways of catecholamines in the formation of lipid peroxides and the genesis of heart diseases. Advances in Experimental Medicine and Biology. 161: 391-401

Turner JF, Bovaris A. 1980. Generation of superoxide anion by the NADH dehydrogenase of bovine heart mitochondria. Biochemical Journal 191: 421-427.

Woodward B, Zakaria M. 1984. Effects of some free radical scavengers on reperfusion-induced arrhythmias in the isolated rat heart. Journal of Molecular and Cellular Cardiology, 16: 497-517.

DIENE CONJUGATION IN
THE CLINICAL MEASUREMENT OF FREE-RADICAL ACTIVITY

T. L. Dormandy

and

D. G. Wickens

Department of Chemical Pathology, Whittington Hospital

Highgate Hill, London N19 5NF, UK

ABSTRACT. Diene conjugation has long been an established but imprecise marker of free-radical activity in biological systems. The main diene-conjugated compounds in human tissues and tissue fluids have now been identified and high-performance liquid chromatographic (HPLC) methods have been developed for their specific measurement. Significant abnormalities have been detected in the serum of chronic alcoholics and in lipolytic states. In tissues the abnormal molar ratio between linoleic acid and its diene-conjugated isomer may prove to be the most sensitive biochemical marker of premalignancy.

INTRODUCTION

Although the key role of free-radical reactions in many biological processes is no longer in doubt, methodology still limits the application of this knowledge to clinical diagnosis and management (1). Electron-spin-resonance (ESR) spectroscopy, the only direct method for detecting free radicals as such, has made great strides in recent years ; but it is still a long way from becoming a "routine" procedure. At the other extreme, long-established methods of measuring "free-radical products" such as TBA reactivity ("malonyldialdehyde"), have become simple kit tests but their lack of specificity is increasingly apparent. The present paper reviews recent and current developments in the measurement of diene conjugation which may become the method of choice in diagnosis of certain diseases.

THE CHEMISTRY OF DIENE CONJUGATION

Among the biological bulk constituients of the body polyunsaturated lipids are the most susceptible to free-radical attack. The initiating event in their free-radical-mediated breakdown is the abstraction of a single electron from a carbon atom situated between two double bonds. In the great majority of naturally occurring polyunsaturated lipids these double bonds are separated from each other by at least two single bonds. The abstraction of a single electron not only converts the molecule into a free radical but also causes a shift in the position of double bonds. They close in on the carbon atom carrying the unpaired electron and become separated by only one single bond. In chemical parlance the hydrocarbon chain becomes diene conjugated. The life-span of the diene-conjugated free radical itself is of course almost undetectably short ; but the diene-conjugated bond sequence, -C=C-C=C-, is retained by many of its more stable products. This has considerable practical importance.

Even before Farmer and his group established the molecular mechanism of free-radical autoxidation (2-4) Gillam and others had noted that polyunsaturated lipids exposed to air or undergoing alkali isomeridation develop an absorption peak in the ultraviolet spectrum around 230 nm (5,6). The peak was soon identified as a function of the diene-conjugated bond sequence (7). It was easily measurable and rapidly became a standard method for assessing free-radical damage in the oil, food and rubber industry. It is still widely used.

DIENE CONJUGATION ON BIOLOGICAL SYSTEMS

In biochemistry free-radical reactions were virtually ignored until the nineteen fifties ; and most early workers used TBA reacitivty for their detection. During the nineteen sixties, however, monitoring changes in diene conjugation emerged as an additional potentially useful experimental approach. It helped to confirm the key role of free radicals in liver damage caused by carbon tetrachloride and other halogenated carbon compounds (8-10) ; it provided information about the effect of ozone and nitrogen dioxide in the lungs (11-13) ; and it could be applied to the study of brain and red-cell lipids (14,15). By and large the measurement correlated well with other indirect evidence of free-radical activity (16-18) - e.g., TBA reactivity, oxygen uptake and the evolution of small-molecular alkanes - though there were inconsistencies both between different methods and between the biochemical findings and functional organ failure (19,20). A number of modifications widened the scope and improved the precision of the technique (21,22).

TOTAL DIENE CONJUGATION IN MAN

In 1972 Di Luzio showed that there is a considerable amount of diene-conjugated material in human serum and that this could be influenced by the administration of large doses of tocopherol (23). Shaw *et al.* used the measurement (inevitably interpreting the results as "lipid peroxidation") in studying the possible relevance of free-radicals to tissue damage in chronic alcoholics (24) ; and it was one of the free-radical parameters explored by Wickens *et al.* in the serum of women with preeclamptic toxaemia (25) and by Lunec *et al.* in the synovial fluid and serum of patients with inflammatory and degenerative arthritis (26). In all these studies but especially in the clinical series it was the "statistical significance" of the results, not the lack of it, which engendered dissatisfaction.

Even in simple lipid systems the measurement of diene conjugation by uv spectroscopy is a generic measurement of a characteristic bond sequence : it provides no information about the actual compounds which incorporate this sequence in their structure. In biological material the lipids exposed to free-radical attack are far more heterogeneous and the difficulties in interpreting results multiply. In human pathology the complexity of the disease processes and the restricted scope for manipulating experimental conditions add to the uncertainty. One need only recall that different factors govern the composition and determine the significance of the main serum lipid classes - triglycerides, cholesterol esters and phospholipids. Free fatty acids do not normally contribute significantly to the total but can do so in abnormal states. The diet, meals, smoking and social drinking, all of which affect different blood lipids differently, may be almost impossible to control. Most chronically ill patients, moreover, and a fast-growing proportion of the professedly fit consume drugs which can interfere with or demolish the value of spectroscopic measurements. The fact that, despite these handicaps, the results were often "suggestive" (though virtually useless, at least in isolation, as the basis of a diagnostic test) underlined the need for developing the method further. In particular the main diene-conjugated compound or compounds clearly needed to be identified and a methodology had to be developed for measuring them individually in different molecular combinations. Some of the results of these studies can now be summarised.

OCTADECA-9,11-DIENOIC ACID (18:2(9,11))

Identification

Over 95% of diene conjugation in human serum, tissue fluids and tissues - abnormal as well as normal - is due to a single fatty acid. This has now been identified as octadeca-9(cis), 11(trans)-dienoic acid (18:2(9,11)). It is a simple isomer of linoleic acid (18:2(9,12)), not a peroxide, hydroxy acid or aldehyde : indeed, it contains no oxygen outside the terminal carboxyl group (27,28). It is present in an esterified form in all the main serum-lipid classes ; and in lipolytic states it represents a variable but often a relatively high proportion of the free (i.e., non-esterified) fatty acids (29). Its concentration, both absolute and relative to linoleic acid, varies independently in the different serum and tissue lipids. (This can be a pitfall in the interpretation of total diene-conjugation.) A range of relatively simple HPLC methods has been developed to measure the molar concentration of the compound quickly and accurately in all the main lipid classes (30). Often the results are best expressed as a "molar ratio" (M%) - 18:2(9,11) x 100 / 18:2(9,12).

Origin

Paradoxically, whereas diene conjugation measured as a simple uv peak (often rising from a distinctly meandering base-line) had been widely accepted as a reasonable free-radical marker, the specific measurement of 18:2(9,11) has raised doubts. The main reason has been the non-peroxide nature of the compound. Although as early as 1957 Chipault et al. suggested that peroxidation may not be the invariable sequel of a free-radical attack on a polyunsaturated lipid (31) in biological studies the notion has remained virtually unchallenged. This is remarkable since it is based on a model constructed to explain a purely non-biological process. Farmer and his colleagues were the first to explain the auto-catalytic nature of lipid autoxidation (as well as a number of other experimental findings) by postulating the addition of dioxygen to the methylenic carbon atom of lipid free radicals to generage lipid-peroxy free radicals (2-4). The accompanying shift in double bonds involved the formation of an intermediate hybrid radical. Although in detail their original concept has been modified (32), its essential correctness is now beyond reasonable doubt. Nor does the identification of 18:2(9,11) as the main diene-conjugated compound in human tissues contradict it.

The non-peroxide 18:2(9,11) can be generated in vitro by exposing 18:2(9,12) to free-radical activity but only in the presence of a protein. Much circumstantial evidence suggests, moreover, that it requires close molecular proximity between the reducing group, almost certainly a thiol, and the lipid free radical. Such a model was not, of course, envisaged by Farmer and his collaborators ; but it is a situation which almost certainly prevails in the living. Ivanov recently outlined the theoretical basis of a "relay" mechanism in highly organised membranes which would allow the rapid lateral spread of diene-conjugated carbon-centred (i.e., non-peroxy) free radicals in preference to the formation of the oxygen-centred (i.e., peroxy) species (33). That such a mechanism may occur or that it is likely to occur does not of course mean that it does occur ; and the experimental evidence against it has to be assessed.

It is possible to expose a more-or-less random selection of biological systems to a similarly random selection of free-radical-generating mechanisms in vitro and demonstrate no increase in the concentration of 18:2(9,11) (34). Yet to conclude from this that 18:2(9,11) is not a free-radical product is like interpreting the absence of a specific enzyme as evidence that a biological process is non-enzymic. There are many ways of generating free radicals (or even one particular free radical) and an even wider choice of biological model systems. If the exposure of the model to free radical activity is monitored by a non-specific marker - TBA reactivity, for example, measures at least twenty peroxidation products and probably much else besides - then the chances of detecting an effect are good. But if the marker is a compound which is generated in vivo by a specific reaction in a specific site under specific conditions, then not demonstrating an effect is no evidence one way or the other. (This is as true of individual small-molecular alkanes as of any specific diene conjugate (35).) The principle has a mundane corrolary.

With the quickening interest in free radicals as possible causes of human disease free-radical biochemists are increasingly asked to establish whether free-radicals reactions are or are not involved in a clinical situation or syndrome. If the answer is required in such general terms, it is obviously better to use as non-specific a free-radical marker as possible. Whether or not such an answer is worth having in the long run is another matter. The role of free radicals in most biological processes is no longer in doubt ; and the idea that this in itself is significant may be misleading.

A more perplexing question looming over the free-radical origin of 18:2(9,11) is that of stereospecificity. On theoretical grounds one would expect the shift of double bonds due to a free-radical attack to yield not one but several diene-conjugated stereoisomers : in particular one would expect it to yield a series of 10,12 as well as 9,11 compounds. This is indeed what happens when linoleic acid and protein are exposed to free-radical activity in vitro. In tissues and tissue fluids, by contrast, diene conjugation is entirely the function of the 9(cis),11(trans) configuration (28). One possible but experimentally still unverified explanation is a closely organised membrane structure in which the steric relationship between the lipids and proteins (if the reducing agents are proteins) would precisely determine the outcome of their interaction.

Although neither of the main alternative to a free-radical mechanism can be dismissed, they are even more open to objection. As pointed out by Iversen _et al_. (30), an enzyme is known to be produced by certain anaerobic microorganisms in the bovine rumen which is capable of catalysing the conversion of 18:2(9,12) to 18:2(9,11) (36). Despite attempts to do so, no such enzyme has been demonstrated in man. One cannot of course object to the description of a stereospecific interation of a lipid free radical and a membrane protein as "enzymic" ; but the label is not particularly helpful.

The second alternative explanation is dietary, based on the relatively high concentration of octadeca-9,11-dienoic acid in milk and milk products (37). In this connection one has to distinguish between base-line levels and abnormal variations as well as between the different molecular combinations in which 18:2(9,11) exist in the body. It is unproven but not unlikely, for example, that long-term dietary habits in different populations or even in different individuals are significant variables in determining the fasting level of phospholipid-esterified 18:2(9,11) in serum. It is highly unlikely, on the other hand, that they could account for the precipitous changes which occur in chronic alcoholics on alcohol withdrawal. It is even more unlikely that they could explain the differences between the concentration of the compound in normal and in premalignant cervical cells.

Physicochemical and biological properties

It is unprofitable but interesting to speculate why vulnerable (and expensive) unsaturated and polyunsaturated lipids account for such a high proportion of body fat or why the double bonds in the vast bulk of polyunsaturated fatty-acids residues conform to the cis-cis steric configuration. Whatever other roles unsaturated and polyunsaturated lipids may have, flesh would set solid (as Hamlet lamented and as happens in rigor mortis) if the degree of unsaturation fell below a critical level ; and normal membrane function would cease if too many fatty acid residues would develop a kink in their hydrocarbon chain. It is often forgotten that even seemingly trivial structural changes sometimes profoundly alter the basic physical and therefore biological properties of molecules. This is certainly true of the shift of one double bond in the 18-carbon chain of linoleic acid. The diene-conjugated biological isomer, for example, 18:2(9,11), is a solid at room temperature in contrast to 18:2(9,12) which is a liquid ; and a cis-trans orientation could seriously disrupt the function of a membrane based on aligned cis-cis isomers (38,39).

18:2(9,11) IN SERUM

A significantly increased level of phospholipid-esterified 18:2(9,11) which could not be attributed to malnutrition of cirrhosis was demonstrated by Fink et al. (40,41) in the serum of chronic alcoholics. Even more striking was the rapid return to normal on alcohol withdrawal. In non-addicts, by contrast, an acute alcohol load had no significant effect. The findings as a whole pointed to a two-stage abnormality : first, the slow induction of a free-radical-dependent detoxifying mechanism during the development of the addiction ; and second, the triggering of this mechanism by an acute alcohol load. The fact that 18:2(9,11) is not a peroxide eliminates the apparent contradiction between the increased free-radical activity suggested by these results and the diminished susceptibility to peroxidation of red-cell lipids observed by Clemens et al. (42). The alcohol-dependent increase in phospholipid-esterified 18:2(9,11) in serum has recently been confirmed in a comparative study of chronic abusers and volunteers from the teetotal Church of Jesus Christ Latter Day Saints (Mormons) (43). High concentrations of phospholipid-esterified 18:2(9,11) have also been demonstrated by Crump et al. (44) in four cases of paraquat poisoning. The significance of slightly or moderately raised concentrations in about 20 % of unselected hospital patients (including the majority of patients with primary biliary cirrhosis) remains to be explored.

Partly for methodological reasons and partly because free fatty acids normally represent only a negligible fraction of serum lipids, an increase in the concentration of non-esterified 18:2(9,11) may be overlooked or misinterpreted. Such an increase has recently been described in patients undergoing cardiopulmonary by-pass surgery or renal haemodialysis (45,46). This is almost certainly the result of heparinisation (47) related to the lipolysis induced by the drug both in plasma and in tissues. The reason why free 18:2(9,11) increases out of proportion to the increase in free 18:2(9,12) remains to be established. A similar increase in free fatty acids may account for the abnormal concentration of 18:2(9,12) reported in some patients in diabetic coma (48).

18:2(9,11) IN BILE

Braganza *et al.* (49) have demonstrated a significantly higher level of phospholipid-esterified 18:2(9,11) in the bile of patients with pancreatic disease compared to patients undergoing endoscopic examination for non-pancreatic disorder. There was a corresponding increase in free-fatty-acid 18:2(9,11) in duodenal juice. The findings led Braganza to raise the provocative question whether the pancrease might be the "victim" of hepatic detoxification (50). She envisages the possibility that a free-radical-dependent detoxifying mechanism in the liver, perhaps involving a cytochrome system, may generate products which could be toxic on being refluxed into the pancreatic duct system.

18:2(9,11) IN CERVICAL PRECANCER

In 1985 the methodology for measuring 18:2(9,11) was adapted first to the study of human biopsy material and then exfoliated cells (51,52). This was prompted largely by the possibility that the measurement might become a useful diagnostic tool in cervical precancer (cervical intra-epithelial neoplasia or CIN).

The cytological method on which the diagnosis of CIN currently rests has been described both as a triumph and as a disaster. There is truth in both descriptions. Potentially cervical cytology based on the Papanicolaou technique is the nearest available approach to the diagnosis of malignancy at a stage when it is curable with virtual certainty. On the other hand, since CIN is asymptomatic the method has to be applied as a screening procedure in apparently well women. Cytology is one of the most labour-intensive laboratory procedures : it requires specially trained staff and it is seemingly impossible to automate. The number of women "at risk" who should theoretically be screened at reasonable intervals to ensure effective prevention is of the order of 10-15 million in England and Wales. In other words, the means and the objective of the programme are incompatible. Cervical cytology, moreover, has a rather horrifying false-negative rate, variously estimated to be between 5 and 30 % (53).

In contrast to microscopic cytology the automated HPLC measurement of phospholipid-esterified 18:2(9,11) and 18:2(9,12) is quick, reproducible and non-observer dependent. The results are best expressed as a molar ratio (M%) - 18:2(9,11) x 100 / 18:2(9,12). The concentration of 18:2(9,12) provides a reference measurement which eliminates the need for a cell count or the chemical estimation of protein or DNA : it is not significantly affected by pre-malignant change. The difference in M% between different groups of patients is, in other words, the function of the concentration of 18:2(9,11). The Table shows the results in a recently completed study in which the biochemical method was compared to the Papanicolaou technique (54).

Diagnosis	n	Molar ratio	Significance*
Normal	40	1.80 (0.47)	-
CIN 1	40	2.89 (1.31)	$p \ll 0.0001$
CIN 2	38	3.06 (1.42)	$p \ll 0.0001$
CIN 3	81	3.32 (1.26)	$p \ll 0.0001$
Invasive Cancer	3	5.25	-

* - Mann-Whitney test against normal.

TABLE. Mean (SD) molar ratios of 18:2(9,11) to 18:2(9,12) in exfoliated cervical cells.

In terms of sensitivity - i.e., the incidence of false - negatives - the former is at least comparable and possibly superior to the latter. To assess their comparative specificity - i.e., the incidence of false positives - and positive prognostic value a multicentre trial is proceeding.

The increased concentration of 18:2(9,11) in at least one kind of precancer and even more in invasive cancer raises a number of questions. On the face of it the findings seem to contradict much earlier work related to free radicals and neoplasia. In particular strong evidence based on a wide range of experimental systems suggests that malignant cells have a markedly diminished susceptibility to peroxidation or, to formulate the same message differently, that they are more highly protected against free-radical-mediated peroxidation than are normal cells (55). This is consonant with the observations of other workers, notably Benedetto et al. (44), who measured ESR signals in both normal and cancerous cervices. A clear signal was obtained from normal organs and could be identified with reasonable certainty as that of a lipid peroxy free radical. The signal was attenuated or absent in malignant tissue (55). The contradiction between these observations (all pointing to a diminished free-radical-mediated peroxidation) and the increased concentration of 18:2(9,11) is, in fact, only apparent : indeed, it is conceivable that they are causally linked.

Although 18:2(9,11) is almost certainly a free-radical reaction product, it is not a peroxide ; and the carbon-centred free radical which must be presumed to be its immediate precursor would almost certainly be undetectable by the ESR method used for the detection of the lipid peroxy signal. One can speculate that 18:2(9,11) may represent a block in and a deflection from the normal peroxidation pathway after the initial free-radical attack on 18:2(9,12). This could be linked to the recent finding of a marked decrease in active thiol groups in malignant cells (56).

References

1. T. L. Dormandy: Lancet, 2, (1983) 1010.
2. E.H. Farmer and A. Sundralingham : J. Chem. Soc. 121, (1942) 1940.
3. E.H. Farmer : Trans. Faraday Soc. 541, (1943) 541.
4. E.H. Farmer, H.P. Koch and D.A. Sutton : J. Chem. Soc. 541, (1943) 1940.
5. A.E. Gillam, I.M. Heilbron and R.A. Morton: Biochem. J. 25, (1931) 30.
6. J.H. Mitchell, H.R. Kraybill and F.P. Scheile : Ind. Eng. Chem. Anal. 15, (1943) 1.

7. J.L. Bolland and H.P. Koch : J. Chem. Soc. 445, (1945) 1940.

8. R.O. Recknagel and A.K. Ghoshal : Lab. Invest. 15, (1966) 132.

9. R.O. Recknagel and E.A. Glende : in Methods in Enzymology (ed. L. Packer) Academic Press, New York, 1984.

10. T.F. Slater : Free Radical Mechanisms in Liver Injury. Pion, London, 1972.

11. B.D. Goldstein, C. Lodi, C. Collinson and O.J. Balchum : Arch. Environ. Health 18, (1969) 631.

12. M.G. Mustafa, A.J. de Lucia, G.K. York and C.E. Cross : J. Lab. Clin. Med. 82, (1973) 357.

13. K. Kyei-Aboagye, M. Hazucha and M.E. Avery : Biochem. Biophys. Res. Commun. 54, (1973) 907.

14. S. Rehncrona, D.S. Smith, B. Akesson, E. Westerberg and B.K. Siesjo : J. Neurochem. 34 (1980) 1630.

15. J.I. Dodge and G.B. Phillips : J. Lipid Res. 7, (1966) 387.

16. M. Sagai and A.L. Tappel : Toxicol. Appl. Pharmacol. 49 (1979) 283.

17. L.K. Dahle, E.G. Hill and R.T. Holman : Arch. Biochem. Biophys. 98, (1962) 253.

18. J. M. C. Gutteridge, P.J. Kelly and D. Armstrong : Biochim. Biophys. Acta. 711, (1982) 46.

19. M. Comporti, C. Saccoci and M.U. Dianzani : Gastro-enterology, 50 (1966) 392.

20. A. Benedetti, A.G. Casini, M. Ferrali and M. Comporti : Chem-Biol. Interact. 17, (1977) 151.

21. R.L. Waller and R.O. Recknagel : Lipids, 12 (1977) 914.

22. F.P. Corongiu and A. Milia : Chem-Biol. Interactions, 44 (1983) 289.

23. N.R. Di Luzio : J. Agr. Food Chem. 20, (1972) 486.

24. S. Shaw, K.P. Rubin and C.S. Lieber : Dig. Dis. Sci. 28, (1983) 585.

25. D.G. Wickens, M.H. Wilkins, J. Lunec, G. Ball and T.L. Dormandy : Ann. Clin. Biochem. 18, (1981) 158.

26. J. Lunec, S.P. Halloran, A.G. White and T.L. Dormandy : J. Rheumatol. 8, (1981) 233.

27. P. Cawood, D.G. Wickens, S.A. Iversen, G.M. Braganza and T.L. Dormandy : FEBS Lett. 162, (1983) 239.

28. S.A. Iversen, P. Cawood, M.J. Madilgan, A.M. Lawson and T.L. Dormandy : Life Chem. Rep. 3, (1985) 45.

29. D.G. Wickens, J.F. Griffin, E.H. Maher, J.R. Curtis and T.L. Dormandy : Free Radical Res. Comms. 1987, in press.

30. S.A. Iversen, P. Cawood and T.L. Dormandy : Ann. Clin. Biochem. 22, (1985) 137.

31. J.R. Chipault, O.S. Privett, G.R. Mizuno, E.C. Nickell and W.O. Lundberg : Ind. Eng. Chem. 49 (1957) 1713.

32. S. Bergstrom : Ark. Kem. Mineral. Geol. 21A (1945) 1.

33. I.I. Ivanov : J. Free Rad. Biol. Med. 1, (1986) 247.

34. S. Thompson and M.T. Smith : Lancet 2, (1985) 774.

35. M. R. Clemens, H Einsele, H. Remmer and H.D. Waller : Clin. Chim. Acta. 145, (1985) 283.

36. P.E. Hughes and S. B. Tove : J. Biol. Chem. 255, (1980) 1802.

37. P.W. Parodi : J. Dairy Sci. 60, (1977) 1550.

38. R.T. Holman and J.J. Ramm : In Progress in the Chemistry of Fats and other Lipids (R.T. Holman, ed.), vol. 9, pp. 13-90. Pergamon, Oxford, 1966.

39. K.S. Markley : Fatty Acids, their Characteristics and Properties : Vol. 1. Wyley, New York, 1948.

40. R. Fink, D.H. Marjot, M.R. Clemens, P. Patsalos, P. Cawood, S.A. Iversen and T.L. Dormandy : Lancet 2, (1985) 291.

41. R. Fink, D.H. Marjot, M.R. Clemens, P. Patsalos, P. Cawood, S.A. Iversen and T.L. Dormandy : Lancet 2, (1985) 291.

42. M.R. Clemens and H. Einsele : in Free Radicals (C. Rice-Evans, ed.), pp. 127-131. Richelieu, London 1986.

43. J. Szebeni, C. Eskelson, R. Sampliner, B. Hartman, J. Griffin and T.L. Dormandy : Alcoholism 10, (1986) 647.

44. B. J. Crump, D.I. Thurnham, R.D. Situnayake and M. Davis : Lancet 2, (1985) 956.

45. C.R.K. Hind, J. Griffin, H.R. Drake, H.M. Jones, T. Treasure and T. L. Dormandy : Clin. Sci. 71, (1986) 77.

46. E.R. Maher, J. Griffin, D.G. Wickens, J.R. Curtis and T.L. Dormandy : Clin. Sci. 71, (1986) 78.

47. E.R. Maher, D.G. Wickens, J. Griffin, P. Kyle, J.R. Curtis and T.L. Dormandy : Nephrol. Dial. Transpl. In press.

48. K. Harrison, P. Cawood, A. Iversen and T.L. Dormandy : Life Chem. Rep. 3 (1985) 45.

49. G. Braganza, D.G. Wickens, P. Cawood and T.L. Dormandy : Lancet, 2, (1983) 375.

50. G. Braganza : Lancet, 2, (1983) 100.

51. S.K. Tay, J.F.A. Griffin, D.G. Wickens, A. Singer and T.L. Dormandy : Clin. Chim. Acta, 1987, in press.

52. J.F.A. Griffin, S.K. Tay, D.G. Wickens, A. Singer and T.L. Dormandy : Clin. Chim. Acta. 1987, in press.

53. R.M. Richart and B.A. Barron : Cancer 47, (1981) 1176.

54. G.W. Burton, K.H. Cheeseman, K.U. Ingold and T.F. Slater : Biochem. Soc. Trans. 11, (1983) 261.

55. C. Benedetto, A. Bocci, M.U. Dianzani, B. Ghiringello, T.F. Slater, A. Tomas and V. Vannini : Cancer Res. 41, (1981) 2946.

56. G. Nohammer, F. Bajardi, C. Benedetto, E. Schaeustein and T.F. Slater : Br. J. Cancer, 53 (1986) 217.

CONVERSION OF RAT XANTHINE DEHYDROGENASE TO XANTHINE OXIDASE DURING OXIDATIVE STRESS.

A. Bindoli, L. Cavallini, M.P. Rigobello, M. Coassin and F. Di Lisa

Centro Studio Fisiologia Mitocondriale, C.N.R. and Istituto di Chimica Biologica, Via F. Marzolo 3, 35131 Padova (Italy).

ABSTRACT

The enzyme "xanthine oxidase" is one of the best characterized sources of superoxide anion and hydrogen peroxide. "In vivo" it mainly acts as a dehydrogenase which, by reducing NAD^+, appears to be the physiologic form. Nevertheless under a variety of conditions the enzyme can undergo a conversion to an oxidase which delivers the electrons to oxygen to form superoxide and hydrogen peroxide. The transformation xanthine dehydrogenase ⟶ xanthine oxidase is irreversible when it is induced by a proteolytic attack or reversible when the SH groups of the enzyme have been oxidized.

In the present study the oxidative stress induced by ischemia and ischemia followed by reperfusion was compared to that induced by hydrogen peroxide or diamide in normoxic conditions. In particular we intended to characterize the type (reversible or irreversible) of the xanthine dehydrogenase ⟶ xanthine oxidase conversion and the importance of glutathione and protein SH groups in this conversion. In the fresh heart and in the control after normoxic perfusion we detected a 80% of xanthine dehydrogenase and a 20% of xanthine oxidase (5% reversible xanthine oxidase and 15% irreversible xanthine oxidase). There appears to be a considerable increase in reversible xanthine oxidase (from 5% to 15%) after reperfusion following 1 hour of global ischemia; in the same conditions there is a decrease of total glutathione and of total SH groups of about 70% and 25% respectively. After perfusion with hydrogen peroxide or with diamide, a well known thiol oxidizing agent, a very marked increase in reversible xanthine oxidase of about 40% and 60% respectively is apparent. When the infusion of hydrogen peroxide or diamide ends, the reversible xanthine oxidase partially reverts to xanthine dehydrogenase. The changes in the redox state of glutathione and of total thiol groups are then in agreement with the changes of the enzyme. From the reported data it can be concluded that: 1) in the rat heart there is a basal level of reversible + irreversible xanthine oxidase which, in the presence of hypoxanthine and xanthine, contributes to the background production of oxygen free radicals. 2) There is no significant increase of irreversible xanthine oxidase during ischemia nor during reperfusion. 3) Reversible xanthine oxidase increases during the reperfusion that follows an ischemic period bringing the total amount of xanthine oxidase to about 30%. 4) Oxidizing agents like diamide and hydrogen peroxide markedly convert xanthine dehydrogenase to reversible xanthine oxidase. The latter can be reconverted to xanthine dehydrogenase after withdrawing diamide or hydrogen peroxide.

OVERVIEW AND INTRODUCTION

The catabolism of purine nucleotides is accomplished by several enzymes which, ultimately, form uric acid, the final product of purine catabolism in man and primates. The last two steps of the catabolic process, namely the transformation hypoxanthine $\longrightarrow$ xanthine and xanthine $\longrightarrow$ uric acid are catalyzed by the enzyme generally called xanthine oxidase [xanthine-oxygen oxidoreductase, E C (1.2.3.2)]. The enzyme from bovine milk has been the most extensively studied, although it appears to be largely distributed in many different species and tissues (Krenitsky et al., 1974; Parks and Granger, 1986).

The native xanthine oxidase protein from liver and other sources is a dimer having a molecular weight of about 300 000 daltons and each subunit contains an internal electron transport chain formed by FAD, molybdenum, iron and acid labile sulfide (Fig. 1). In the enzyme from animal sources (mammalian and avian) these groups are present in a molar ratio of 1:1:4:4. Within xanthine oxidase the oxidation-reduction potential of the various prosthetic groups, i.e. Mo $\leqslant$ Fe.S $\leqslant$ FAD (Olson et al., 1974), determines the direction of the electron flux from Mo to FAD. Mo is the site of oxidation of hypoxanthine and xanthine while FAD is the site which donates the electrons to the acceptor. The electron acceptor of the xanthine-converting enzyme isolated from mammalian sources is mainly, if not exclusively, NAD^+, which is reduced to NADH and, consequently, the enzyme behaves like a dehydrogenase (EC 1.2.1. 37) considered to be its physiologic form (Stirpe and Della Corte, 1969). Under a variety of heterogenous conditions, first studied by Stirpe and coworkers (Stirpe and Della Corte, 1969; Della Corte and Stirpe, 1972), the enzyme is converted to an oxidase form in which the acceptor is the dioxygen in turn transformed to both O_2^- and H_2O_2. The relative amounts of O_2^- and H_2O_2 produced depend on factors like pH, concentration of oxygen and substrates (Fridovich, 1970). In the milk enzyme, in fact, it has been shown that, at pH 7, only the 20% of oxygen is transformed into the superoxide anion while the remaining is transformed to H_2O_2 (Fridovich, 1970). It has also been shown that the amount of univalently reduced oxygen increased by decreasing the concentration of xanthine.

The xanthine dehydrogenase (XD) $\longrightarrow$ xanthine oxidase (XO) transformation can be operated by many different conditions like proteolysis, heating at 37°C, storage at -20°C, anaerobiosis, treatment with organic solvents and SH groups reagents (Stirpe and Della Corte, 1969; Della Corte and Stirpe, 1972); all these treatments may fall into two categories which are (I) proteolysis and (II) oxidation or binding of thiol groups (Battelli et al., 1973). All these conditions might probably induce a conformational change at the flavin site which, becoming unable to interact with its natural substrate NAD^+, interacts with molecular oxygen. According to the type of the experimental condition used for the transformation of XD to XO, the latter can be of the reversible (XOrev) or irreversible (XOirrev) type. The irreversible type is obtained from the dehydrogenase or from the reversible type by proteolytic treatment (trypsin, chymotrypsin, papain, subtilisin) (Battelli et al., 1973) which determines the cleavage of a polypeptidic fragment not essential for the oxidase activity but necessary to warrant a proper conformation at the flavin site for the interaction with NAD^+; there appears to be a direct relationship between the formation of a stable flavin semiquinone radical (FADH•) and the ability for NAD^+ reduction (Waud and Rajagopalan, 1976). The reversible oxidase (XOrev) can be obtained from the dehydrogenase by oxidation of some sulfhydryl groups to disulphides or by treatment with thiol modifying reagents (Della Corte and Stirpe, 1972; Waud and Rajagopalan, 1976) by sulfhydryl oxidase (Clare et al., 1981) or thiol-transferase (Battelli and Lorenzoni, 1982). The conversion from XD to XO is progressive so that a XD/XO form, intermediate between the dehydrogenase and the oxidase form, and characterized by a partial modification of the SH groups was reported (Kaminski and Jezewska, 1979). The XD/XO form interacts both with NAD^+ and oxygen. With the exception of the intestine (Battelli et al., 1972), the back conversion XOrev ⟶ XD can be catalyzed in other tissues and is obtained with thiol compounds, the most effective being dithioerythritol (DTE), dithiothreitol (DTT) and dihydrolipoic acid while GSH, cysteine, cysteamine and other low molecular weight thiols are scarcely effective (Battelli et al., 1973).

Of the various organs of the rat, the liver and intestine exhibit the highest activity of the xanthine-converting enzyme (Battelli et al., 1972) while the heart appears to have only 13% of the activity found in the intestine. Moreover, comparing the levels reported for other mammals, liver and intestine of man have relatively low values of xanthine oxidase (Parks and Granger, 1986). As far as xanthine oxidase of human heart is concerned, there is a report of just one experiment showing its presence (Krenitsky et al., 1974) while another author does not find any activity (Ramboer, 1969). In our laboratory, in three different measurements on hearts removed after heart transplantation from patients suffering from dilatative cardiomyopathy we did not find any significant activity (not shown).

By the use of immunohystochemical techniques (Jarasch et al., 1981), xanthine oxidase was localized preferentially in the cytoplasm of endothelial cells of the mammary gland, intestine, liver, heart and lung.

Recently there has been a surge of interest on this enzyme as generator of oxygen free radicals since the latter appear to be involved in the pathogenesis of injury provoked by reperfusion following a period of ischemia. Oxygen free radicals appear in fact to play a major role in inducing microvascular and parenchimal damage. The most important sources of free radicals in the infarcting myocardium, recently reviewed by Hearse et al. (1986), are: a) catecholamines which are catabolized by monoamino oxidases producing hydrogen peroxide b) mitochondria that, particularly after an ischemic period, could leak superoxide and hydrogen peroxide c) leucocytes which, after having invaded the myocardium are able to convert oxygen to superoxide by their NADPH oxidase activity and, finally d) xanthine oxidase. The production of superoxide by xanthine oxidase is considered responsible for ischemia-reperfusion disorders appearing in different tissues such as the intestine (Granger et al., 1981), the kidney (Hansson et al., 1983), the heart (Hearse et al., 1986), and the liver (Adkison et al., 1986). The conversion XD⟶XO was reported to occur in several organs during ischemia concomitantly with a marked catabolism of adenine nucleotides which brings to an accumulation of hypoxanthine. The latter acts as a substrate for the enzyme during the reperfusion following the ischemic period, leading to a rapid formation of superoxide and hydrogen peroxide. Since superoxide can dismutate, spontaneously or through the superoxide dismutase (SOD) activity, to hydrogen peroxide, the latter can accumulate. Hydrogen peroxide can either oxidize glutathione through glutathione peroxidase or initiate lipid peroxidation by interaction with myoglobin or with iron released from its stores during ischemia. Glutathione oxidation can secondarily induce the oxidation of protein SH groups.

The accumulation of activated forms of oxygen together with the impairement of the endogenous scavenging systems (GSH, protein SH groups, glutathione peroxidase and phospholipid hydroperoxide glutathione peroxidase (Ursini et al., 1985) can be the beginning of the peroxidative damage of the ischemic/reperfused organs.

In the present work the oxidative stress induced by ischemia and ischemia followed by reperfusion was compared to that induced by hydrogen peroxide and diamide in normoxic conditions. The parameters considered are the conversion XD⟶XO and particularly the type of conversion (reversible or irreversible), the redox state of glutathione and of the protein SH groups. Other parameters which are directly or indirectly indicative of an oxidative stress like formation of malondialdehyde (MDA), and left ventricular pressure developed were also considered.

MATERIALS AND METHODS

Rat heart were perfused at 37°C by the non-recirculating Langendorff procedure with a medium composed by 118 mM NaCl, 25 mM $NaHCO_3$, 4.7 mM KCl, 2 mM KH_2PO_4, 1.2 mM $MgSO_4$, 1.5 mM $CaCl_2$ and 11 mM glucose at pH 7.4; the solution was kept at 37°C and saturated with 95% O_2 and 5% CO_2. Before any experiment the hearts were perfused for 20 minutes to allow hemodynamic and metabolic stabilization of the preparation. Left ventricular pressure (LVP) was measured by introducing into the left ventricular cavity a liquid-filled balloon connected to a pressure transducer. During normoxic perfusion the flow rate was 12 ml/min; in the experiments where total ischemia was induced the flow was reduced to nought. Fractions of the effluent were collected for the determination of glutathione released. At the end of the perfusion experiment the hearts were rapidly removed and homogenized with Ultra Turrax in 10 ml of 0.1 M Tris buffer (pH 8.1), containing 1.5 mM EDTA, 1.5 mM EGTA and 1 mM phenylmethylsulfonylfluoride (PMSF). One ml of the homogenate was saved for the estimation of total sulphydryl groups and malondialdehyde (MDA), while the remaining volume was centrifuged at 105 000 x g for 40 minutes; pellet was discarded and supernatant was eluted through a 10 x 1.5 cm column of Sephadex G-50. This fraction was utilized for the estimation of the various forms of the xanthine-oxidizing enzyme. The assay was performed at 37°C by following the formation of uric acid at 292 nm (εM = 9 900). About 0.2 mg/ml of supernatant protein was incubated in 0.1 M phosphate buffer (pH 7.8) containing 80 μM xanthine and, when requested, 0.3 mM NAD^+, 2 mM DTE, 2 mM pyruvate and 0.1 U/ml of lactate dehydrogenase. The total enzyme activity (XD + XOrev + XOirrev) was measured in the aerobic medium in the presence of NAD^+; pyruvate and lactate dehydrogenase were also added in order to reoxidize the NADH formed that otherwise could inhibit the enzyme activity. The total oxidase activity (XOrev + XOirrev) was measured in the absence of NAD^+. The percentage of the total oxidase activity <u>versus</u> the total enzymatic activity could then be calculated and, by difference, the amount of XD obtained. The activity of XOirrev was estimated in the absence of NAD^+ after preincubating the supernatant at 37°C for 10 minutes in the presence of 10 mM DTE; an aliquot, about 0.4 mg/ml, was withdrawn for the assay to achieve a final concentration of 2 mM DTE. The percentage of XOirrev was obtained from the total enzymatic activity measured as reported above but in the presence of DTE in order to avoid any aspecific inhibitory effect by this reducing compound. Finally the percentage of XOrev was calculated by substracting the % of XOirrev from the % of total oxidase.

Total sulfhydryl groups of the homogenate were titrated by using the Ellman's reagent, 5,5'-dithiobis-(2-nitrobenzoic acid) (DTNB). Homogenate (0.5 mg protein) was incubated in 0.2 M Tris-HCl buffer (pH 8.1) containing 5 mM EDTA and 0.8% SDS to a final volume of 3 ml. The reaction was started by adding DTNB to a final concentration of 2 mM and the increase of absorbance was followed at 412 nm until a constant value was obtained. The concentration of sulfhydryl groups was calculated using εM = 13 600.

Glutathione was essentially measured with the procedure of Tietze (1970) modified for the determination of oxidized glutathione (GSSG) as described by Xia <u>et al.</u> (1985) where reduced glutathione (GSH) was enzymatically trapped by methylglyoxal in the presence of glyoxalase I.

The malondialdehyde formed was determined on homogenate aliquots of 0.3-0.6 mg protein with the method described by Yagi (1978) originally used for the determination of serum MDA. The solution for the final assay was formed by 12% acetic acid, 0.17% thiobarbituric acid (TBA), 0.01% butylated hydroxytoluene (BHT) and 0.25% Nonidet P-40. The suspension was left to react for 1 hour at 95°C, cooled and centrifuged. The absorption of the adduct formed between MDA and TBA was read at 532 nm and the concentration of MDA calculated after substraction of the 580 nm absorption utilizing an εM = 156 000.

Protein of the homogenate were determined by the biuret method (Gornall <u>et al.</u>, 1949), while those of the xanthine oxidase preparation were determined with the method of Lowry <u>et al.</u> (1951).

RESULTS

When perfused hearts are maintained in ischemic conditions (perfusion flow = 0 ml/min) at 37°C for 1 hour and then reperfused with a normoxic medium a massive coronary efflux of glutathione (80% reduced) ensues, as shown in Fig. 2. Fig. 3 shows the effect of total ischemia and subsequent reperfusion on contractile performance of isolated and perfused rat hearts. The reduction of the perfusion flow from 12 to 0 ml/min resulted in a rapid decline of the developed pressure so that contractile activity completely ceased five minutes after the onset of the ischemia. The resting pressure began to rise as early as twenty minutes after ischemia and, during the post-ischemic reperfusion, there was a marked increase of the resting pressure and a poor recovery of the developed pressure (less than 20% of the control value). The distribution of the various forms of the xanthine-converting enzyme in the above reported conditions is shown in Tab. 1. After 1 hour of ischemia the dehydrogenase activity is poorly affected and decreases from 80% to 75%; a simultaneous small increase of the reversible form (4%) is observed while the irreversible form does not significantly change. When ischemia is followed by 1 hour of reperfusion there is a significant increase (9%) of only the reversible form; two hours of reperfusion do not determine any substantial increase with respect to the values found after 1 hour (data not reported). The lack of conversion XD ⟶ XOirrev during ischemia indicates that probably during ischemia there is no involvement of cytosolic proteases. Only if extreme experimental conditions, like autolysis for 18 hours at room temperature, are used it becomes possible to find a significant conversion of xanthine dehydrogenase which is converted 42% in XOirrev and 45% in XOrev. Glutathione was almost completely lost from the autolyzing heart and recovered in the medium partially in the oxidized form (31%).

In Tab. 2 MDA, formation, total SH groups and glutathione content after ischemia and ischemia followed by reperfusion are reported. MDA content, even though very low, appears to increase after ischemia. There are no significant alterations in the concentration of total SH groups and glutathione after the period of ischemia while they are strongly decreased when reperfusion follows the ischemic period. After 1 hour of reperfusion total glutathione is decreased to about a third of that present in the control and about 25% of this residue is in the oxidized form.

Normoxic perfusion in the presence of hydrogen peroxide or diamide were carried out in order to understand if some of the damaging effect observed during ischemia and ischemia followed by reperfusion could be partly due to the accumulation of H_2O_2 or to the oxidation of glutathione. Treatment of the heart with thiol oxidizing agents can also give information about the extent of reversible conversion of the xanthine-converting enzyme.

Under aerobic conditions, the addition of H_2O_2 or diamide (Fig. 4) to the perfusion medium induced alterations of the mechanical functions. As soon as hydrogen peroxide was administered, an initial increase in the heart rate was observed, and the developed pressure was maintained at a constant level even though quite erratic and lasted also when the oxidant was withdrawn. When diamide was added, there was a slow decline of contractile activity with no major changes in the resting pressure. Under the latter conditions, even after 1 hour, low values of developed pressure were still maintained; nevertheless the contractile activity was resumed almost completely when the infusion of diamide was suspended.

The effects of hydrogen peroxide and diamide on the xanthine-converting enzyme activity are reported in Tab. 3. About 40% of the xanthine dehydrogenase is transformed into reversible oxidase after perfusion in the presence of hydrogen peroxide; when hydrogen peroxide is removed from the perfusion medium, the reversible oxidase is extensively reconverted to the dehydrogenase. The transformation XD ⟶ XO is more dramatic when diamide is used instead of hydrogen peroxide, since in this case, almost 60% of the dehydrogenase is transformed into the oxidase. Also with diamide the enzyme reconverts to the native form upon withdrawal of the reagent from the perfusion medium. Both with diamide and hydrogen peroxide, the transformation affects only the reversible form of the oxidase while the irreversible form remains constant at the basal level of about 15%.

Tab. 4 shows that hydrogen peroxide but not diamide can slightly increase MDA content at a level close to that found after ischemia. Total SH groups are extensively oxidized during the perfusion with hydrogen peroxide and diamide, and a decrease of 25% and 35% respectively is apparent (Tab. 4); the decrease in glutathione is proportionally greater since about 50% of it is lost from the heart after 30 minutes of perfusion in the presence of hydrogen peroxide or diamide; the amount of glutathione lost was recovered in the pooled perfusate (Fig. 5 and 6). The fraction remaining in the heart is about 50% in the oxidized form after perfusion with either hydrogen peroxide or diamide (Tab. 4). The reperfusion with the medium without the oxidant determines an increase of both the total sulfhydryl groups and of reduced glutathione, the reduced/oxidized ratio of which reaches a value close to that of the control.

DISCUSSION

Current literature dealing with xanthine oxidase reports that in most tissues this enzyme is present "mainly, if not exclusively" as xanthine dehydrogenase; the ratio XD/XO existing "in vivo" has not been clearly defined. From our data it appears that an average amount of 15% XOirrev is always present in the rat heart tissue and that this amount does not significantly increase after ischemia, ischemia followed by reperfusion or after oxidative stress induced by oxidizing agents like H_2O_2 or diamide. This amount of XOirrev corresponds, in terms of mU, to about 10 mU/g wet weight; consequently when hypoxanthine concentration increases as during ischemia (Granger et al., 1986; Schosten et al., 1983) a flux of reduced forms of oxygen is produced and could contribute to the well established reperfusion injury.

The basal level of XOirrev can be found even when the homogenization is carried out in the presence of DTT (not reported), EDTA, EGTA and PMSF in order to prevent any reversible or irreversible conversion of the enzyme. The XOirrev, which is always present, could represent a xanthine oxidase with different catalytic properties (Schousten <u>et al.</u>, 1983) or a particular catabolic form of this enzymatic protein.

The activity of XOrev in fresh rat heart is about 5% and after reperfusion following an ischemic period there appears to be a net conversion of XD⟶XOrev. This conversion, which is determined by the oxidation of some SH groups of the enzyme, appears to depend on the production of oxidizing species during reperfusion, a likely candidate being H_2O_2. Concomitantly with the reversible conversion of the enzyme there is a very dramatic decrease of cellular glutathione so that the cell is left without one of the most relevant defence-systems against the oxidative stress. The decrease in glutathione concentration is paralleled by a decrease in the total SH groups, which represent the sum of glutathione and protein thiol groups; this indicates that a consistent number of protein SH groups were transformed to disulfides because of lack of the reducing buffer capability of glutathione. The amount of glutathione which remains in the heart even after severe ischemia followed by reperfusion probably is the fraction contained within the mitochondria, the membrane of which appears then to be damaged secondarily; the bulk of glutathione lost is mainly represented by the cytosolic fraction. The extention of the reperfusion damage is also shown by the decrease in the left ventricular pressure which, after reperfusion, is about 10-20% of the control value.

From the above reported results obtained in an ischemic/reperfused model it appears that the conversion XD⟶XOrev occurs only during the reperfusion period. Perfusion experiments in the presence of H_2O_2 and diamide were then devised in order to: a) establish a relationship between the oxidative stress and the reversible conversion of the enzyme. b) clarify the role of glutathione and protein SH groups in the reversible conversion of xanthine oxidase.

Perfusion with H_2O_2 or with diamide determines a large conversion XD⟶XOrev which is of about 35% and 60% respectively. If the basal level of XOirrev is added to the concentration of XOrev, the amount of total oxidase increases to about 50% and 75% respectively. The different effects of diamide and H_2O_2 on the conversion XD⟶XOrev could be explained by the direct action of diamide upon GSH and protein SH groups, while the action of H_2O_2 is mediated through the oxidation of glutathione. If, after a period of perfusion, these oxidizing reagents are withdrawn from the perfusion medium, the XOrev partly reconverts to XD. The reconversion increases when perfusion time is longer (not shown). A behaviour similar to that of the enzyme is shown by cellular glutathione and protein SH groups; they are oxidized upon the action of diamide and restored to the reduced state upon withdrawal of the reagents. Consequently, it appears that the redox state of glutathione could influence the status of protein thiols like those of xanthine dehydrogenase.

After H_2O_2 or diamide perfusion, the sum of the total pooled glutathione of the perfusates with the amount of the glutathione found in the heart is lower than the amount of the glutathione of the controls; in addition there is an apparent "increase" of the cellular glutathione after the perfusion in the absence of the oxidizing agents. This discrepancy can be explained considering that the oxidizing agents can induce the formation of mixed disulfides between glutathione and protein thiol groups; the reduction of these disulfides determines an intracellular release of GSH.

The conversion XD ⟶ XOrev appears to depend upon the presence of oxidized glutathione and on an enzymatic system. A GSSG-dependent thiol: disulfide oxidoreductase has been extensively characterized in rat liver (Battelli and Lorenzoni, 1982) and found to have a molecular weight of 40 000; this enzyme exhibits an activity also in rat heart even though to a lower extent, being of about a quarter of that present in the liver. This enzyme acts on XD in the presence of GSSG and converts XD into a XOrev.

The sulfhydryl oxidase that could act directly on the SH groups of XD without the intermediation of GSSG is present in the milk but does not appear to be involved in the heart tissue.

It has been reported that XOrev from rat liver cannot be reconverted to XD by GSH (Battelli and Lorenzoni, 1982), nevertheless we were able to get the XOrev partially reconverted to the dehydrogenase after perfusion without the oxidizing agents. The reducing equivalents are supplied by NADPH which, after oxidation, could be reduced both by the pentose phosphate shunt or by the malic enzyme. The latter could have an important role since a special feature of the myocardium is its poor activity of the pentose phosphate pathway (Zimmer <u>et al.</u>, 1984). NADPH can reduce GSSG through glutathione reductase which, in turn, by a thioltransferase can reduce the disulfides of the XOrev to the native dithiols so that the XD activity is recovered. NADPH, instead of acting on GSSG, could reduce thioredoxin, through thioredoxin reductase, which, in turn, can operate the transformation XOrev XD. As pointed out by Mannervik <u>et al.</u>, (1983) the two systems could act complementary and, according to the nature of a particular substrate, the one or the other of the two reducing systems could be operative.

Many papers indicate a protective effect of antioxidants, superoxide dismutase, catalase and allopurinol on ischemic and reperfused rat heart (Guarnieri <u>et al.</u>, 1978; Manning <u>et al.</u>, 1984; Jolly <u>et al.</u>, 1984). In the present research we observed both a marked decrease of sulfhydryl groups during ischemia/reperfusion and an oxidative stress-induced conversion of XD to XOrev which nevertheless can be restored to its original function by the reducing pool mainly represented by glutathione. The recovery of the contractile performance after removal of diamide confirms the capability of the tissue to repair the damage induced by oxidative stress as shown by the heart functional parameter like left ventricular pressure (L.V.P.). Consequently, the infusion of thiols or thiols-delivering agents could limit the injury caused by ischemia and by the action of oxidizing species thereby protecting the myocardium from a potential damage.

The xanthine-converting enzyme appears to be sensitive to the redox state of the cellular glutathione. A decrease in the ratio GSH/GSSG could shift the xanthine dehydrogenase towards the XO form with the consequent production of reduced forms of oxygen, provided that a sufficient concentration of hypoxanthine is present. Heart tissues, compared to other tissues, exhibit a lower activity of xanthine oxidase and consequently the role of this enzyme in the production of free radicals in the heart could be less relevant than in other tissues like the liver and the intestine.

Xanthine oxidase might be both a cause of oxidative stress and a consequence of it. It is a cause since about 20% of the total enzyme is always present in the oxidase form in the rat cardiac tissue. The transformation XD $\longrightarrow$ XO is also a consequence of the oxidative stress since H_2O_2 and other oxidizing agents, directly or through the oxidation of glutathione, can induce the XD $\longrightarrow$ XOrev conversion and, thereby, amplify the damage.

Tab. 1. Conversion of xanthine dehydrogenase to xanthine oxidase during ischemia and ischemia followed by reperfusion.

	Xanthine dehydrogenase	Xanthine oxidase (reversible)	Xanthine oxidase (irreversible)
Control	80.00 ± 1.9 (8)	5.00 ± 0.2 (8)	15.25 ± 0.59 (8)
Ischemia (60 min)	75.25 ± 5.0 (10)	9.00 ± 0.5 (10)	16.00 ± 1.0 (10)
Ischemia (60 min) + Reperfusion (60 min)	67.00 ± 3.5 (10)	18.00 ± 1.2 (10)	15.00 ± 0.6 (10)

Values, expressed as percentage of the total activity, are mean ± S.D. and figures in brackets show the number of experiments.

Tab. 2. Malondialdehyde, sulfhydryl groups and glutathione content of rat heart after ischemia and ischemia followed by reperfusion.

	Malondialdehyde	Total SH groups	GSH + GSSG	GSSG
Control	0.316 ± 0.06(3)	90 ± 9(7)	11.8 ± 1.0(5)	1.1 ± 0.3(3)
Ischemia (60 min)	0.413 ± 0.04(3)	88 ± 3(8)	12.0 ± 0.6(3)	1.9 ± 0.2(3)
Ischemia (60 min) + Reperfusion (60 min)	0.400 ± 0.07(3)	70 ± 6(7)	3.6 ± 1.4(3)	0.9 ± 0.2(3)

Values, expressed as nmol/mg protein, are mean ± S.D. and figures in brackets show the number of estimations, each obtained with a different heart.

Tab. 3. Conversion of xanthine dehydrogenase to xanthine oxidase after perfusion with hydrogen peroxide and diamide

	Xanthine dehydrogenase	Xanthine oxidase (reversible)	Xanthine oxidase (irreversible)
Control	80.00 ± 1.9 (8)	5.00 ± 0.2 (8)	15.25 ± 0.6 (8)
H_2O_2 (30 min)	48.00 ± 4.0 (10)	38.00 ± 4.0 (10)	14.00 ± 0.5 (10)
H_2O_2 (30 min) + H_2O_2 omitted (30 min)	71.50 ± 1.5 (10)	18.00 ± 1.0 (10)	14.00 ± 0.5 (10)
Diamide (30 min)	28.00 ± 4.0 (3)	59.00 ± 3.0 (3)	13.00 ± 1.0 (3)
Diamide (30 min) + Diamide omitted (30 min)	47.00 ± 1.0 (3)	39.00 ± 2.0 (3)	14.00 ± 1.0 (3)

Hydrogen peroxide and diamide are 50 μM and 100 μM respectively. Values, expressed as percentage of the total activity, are mean ± S.D. and figures in brackets show the number of experiments.

Tab. 4. Malondialdehyde, sulfhydryl groups and glutathione content of rat heart after perfusion in the presence of hydrogen peroxide or diamide.

	Malondialdehyde	Total SH groups	GSH + GSSG	GSSG
Control	0.316 ± 0.06(3)	90 ± 9(7)	11.8 ± 1.0(5)	1.1 ± 0.3(3)
H_2O_2 (30 min)	0.380 ± 0.03(3)	63 ± 17(8)	6.2 ± 0.5(3)	3.3 ± 0.2(3)
H_2O_2 (30 min) + H_2O_2 omitted (30 min)	0.395 ± 0.05(4)	78 ± 17(9)	6.8 ± 0.8(4)	1.0 ± 0.1(3)
Diamide (30 min)	0.368 ± 0.04(3)	68 ± 4(3)	5.7 ± 1.6(3)	3.0 ± 1.1(3)
Diamide (30 min) + Diamide omitted (30 min)	0.300 ± 0.05(3)	82 ± 3(3)	7.1 ± 1.2(3)	1.1 ± 0.9(3)

Values, expressed as nmol/mg protein, are mean ± S.D. and figures in brackets show the number of experiments, each obtained with a different heart.

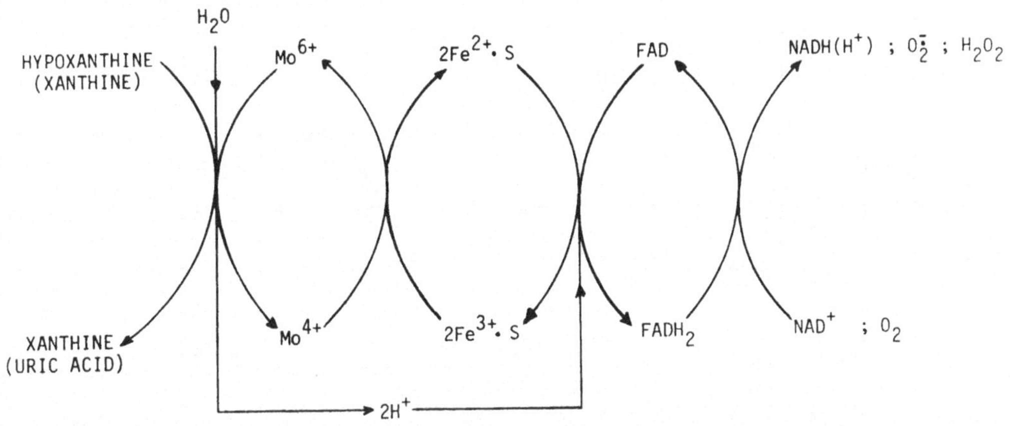

$XANTHINE + H_2O + NAD^+ \longrightarrow URIC\ ACID + NADH + H^+$

$XANTHINE + H_2O + 2O_2 \longrightarrow URIC\ ACID + 2O_2^{\bar{}} + 2H^+$

$XANTHINE + H_2O + O_2 \longrightarrow URIC\ ACID + H_2O_2$

Fig. 1. Mechanism of action of xanthine oxidoreductase.

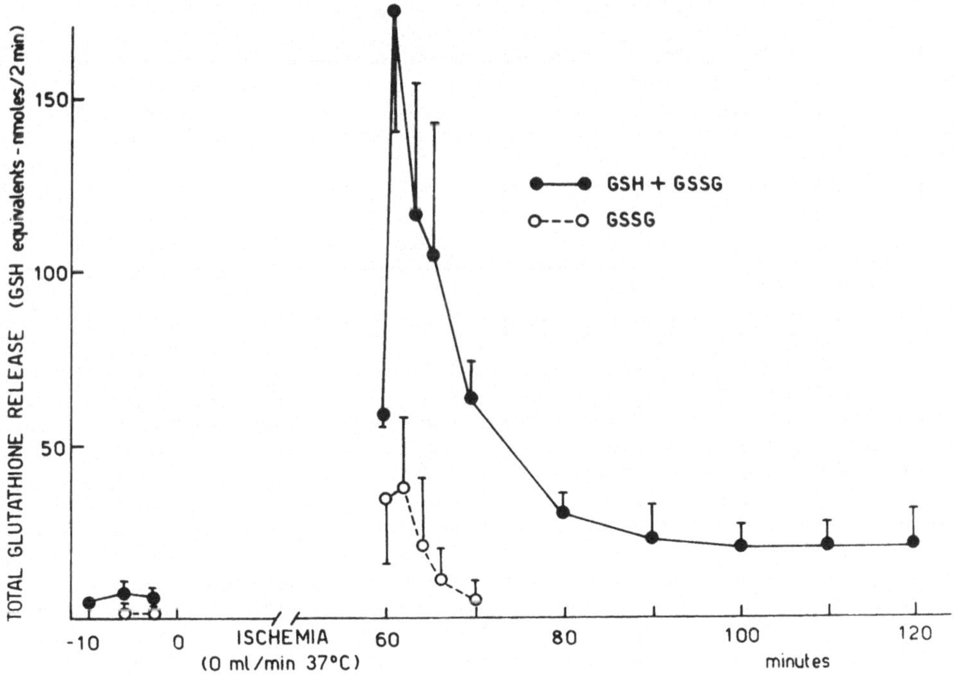

Fig. 2. Time course for release of glutathione from rat heart during reperfusion following global ischemia.

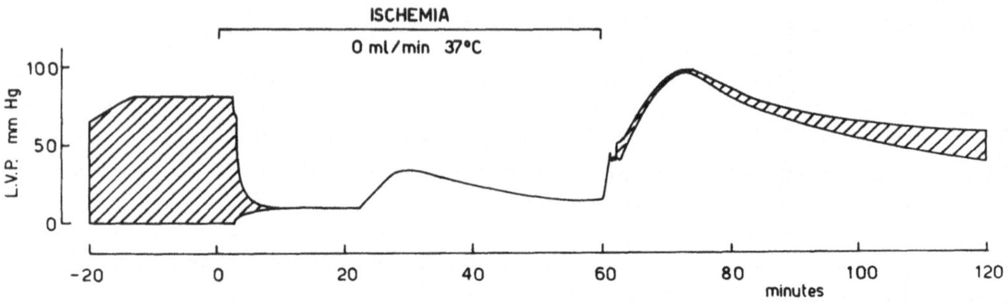

Fig. 3. Time course of left ventricular pressure (L.V.P.) during global ischemia and reperfusion of rat heart.

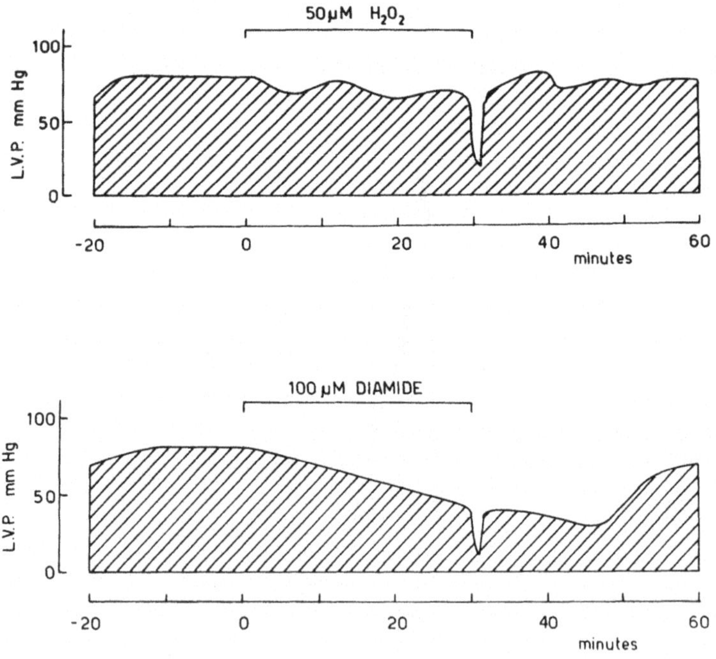

Fig. 4. Time courses of left ventricular pressure (L.V.P.) during perfusion in the presence of hydrogen peroxide and diamide in rat heart.

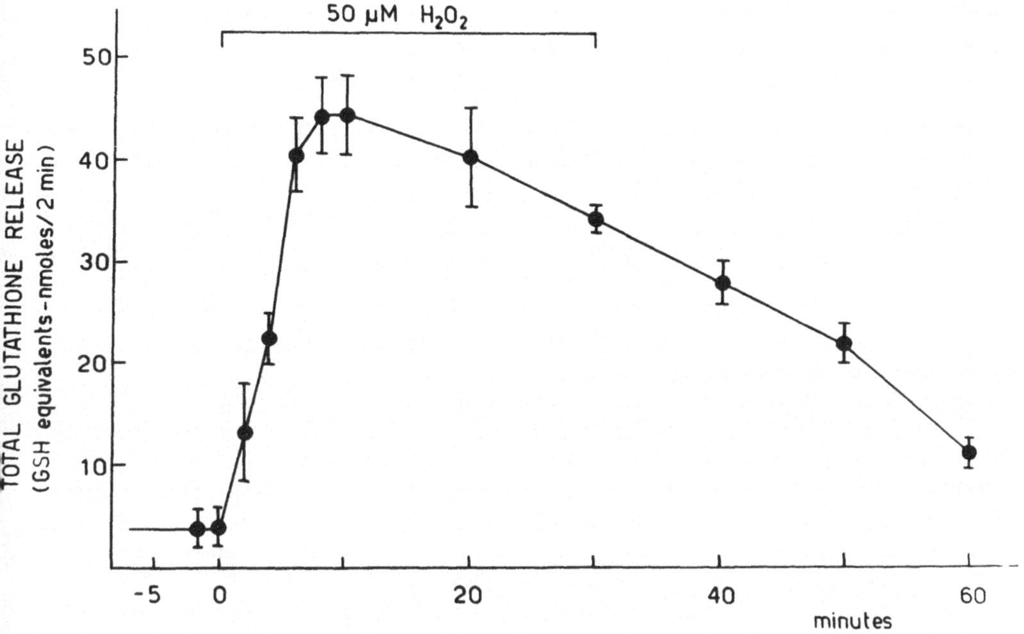

Fig. 5. Time course for release of glutathione from rat heart perfused for 30 minutes with medium containing H_2O_2.

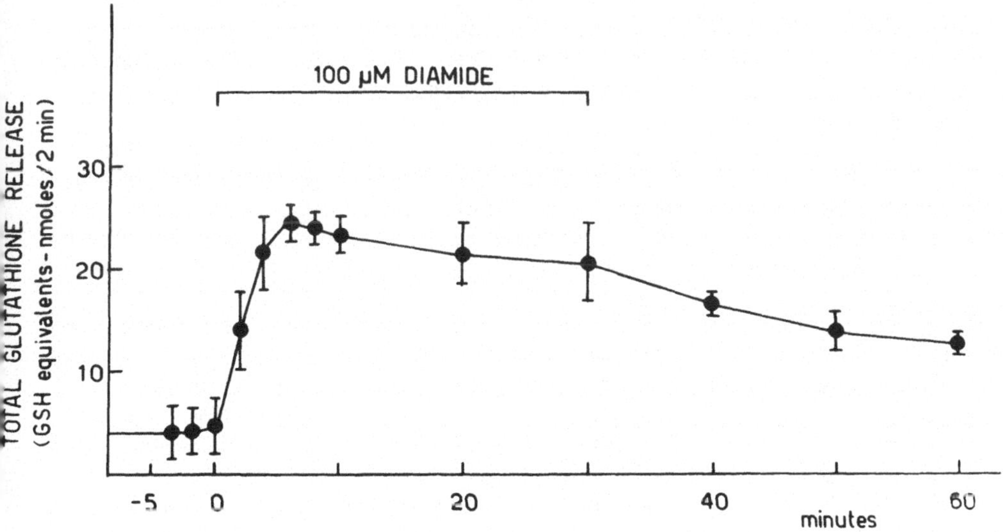

Fig. 6. Time course for release of glutathione from rat heart perfused for 30 minutes with medium containing diamide.

REFERENCES

Adkinson, D., Höllwart, M.E., Benoit, J.N., Parks, D.A., McCord, J.M. and Granger, D.N., 1986. Role of free radicals in ischemia-reperfusion injury to liver. Acta Physiol. Scand., Suppl. 548: 101-107.

Battelli, M.G., Della Corte, E. and Stirpe, F., 1972. Xanthine oxidase type D (dehydrogenase) in the intestine and other organs of the rat. Biochem. J., 126: 747-749.

Battelli, M.G., Lorenzoni, E. and Stirpe, F., 1973. Milk xanthine oxidase type D (dehydrogenase) and type O (oxidase) purification, interconversion and some properties. Biochem. J., 131: 191-198.

Battelli, M.G. and Lorenzoni, E., 1982. Purification and properties of a new glutathione-dependent thiol: disulfide oxidoreductase from rat liver. Biochem. J., 207: 133-138.

Clare, D.A., Blakistone, B.A., Swaisgood, H.E. and Horton, H.R., 1981. Sulfhydryl oxidase-catalyzed conversion of xanthine dehydrogenase to xanthine oxidase. Arch. Biochem. Biophys., 211: 44-47.

Della Corte, E. and Stirpe, F., 1972. The regulation of xanthine oxidase. Involvement of thiol groups in the conversion of the enzyme activity from dehydrogenase (type D) into oxidase (type O) and purification of the enzyme. Biochem. J., 126: 739-745.

Fridovich, I., 1970. Quantitative aspects of the production of superoxide anion radical by milk xanthine oxidase. J. Biol. Chem., 245: 4053-4057.

Gornall, A.G., Bardawill, C.J. and David, M.M., 1949. Determination of serum proteins by means of the biuret reaction. J. Biol. Chem. 177, 751-766.

Granger, D.N., Rutili, G. and McCord, J.M., 1981. Superoxide radicals in feline intestinal ischemia. Gastroenterology, 78: 474-480.

Granger, D.N., Hollwarth, M.E. and Parks, D.A., 1986. Ischemia-reperfusion injury: role of oxygen-derived free radicals. Acta Physiol. Scand, Suppl. 548: 47-63.

Guarnieri, C., Ferrari, R., Visioli, O., Caldarera, C.M. and Nayler, W.G., 1978. Effect of α-tocopherol on hypoxic-perfused and reoxygenated rabbit heart muscle. J. Mol. Cell. Card., 10: 893-906.

Hansson, R.O., Jonsson, O., Lundstam, S., Petterson, S. and Schersten, T., 1983. Effects of free radical scavengers on renal circulation after ischemia in the rabbit. Clin. Sci. 65: 605-610.

Haerse, D.J., Manning, A.S., Downey, J.M. and Yellon, D.M., 1986. Xanthine oxidase: a critical mediator of myocardial injury during ischemia and reperfusion? Acta Physiol. Scand., Suppl. 548: 65-78.

Jarasch, E.D., Grund, C., Bruder, G., Heid, H.W., Keenan, T.W. and Franke, W.W., 1981. Localization of xanthine oxidase in mammary gland epithelium and capillary endothelium. Cell, 25: 67-82.

Jolly, S.R., Kane, W.J.,Bailie, M.B., Abrams, G.D. and Lucchesi, B.R., 1984. Canine myocardial reperfusion injury. Its reduction by the combined administration of superoxide dismutase and catalase. Circ. Res., 54: 277-285.

Kaminski, Z.W. and Jezewska, M.M., 1979. Intermediate dehydrogenase-oxidase form of xanthine oxidoreductase in rat liver. Biochem. J., 181: 177-182.

Krenitsky, T.A., Tutle, J.V., Cattau, E.L. and Wang, P., 1974. A comparison of the distribution and electron acceptor specificities of xanthine oxidase and aldehyde oxidase. Comp. Biochem. Physiol., 49B: 687-703.

Lowry, O.H., Rosebrough, N.J., Farr, A.L. and Randall, R.J., 1951. Protein measurement with the Folin phenol reagent. J. Biol. Chem., 193: 265-293.

Mannervik, B., Axelsson, K., Sundewall, A.C. and Holmgren, A., 1983. Relative contribution of thioltransferase - and thioredoxin - dependent systems in reduction of low molecular mass and protein disulphides. Biochem. J., 213: 519-523.

Manning, A.S., Coltart, D.J. and Hearse, D.J., 1984. Ischemia and reperfusion-induced arrhythmias in the rat. Effect of xanthine oxidase inhibition with allopurinol. Circ. Res., 55: 545-548.

Olson, J.S., Ballou, D.P., Palmer, G. and Massey, V., 1974. The mechanism of action of xanthine oxidase. J. Biol. Chem., 249: 4363-4382.

Parks, D.A. and Granger, D.N., 1986. Xanthine oxidase: biochemistry, distribution and physiology. Acta Physiol. Scand., Suppl. 548: 87-99.

Ramboer, C.R.H., 1969. A sensitive and nonradioactive assay for serum and tissue xanthine oxidase. J. Lab. Clin. Med., 74: 828-829.

Schousten, B., De Jong, J.W., Harmsen, E., De Tombe, P.P. and Achterberg, P.W., 1983. Myocardial xanthine oxidase/dehydrogenase. Biochim. Biophys. Acta, 762: 519-544.

Stirpe, F. and Della Corte, E., 1969. The regulation of rat liver xanthine oxidase. Conversion in vitro of the enzyme activity from dehydrogenase (type D) to oxidase (type O). J. Biol. Chem., 244: 3855-3863.

Tietze, F., 1969. Enzymatic method for quantitative determination of nanograms amounts of total and oxidized glutathione. Anal. Biochem. 27: 502-522.

Ursini, F., Maiorino, M. and Gregolin, C., 1985. The selenoenzyme phospholipid hydroperoxide glutathione peroxidase. Biochim. Biophys. Acta, 839: 62-70.

Waud, W.R. and Rajagopalan, K.V., 1976. The mechanism of conversion of rat liver xanthine dehydrogenase from a NAD^+-dependent form (type D) to an O_2 dependent form (type D). Arch. Biochem. Biophys., 172: 365-379.

Xia, Y., Hill, K.E. and Burk, R.F., 1985. Effect of selenium-deficiency on hydroperoxide-induced glutathione from the isolated perfused rat heart. J. Nutr., 115: 733-742.

Yagi, K., 1984. Malondialdehyde assay for blood plasma or serum. Methods Enzymol., 105: 328-331.

Zimmer, H.G., Ibel, H., Suchner, U. and Schad, H., 1984. Ribose intervenction in the cardiac pentose phosphate pathway is not species-specific. Science, 233: 712-714.

CARDIAC CELL BREAKDOWN AT REOXYGENATION: ABSENCE OF CHANGES IN XANTHINE OXIDASE AND EFFECTS OF CALCIUM CONCENTRATION

James P. Kehrer[1]

Institut für Physiologische Chemie I, Universität Düsseldorf, Düsseldorf, Federal Republic of Germany.

ABSTRACT

The formation of oxygen radicals has been hypothesized as a factor responsible for cellular injury and enzyme release following reoxygenation of hypoxic or ischemic tissue. One purported source of such radicals is the metabolism of hypoxanthine and xanthine by xanthine oxidase. Xanthine oxidase (O form) has been suggested to be formed *in vivo* by limited proteolysis of xanthine dehydrogenase (D form) during the hypoxic period (Granger *et al.*, 1981). We measured the activities of xanthine oxidase in both fresh and isolated rat heart tissue perfused (Langendorff) with Krebs-Henseleit medium containing 10 mM glucose. Hearts were equilibrated for 30 min followed by 30 or 60 min of hypoxia and 30 min of reoxygenation. Total xanthine oxidase activity in the O form was 32 and 37% in fresh and perfused rat heart, respectively. This value was unchanged following 60 min of hypoxia and 30 min of reoxygenation. Perfusion with medium containing 250 μM allopurinol completely inhibited cardiac xanthine oxidase but had no effect on the release of lactate dehydrogenase (LDH) upon reoxygenation after 30 or 60 min hypoxia even when rats had been pretreated for 48 hr with 30 mg/kg/day allopurinol. Superoxide dismutase (50 units/ml), catalase (200 units/ml), or the antioxidant cyanidanol (100 μM) also had no effect on LDH release upon reoxygenation. Enzyme release upon reoxygenation was a calcium-dependent process. Removing calcium from the medium at the onset of hypoxia prevented LDH release at reoxygenation. However, removing calcium after 50 min of hypoxia initiated LDH release without reoxygenation. Perfusion with 1 or 5 mM cystamine 10 min before reoxygenation, or 0.5 or 5 mM cyanide 5 min before reoxygenation, significantly decreased LDH release. LDH release commenced immediately upon withdrawal of cyanide. Analyses of cardiac ATP/ADP and creatine phosphate/creatine ratios revealed some increases 4 min after reoxygenation or removal of cyanide. However, increases in these ratios were also measured following treatment with cystamine, which inhibited LDH release, and were not evident during hypoxic calcium-free perfusions which stimulated LDH release. These data demonstrate that xanthine dehydrogenase is not converted to xanthine oxidase in hypoxic tissue of the isolated-perfused rat heart, and that the release of intracellular enzymes upon reoxygenation in this experimental model is probably mediated by factors other than reactive oxygen species. LDH release was triggered, without reoxygenation, by removing calcium after 50 minutes of hypoxia and was inhibited by cyanide or cystamine. This suggests that, following an early calcium-dependent change, reoxygenation induces enzyme release as the resynthesis of ATP permits cells to decrease elevated intracellular calcium levels toward normal.

[1]on leave from the Division of Pharmacology and Toxicology, College of Pharmacy, The University of Texas at Austin, Austin, Texas, U.S.A.

INTRODUCTION

Reoxygenation injury in the heart, also known as the "oxygen paradox", was originally described by Hearse *et al.* (1973) as the abrupt release of cytoplasmic constituents, including a variety of soluble enzymes, upon reoxygenation of the myocardium following a sustained period of hypoxic perfusion. Massive ultrastructural damage accompanies this release and a similar phenomenon occurs following ischemic episodes (Hess and Manson, 1984). The mechanism(s) underlying the sudden release of intracellular constituents at reoxygenation is not known but may involve either the direct production of additional cardiac damage sufficient to cause cell breakdown or be a distinct, indirect, process that leads to the breakdown of a population of cells damaged during the preceeding hypoxic period.

The possibility that oxygen radicals are formed following the sudden influx of oxygen at reperfusion has received much attention as a possible mechanism of cellular injury and breakdown. The formation of such radicals has not yet been demonstrated although activated species of oxygen have been indirectly implicated in reperfusion injury in small intestine, stomach, liver, pancreas, kidney, heart, skin and brain (Granger *et al.*, 1986).

A mechanism by which oxygen radicals may arise following reoxygenation of ischemic tissue has been proposed (Granger *et al.,* 1981). During ischemia there is a rapid breakdown of ATP to hypoxanthine. This is accompanied by an influx of Ca^{2+} which, this hypothesis suggests, may activate a latent protease. This protease would act on xanthine dehydrogenase (D form) converting it to xanthine oxidase (O form). Upon reoxygenation, the formation of superoxide anions would then occur as hypoxanthine was metabolized to urate by the action of xanthine oxidase. However, the postulated D to O conversion during hypoxia or ischemia appears not to have been well studied although the group which proposed this hypothesis has reported that the conversion occurs in various tissues of the rat (Roy and McCord, 1983) and in ischemic dog heart (Chambers *et al.,* 1985).

One purpose of the present study was to assess these two enzymatic activities in freshly isolated and perfused rat heart tissue. In addition, experiments were designed to assess the calcium- and energy-dependence of enzyme release at reoxygenation. Previous work has shown that mitochondrial respiration at reoxygenation is necessary for enzyme release (Ganote *et al.*, 1976; Ganote *et al.*, 1980) and that calcium is important in this process as well (Hearse, 1977). The results of the present study demonstrate that, in contrast to previous reports, the D to O conversion did not occur in hypoxic-reoxygenated rat myocardium, although there was a substantial percentage of total xanthine oxidase activity present normally in the O form. Allopurinol, an inhibitor of xanthine oxidase, and other antioxidants did not prevent the release of lactate dehydrogenase (LDH) during the reoxygenation of myocardial tissue subjected to 30 or 60 minutes of hypoxia. LDH release was triggered, without reoxygenation, by removing calcium after 50 minutes of hypoxia and was inhibited by cyanide or cystamine.

MATERIALS AND METHODS

Dithioerythritol, phenylmethylsulfonyl fluoride (PMSF), NAD^+, allopurinol, xanthine, cystamine, creatine kinase and superoxide dismutase (SOD) were obtained from Sigma (St. Louis, MO). Catalase, glyceraldehyde-3-phosphate dehydrogenase, 3-phosphoglycerate kinase, myokinase, pyruvate kinase, lactate dehydrogenase (LDH), pyruvate, and NADH were obtained from Boehringer (Mannheim, FRG). Cyanidanol was obtained from Fluka (Buchs, Switzerland). All other chemicals used were of reagent grade.

Male Wistar rats, 160-230 g, fed on stock diet (Altromin), were used. The rats were anesthetized with pentobarbital and heparinized with 200 IU heparin through the inferior vena cava. Hearts were rapidly removed and placed into ice-cold Krebs-Henseleit bicarbonate solution containing 2.5 mM $CaCl_2$ and 10 mM glucose. Hearts were perfused with the same solution by the method of Langendorff (1895) with a constant pressure of 80 cm water at 36°C as described previously (Ishikawa and Sies, 1984). The standard perfusion medium was equilibrated with 95% O_2, 5% CO_2 and all hearts were allowed to stabilize for 30 min with this medium before initiating hypoxia. Hypoxic perfusions were performed for 30 or 60 min by equilibrating the same perfusion medium with 95% N_2, 5% CO_2 .

Samples of the coronary effluent were collected continuously for determination of oxygen concentration and at selected intervals for the determination of coronary flow rates and LDH release. LDH activity, at 25°C, was determined spectrophotometrically at 340 nm in 100 mM triethanolamine HCl buffer, pH 7.6, containing 0.15 mM NADH, 1 mM EDTA, and 1.5 mM pyruvate. Enzyme activity is expressed as units/g wet or dry heart weight where 1 unit (U) is that which oxidizes 1 μmol NADH per minute.

Xanthine oxidase activity was measured in the 27,000 x *g* supernatant fraction of heart tissue homogenized in 0.05 M potassium phosphate buffer, pH 7.8, containing 1 mM PMSF and 10 mM dithioerythritol (Chambers *et al.*, 1985; Della Corte and Stirpe, 1972). Whole hearts were homogenized within 15 seconds of removal from the perfusion apparatus or the rat's body. These latter hearts (fresh controls) were briefly perfused with oxygenated Krebs-Henseleit solution *in situ* to remove all blood. The reaction mixture contained 60 μM xanthine, and urate production was monitored at 293 nm in the absence of NAD^+ to determine the oxidase activity and in the presence of 0.67 mM NAD^+ to determine the oxidase plus dehydrogenase activity. Reaction rates were corrected for nonspecific absorbance changes by subtracting any residual activity measured in the presence of 167 μM allopurinol (less than 15% of the enzymatic rate). Enzyme activity was calculated as nmol urate formed/min/mg protein using an extinction coefficient of 12.6 $mM^{-1}cm^{-1}$ for urate. Protein was determined by the microbiuret method (Itzhaki, and Gill, 1964).

ATP, ADP, creatine phosphate and creatine were determined in heart tissue freeze-stopped using aluminum tongs precooled with liquid nitrogen. The frozen heart tissue was pulverized in a mortar and pestle and approximately 250 mg of powder was extracted with 1.0 ml 1 M perchloric acid containing 2 mM EDTA. The mixture was centrifuged, the supernatant rapidly neutralized with 6 M KOH/1 M triethanolamine HCl, and the samples stored at -20°C until analyzed by conventional enzymatic procedures (Lowry and Passoneau, 1972). The protein content of the pellet was determined by method of Lowry *et al.* (1951).

Data are expressed as mean ± S.E. Multiple groups were analyzed by one way analysis of variance, and comparisons between groups were done with Newman-Keuls test (Zivin and Bartko, 1976). The variances of creatine phosphate/creatine ratios and total LDH release from 92-100 minutes were found to be heterogeneic by Cochran's test. Additional analyses indicated that the means were directly proportional to the standard deviations (creatine phosphate/creatine) or proportional to the variances (LDH release). These data were, therefore, transformed by taking their natural logarithm or square roots, respectively, before statistical analyses (Zivin and Bartko, 1976).

RESULTS

There were no significant changes in the percentage of xanthine oxidase activity in the O form in myocardial tissue following a 2 hr perfusion with oxygenated Krebs-Henseleit solution, compared to fresh heart tissue (Table 1). Perfusing the myocardium for 30 min with oxygenated medium followed by 60 min with hypoxic medium and a subsequent 30 min of reoxygenation also had no significant effect on this percentage. Freshly isolated rat liver and heart tissue contained approximately the same specific activity (per mg protein) of the O form of xanthine oxidase. In contrast, the specific activity of the D form was five-fold higher in liver than in heart (Table 1). The percentage in the O form was unaffected by freezing liver homogenates for 24 hours before assay if dithioerythritol and PMSF were present in the buffer. In the absence of these agents, the percentage in the O form increased to 41% (Table 1).

All perfused hearts released an increased amount of LDH after 15 minutes of hypoxia. This release gradually declined, but remained elevated above nonhypoxic hearts, to 90 min (Fig. 1). Within 2 min of reoxygenation after either 30 or 60 min of hypoxia the release of LDH activity into the coronary effluent was significantly increased (Fig. 1). Hearts perfused with oxygen saturated Krebs-Henseleit medium for 2 hr released less than 10 mU of LDH/min/g wet heart during this period (Fig. 1).

Perfusion of heart tissue with medium containing 250 μM allopurinol completely inhibited xanthine oxidase activity, but had no effect on LDH release upon reoxygenation after 30 or 60 min of hypoxia (Fig. 2). Pretreatment with allopurinol at 30 mg/kg/day for 2 days before perfusing with allopurinol-containing medium was also unable to block LDH upon reoxygenation after 30 min of hypoxia.

Table 1
Xanthine Oxidase Activity In Rat Heart And Liver

Sample	O Form[1]	D + O Form[1]	% O Form
fresh heart	0.25 ± 0.02 (7)	0.79 ± 0.05 (7)	31.8 ± 1.7 (7)
oxygenated heart[2]	0.34 ± 0.06 (4)	0.93 ± 0.13 (4)	36.6 ± 2.8 (4)
reoxygenated heart[3]	0.36 ± 0.05 (4)	1.04 ± 0.09 (4)	34.8 ± 4.6 (4)
fresh liver[4]	0.37 ± 0.08 (3)	2.95 ± 0.47 (3)	12.3 ± 1.2 (3)
liver after 24 hr[5]	0.37 ± 0.01 (2)	2.77 ± 0.33 (2)	13.8 ± 1.8 (2)
liver after 24 hr without inhibitors[6]	1.06 ± 0.17 (2)	2.57 ± 0.47 (2)	41.5 ± 1.0 (2)

[1]Data are expressed as nmol urate formed/min/mg protein ± S.E. Values in parentheses = n.
[2]Hearts were perfused for 2 hours with oxygenated medium.
[3]Hearts were perfused for 30 min with oxygenated, 60 min with hypoxic, and 30 min with oxygenated medium.
[4]Livers were homogenized in buffer containing dithioerythritol and PMSF and assayed immediately.
[5]Livers were homogenized in buffer containing dithioerythritol and PMSF, frozen for 24 hours, thawed and assayed.
[6]Livers were homogenized in buffer without dithioerythritol and PMSF, frozen for 24 hours, thawed and assayed.

Table 2

Total Cardiac LDH Release[1]

Treatment		% of Total Cardiac LDH Released: 92-100 min	0-120 min[2]
O_2 control		0.05	0.4
Hypoxia-reoxygenation		8.2	20
NaCN	0.5 mM	2.9	24
	5.0 mM	0.6	32
Cystamine	1 mM	3.3	12
	5 mM	1.8	17
Calcium-free	30 min	0.2	5
	80 min	27.3	54
	80 min[3]	19.8	58
25 μM Calcium	80 min[3]	12.4	39

[1]Fresh heart tissue, perfused for 5 min to remove all blood, contained 1227 ± 52 units LDH/g dry wt (n = 3).
[2]LDH release, measured at selected time points, was extrapolated to the entire 2 hr period of perfusion. Except for O_2 control, hypoxia was initiated after 30 min. Reoxygenation occurred at 90 min except where indicated.
[3]Not reoxygenated.

Superoxide dismutase (50 U/ml) or catalase (200 IU/ml), beginning at the time of hypoxia and continuing throughout the remainder of the perfusion, had no significant effect on LDH release upon reoxygenation after 60 min of hypoxia (Fig. 2). The antioxidant cyanidanol (100 μM), added to the perfusate from 15 to 120 min, also failed to provide statistically significant protection (Fig. 2).

In a separate series of experiments, the oxygen-induced release of LDH was completely prevented by the infusion of 5 mM sodium cyanide from 5 min before to 10 min after reoxygenation (Figs. 3 & 4). Complete inhibition was also obtained with 1 mM cyanide (not shown) and a smaller, but still significant, inhibition was seen with 0.5 mM cyanide. With both doses, LDH release commenced upon removal of cyanide (Fig. 3).

Perfusion with calcium-free medium throughout hypoxia and reoxygenation prevented any increase in LDH release above the levels normally seen during hypoxia (Fig. 4). However, if the calcium-free period was begun after 50 min of hypoxia, LDH release was stimulated within 5 min even without reoxygenation (Fig. 4). LDH release was also initiated without reoxygenation if the perfusion medium contained only 25 μM calcium after 50 min of hypoxia (Fig. 4). However, perfusion with 250 μM calcium was unable to initiate LDH release (data not shown). The amount of LDH released from hearts perfused with calcium-free medium after 50 min of hypoxia was unaffected by reoxygenation.

The quantity of LDH released from 92-100 min of perfusion without reoxygenation in hearts made calcium-free after 50 min hypoxia was significantly greater than that obtained upon reoxygenation of control hearts in the presence of 2.5 mM calcium (Fig. 4). During these 9 min, almost 20% of the total cardiac content of LDH was released, compared to only 8% in reoxygenated controls (Table 2). During the entire 2 hr perfusion period, 58% of the total cardiac LDH content was released from calcium-free hearts while oxygenated and reoxygenated controls released only 0.4 and 20%, respectively (Table 2).

The infusion of 1 or 5 mM cystamine from 10 min before to 10 min after reoxygenation significantly decreased the oxygen-induced release of LDH (Fig. 4). Upon removal of cystamine, there was a small increase in LDH release such that by 2 hr of perfusion the total release approached that seen in hypoxic-reoxygenated hearts (Table 2).

The ATP/ADP ratio was significantly decreased following 60 min of hypoxia in all treatment groups, compared to hearts perfused with oxygenated medium (Table 3). Increases in this ratio 4 min after reoxygenation were small and variable. Creatine phosphate/creatine ratios also decreased significantly following 60 min of hypoxia (Table 3). There were, however, consistent increases in this ratio following reoxygenation or removal of cyanide. Interestingly, ATP/ADP and creatine phosphate/ creatine ratios in hearts made calcium-free at 30 min were not significantly different from oxygenated controls.

Oxygen uptake was identical in all treatment groups before hypoxia. Uptake rapidly returned to control levels upon reoxygenation and then exhibted a gradual decline (Fig. 5). Oxygen uptake was diminished following reoxygenation during cyanide infusion and increased after its removal. Cystamine also inhibited oxygen uptake, although there was no increase after its removal from the perfusion medium. There were no drug treatment-related effects in coronary flow evident between the various groups (data not shown). Coronary flow increased in response to hypoxia in all experiments.

DISCUSSION

D to O conversion of xanthine oxidase

The D to O conversion of xanthine oxidase has been extensively studied in liver tissue (Battelli, *et al.*, 1972; Della Corte and Stirpe, 1972; Stirpe and Della Corte, 1969). Although this process can occur both reversibly by sulfhydryl oxidation and irreversibly by proteolysis, only the irreversible process was measured by including PMSF and dithioerythritol in the homogenization buffer. The D to O conversion could be observed in frozen and thawed liver homogenates, as reported previously, when these agents were omitted (Della Corte and Stirpe, 1972; Stirpe and Della Corte, 1969). In the current study, xanthine oxidase did not undergo an irreversible D to O conversion following hypoxia and reoxygenation of perfused rat heart tissue (Fig. 1, Table 1). This contrasts with previous observations in rat heart suggesting nearly 100% is found as type O within 15 min (Granger *et al.*, 1986) and to results in dog heart where the percentage in the O form increased from 10 to 33% following ischemia (Chambers *et al.*, 1985).

Battelli *et al.* (1972) originally reported that all xanthine oxidase activity in rat heart tissue was in the D form. This finding conflicts with the results presented here and a recent report on rats from Oei *et al.* (1986), both of which indicated that 24% is normally in the O form. Thus, at least in the rat, a significant level of oxidase activity is normally present. Importantly, the specific activity of the O and the D forms in heart and liver were similar in the work presented here and by Oei *et al.* (1986) and were higher than the maximum of 10% previously reported in healthy tissue by some of the same workers (Granger *et al.*, 1981; Roy and McCord, 1983).

Effects of allopurinol

Xanthine oxidase could still be involved in reoxygenation injury even though the conversion did not occur since it is present initially at appreciable levels. However, completely inhibiting xanthine oxidase activity with allopurinol had no effect on the release of LDH following reoxygenation of hypoxic heart tissue. This contrasts with reports in rats, dogs and rabbits (Grisham *et al.*, 1986; Myers *et al.*, 1985; Myers *et al.*, 1986; Peterson *et al.*, 1985), but is in agreement with other results that allopurinol has no beneficial effects against reperfusion injury in dogs (Reimer and Jennings, 1985; Shatney *et al.*, 1976). Comparison among these studies must, however, be done with caution. With only one exception that directly conflicts with the current results (Grisham *et al.*, 1986), protection was observed using models of ischemia rather than hypoxia. Hypoxia mimics ischemia in producing a rapid depletion of energy reserves but there are dramatic differences in the rate of removal of metabolic byproducts. Nevertheless, although the hypothesized accumulation of hypoxanthine may occur during complete ischemia, collateral flow is sufficient to wash out purines from the ischemic area in partially occluded models of ischemia and reperfusion (Hearse *et al.*, 1986). Cell breakdown still occurs at reperfusion or reoxygenation in these models, however, suggesting that accumulation of hypoxanthine is unneccesary.

Interestingly, reports of allopurinol's effectiveness in ameliorating reperfusion injury have largely involved animals which were pretreated for 24-48 hours before ischemia or hypoxia (Chambers *et al.*, 1985; Grisham *et al.*, 1986; Peterson *et al.*, 1985). Pretreatment is believed necessary for the metabolism of allopurinol to oxypurinol, the actual inhibitory species. However, allopurinol failed to prevent reoxygenation-induced release of LDH in the present study even when animals were pretreated and the drug was present throughout the perfusion period. Therefore, the ability of allopurinol to protect under certain conditions may involve some other mechanism such as enhancing electron transport (Peterson *et al.*, 1986) or decreasing arrhythmias (Hearse *et al.*, 1986). These actions could explain some of the reported functional improvement and may also increase the reduction of dyes used to assess infarct size thereby producing misleading results regarding the protective ability of allopurinol.

Models of Reoxygenation Injury

A variety of *in vivo* and *in vitro* model systems have been used to study reoxygenation injury in the heart. Unfortunately, there has been no standard perfusion temperature or time of oxygen deprivation, and the conflicting results obtained following treatment with various substances are difficult to explain. Both perfusion temperature and the period of hypoxia or ischemia are critical variables for the massive release of intracellular enzymes upon reoxygenation (Hess and Manson, 1984; Reimer and Jennings, 1985). Studies examining reperfusion injury at lower temperatures or with shorter times of hypoxia may not, therefore, be examining the same molecular events as those at higher temperatures and longer times of hypoxia. Furthermore, *in vivo* studies permit normal physiological responses, such as the infiltration of leukocytes, which may play a prominent role in radical generation during reperfusion injury (Lucchesi and Mullane, 1986).

The absence of any D to O conversion in heart and the inability of allopurinol to provide protection indicate that neither this conversion, nor xanthine oxidase activity is involved in cellular breakdown upon reoxygenation of hypoxic isolated-perfused rat heart tissue. The positive results with antioxidants in some, but not all, models of reoxygenation injury are suggestive that oxygen radicals are involved in some aspect of this process. Superoxide dismutase or catalase have been reported to block the oxygen paradox in isolated perfused rat heart (Grisham *et al.*, 1986) while catalase, allopurinol, or desferoxamine, but not superoxide dismutase, were reportedly protective in rabbit hearts (Myers *et al.*, 1985). This latter report indicated there was no functional recovery and also found no difference whether these substances were present only during the hypoxic period or also during reoxygenation. Evidence of functional improvement in reperfused hearts has been obtained following treatment with SOD even though the release of intracellular enzymes was not altered (Shlafer *et al.*, 1982). Additional studies have demonstrated protective effects on cardiac function, arrhythmias or infarct size with these substances in other models of reperfusion injury (Bernier *et al.*, 1986; Gaudel and Develleroy, 1984; Jolly *et al.*, 1984; Otani *et al.*, 1986).

Together, these reports suggest factors in addition to oxygen radicals are involved. This is also supported by the data presented here indicating no signficant protection from cell breakdown with SOD, catalase and the naturally occurring flavonoid antioxidant cyanidanol which is water-soluble and should function as an effective radical scavenger in biologic systems (Slater and Eakins, 1975). Thus, reoxygenation may trigger the release of intracellular enzymes from cells damaged during hypoxia without the intervention of radicals (Kehrer and Sies, 1987).

Calcium- and energy-dependence of enzyme release

The mechanisms underlying the sudden release of intracellular enzymes upon reoxygenation of blood-free isolated perfused heart tissue after episodes of ischemia or hypoxia remain unclear. A variety of evidence is available, however, suggesting that calcium is a critical mediator of hypoxic tissue injury (Cheung *et al.*, 1986). The fact that LDH release was prevented when the perfusion medium was made calcium-free at the time of hypoxia suggests there is some early calcium-dependent change which causes cell-breakdown at reoxygenation. However, it is also possible that a severe energy deficiency does not develop in heart tissue when the calcium-free perfusion begins with the onset of hypoxia. The ATP/ADP and creatine phosphate/creatine ratios after 60 min of hypoxia in these calcium-free hearts were not significantly different from oxygenated controls. After reoxygenation, the creatine phosphate/ creatine ratio was actually greater than controls, perhaps because of the absence of any demands for contraction.

The detrimental effect of calcium-free perfusions after 50 min of hypoxia is more difficult to explain. Removing calcium from the medium at this time resulted in a dramatic breakdown of myocardial cells and the release of almost 60% of total cardiac LDH. Hearts perfused in this manner appeared pale from loss of myogobin. The ATP/ADP and creatine phosphate/creatine ratios were unchanged during hypoxia despite the complete lack of contractile activity and the release of LDH. Thus, it would appear that LDH release is not directly dependent on the resynthesis of high-energy phosphates. This is further supported by the increased creatine phosphate/creatine ratio after reoxygenation of cystamine treated hearts despite the decreased release of LDH.

The mechanism by which cystamine prevents cell breakdown is not clear. This disulfide, which is poorly taken up by hepatocytes, oxidizes membrane sulfhydryls (Thor *et al.*, 1985) and will inhibit plasma membrane calcium ATPase (Nicotera, 1986). Although these effects have not been confirmed in myocytes, in hepatocytes this is followed by increased intracellular calcium and ultimately cell death. The inhibition of LDH release seen in the present study appears to conflict with this finding. However, if one assumes that calcium ATPase is inactive during hypoxia from a lack of ATP, the absence of any enhanced LDH release might be expected. Oxygen uptake is substantial at reoxygenation, and the failure to measure increased ATP/ADP may be explained by rapid ATP utilization by plasma membrane calcium ATPase to extrude the abnormally high intracellular content of calcium. Blockade of this action by cystamine may explain the ability of this agent to prevent membrane lysis. It is possible that some change takes place early during hypoxia which triggers membrane breakdown when intracellular calcium declines to some critical level. This level can be achieved by reoxygenation or perfusion with medium containing a reduced content of calcium.

The hypothesis described above accounts for the ability of inhibitors of mitochondrial respiration to prevent LDH leakage as well as the effects of cystamine and calcium-free perfusions. Nevertheless, a decrease in intracellular calcium at reoxygenation has not been demonstrated and it remains possible that cell breakdown upon perfusion of hypoxic heart tissue with calcium-free medium is a separate phenomenon. In fact, data are available showing that intracellular calcium rapidly increases upon reoxygenation (Poole-Wilson *et al.*, 1984). However, calcium would be expected to rapidly accumulate in various subcellular organelles as the plasma membrane is disrupted. Although some evidence suggests calcium accumulation can occur without such disruption (Poole-Wilson *et al.*, 1984), the unanswered question is whether this is preceeded by decreased calcium levels.

The massive ultrastructural damage and enzyme leakage which occurs upon the readmission of calcium following a period of aerobic calcium-free perfusion is known as the calcium paradox. The oxygen and calcium paradoxes show both similarities (Hearse *et al.*, 1978; Hess and Manson, 1984) and differences (Nayler and Elz, 1986). In the current

Table 3

Cardiac ATP/ADP and Creatine Phosphate/Creatine Content[1]

		Time (min)					
		ATP/ADP			creatine phosphate/creatine		
Treatment		90	94	104	90	94	104
O_2 Control		3.5 ± 0.3†	-	-	0.34 ± 0.06†	-	-
Hypoxia-reoxygenation		1.0 ± 0.1*	1.7 ± 0.4	-	0.05 ± 0.01*	0.41 ± 0.17†¶	-
NaCN	0.5 mM	0.7 ± 0.1*	0.9 ± 0.1*	1.3 ± 0.3*	0.02 ± 0.002*	0.09 ± 0.02¶	0.26 ± 0.10†¶
	5.0 mM	0.9 ± 0.1*	0.8 ± 0.1*	1.1 ± 0.1*	0.01 ± 0.01*†	0.02 ± 0.01*	0.16 ± 0.03¶
Cystamine	5.0 mM	1.2 ± 0.1*	1.8 ± 0.7	-	0.11 ± 0.02	0.43 ± 0.30†	-
Calcium Free	30 min	2.9 ± 0.2†	3.8 ± 1.1†	-	0.27 ± 0.09†	2.51 ± 0.95*†¶	-
	80 min	1.6 ± 0.4*	2.0 ± 0.3	-	0.14 ± 0.05	0.83 ± 0.22†¶	-
	80 min[2]	-	1.0 ± 0.1*	-	-	0.07 ± 0.003*	-

[1]Data are expressed as mean ± S.E. N = 3 for all data except hypoxia-reoxygenation at 90 min where n = 4. Except for O_2 controls, hypoxia was initiated at 30 min. Reoxygenation occurred at 90 min except where indicated.

[2]Not reoxygenated

* Significantly different from control O_2 ($p < 0.05$).

†Significantly different from hypoxia-reoxygenation 90 min ($p < 0.05$).

¶Significantly different from the corresponding 90 minute value ($p < 0.05$).

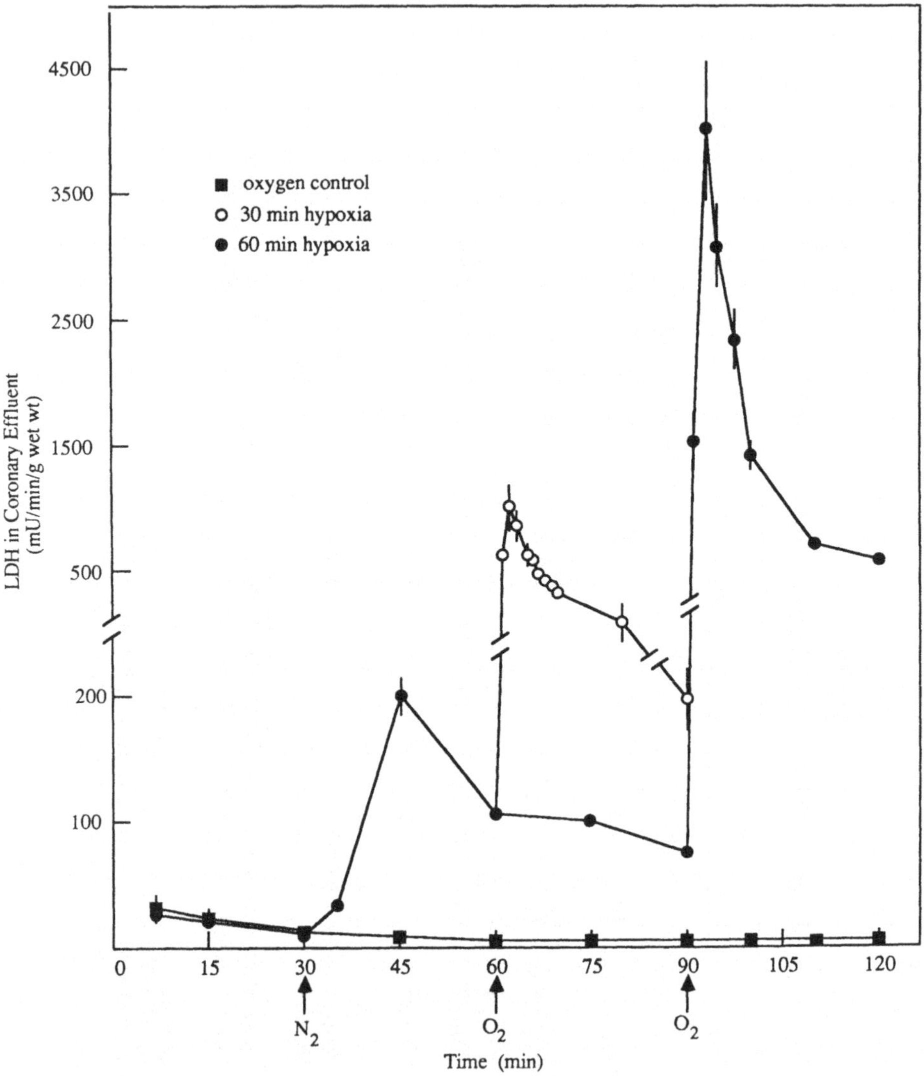

Figure 1: LDH released into the coronary effluent from isolated perfused hearts. Control hearts were perfused with oxygenated Krebs-Henseleit solution throughout. Hypoxia and reoxygenation were performed at the indicated times. N values ranged from 4-6 for each treatment. LDH release did not differ up to the time of reoxygenation and the data up to 60 min from all hypoxic hearts were, therefore, pooled. Data are expressed as mean ± S.E.

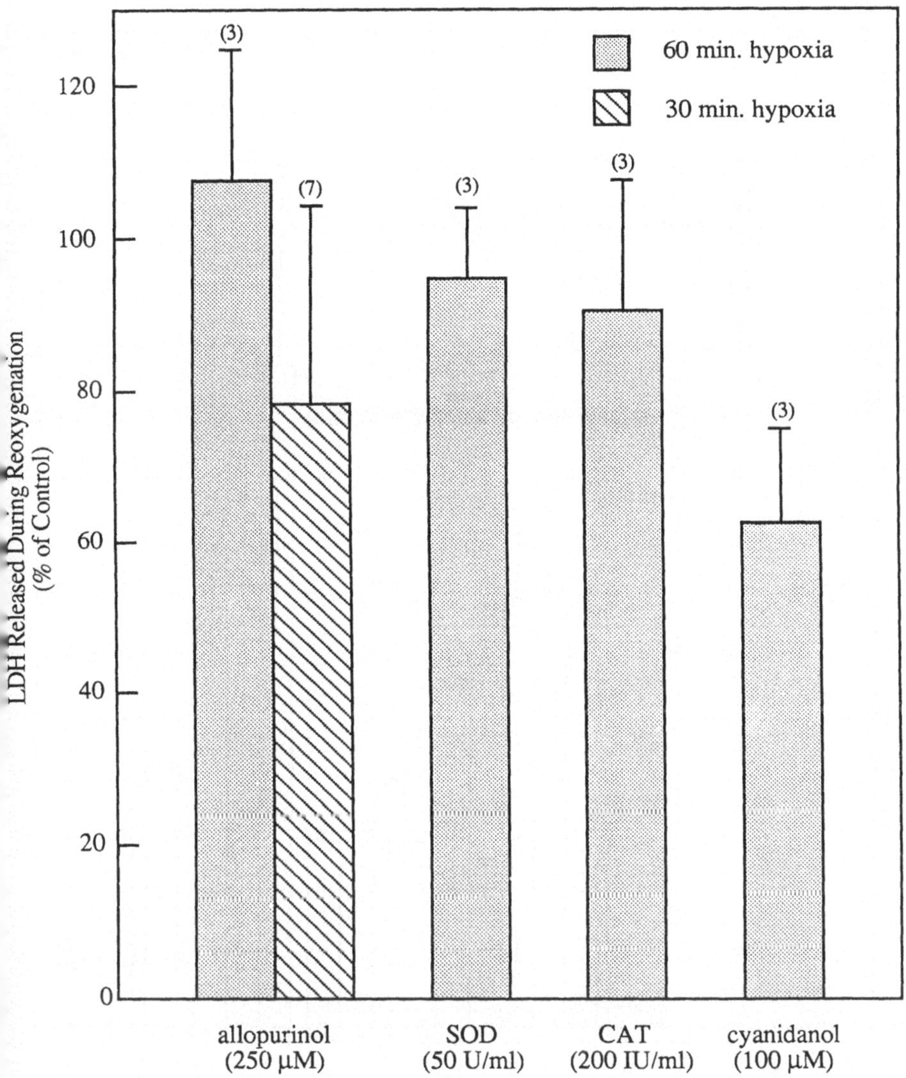

Figure 2: LDH released upon reoxygenation following treatment with various antioxidants. Allopurinol was present throughout the perfusion. Superoxide dismutase (SOD) and catalase (CAT) were added at the onset of hypoxia and cyanidanol was added 15 min before hypoxia. LDH release was measured during 10 min of reoxygenation. Control LDH release after 30 and 60 minutes of hypoxia averaged 611 $\pm$ 161 (n = 7) and 2474 $\pm$ 615 mU/min/g wet heart (n = 4), respectively. Data are expressed as mean $\pm$ S.E. Values in parentheses = n. There were no significant differences from hypoxic control values with any treatment ($p > 0.05$).

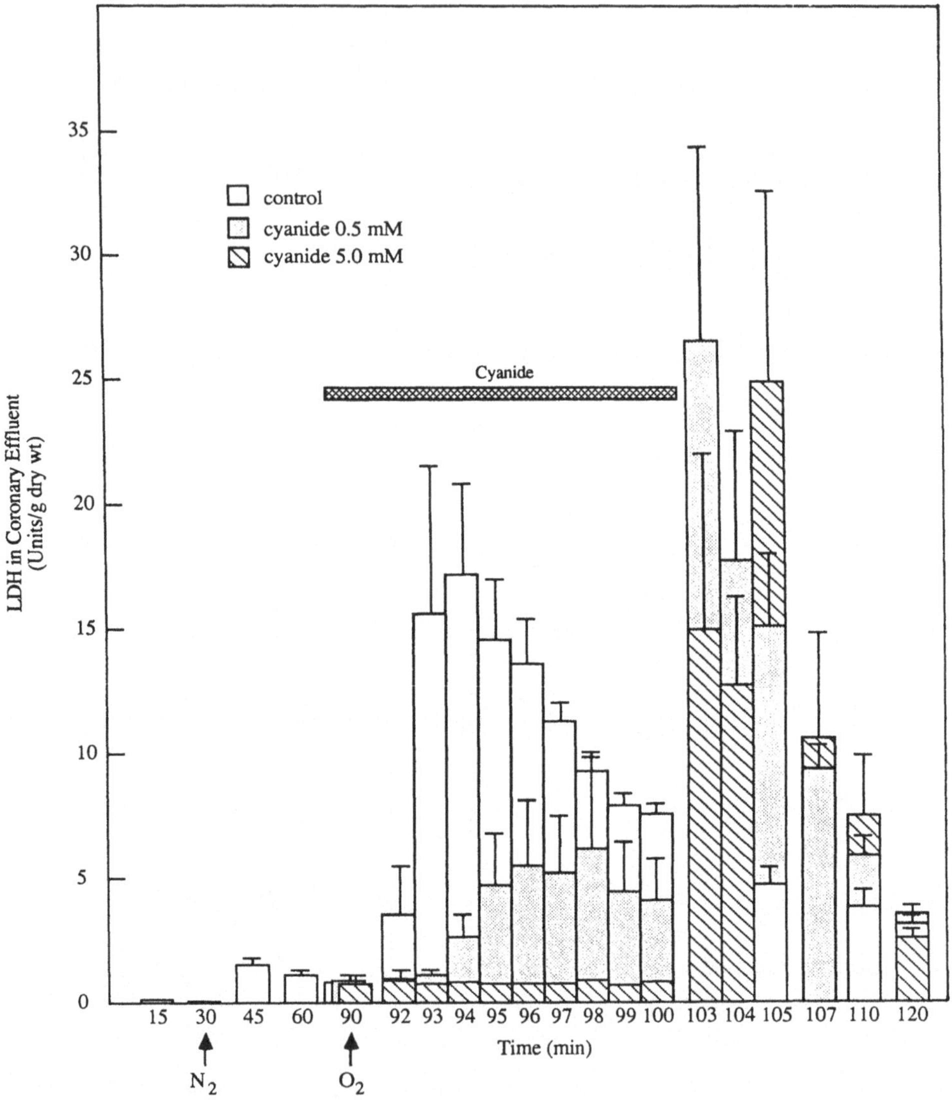

Figure 3: LDH released into the coronary effluent from isolated hearts perfused with sodium cyanide from 85 to 100 min. All hearts were subjected to hypoxia from 30 to 90 min and reoxygenated from 100 to 120 min. N values were 3-4 for all times and treatments. LDH release did not differ up to the time of cyanide infusion and the data up to 60 minutes from all hearts were, therefore, pooled. Data are expressed as mean ± S.E.

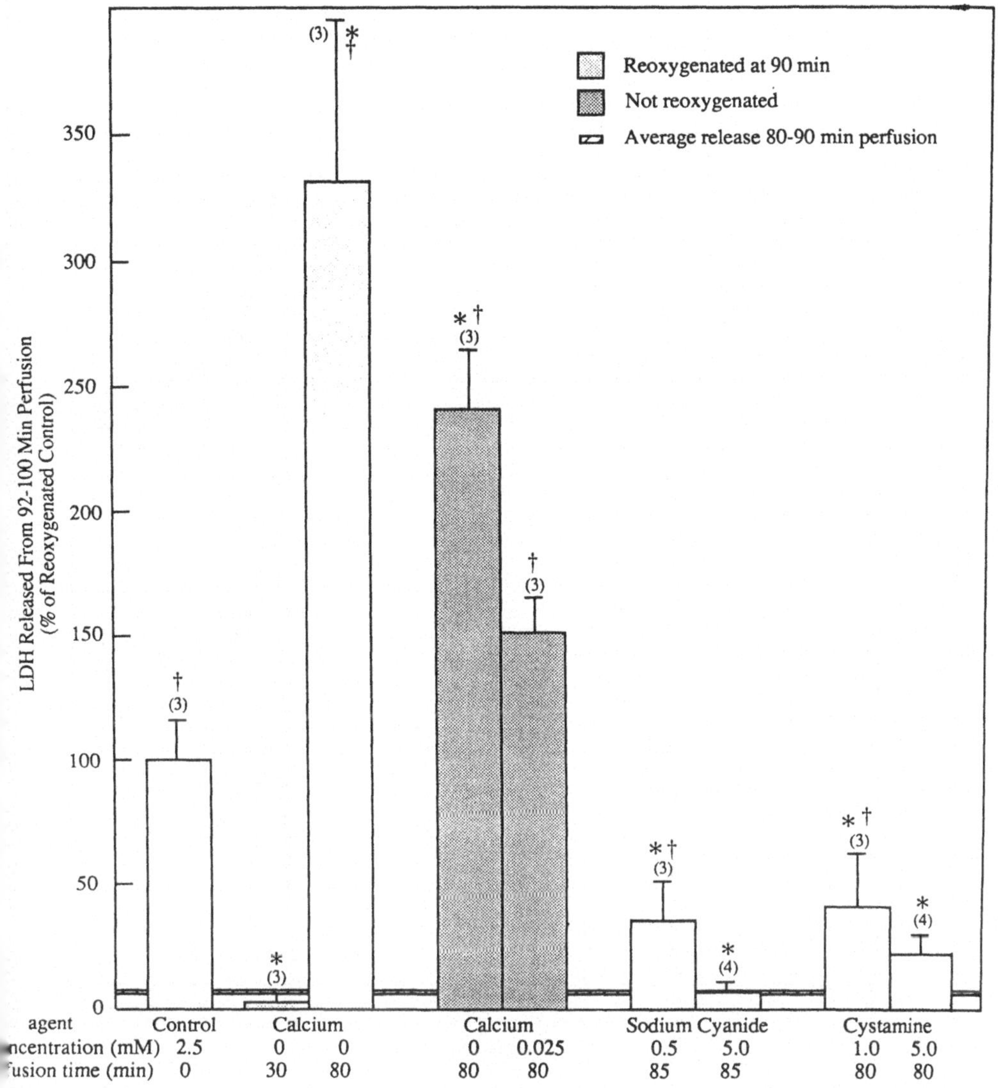

Figure 4: LDH released into the coronary effluent between 92-100 min of perfusion. All hearts were subjected to hypoxia at 30 min. Where indicated, reoxygenation occurred at 90 min. Sodium cyanide and cystamine were infused at the concentrations and times indicated in medium containing 2.5 mM calcium. Hearts subjected to hypocalcemia were infused with medium containing 2.5 mM calcium until the indicated times. Control hearts released 0.73 ± 0.09 and 11.2 ± 1.9 U/min/g dry wt from 80-90 and 92-100 minutes, respectively. Values in parentheses = n. Data are expressed as mean ± S.E. * Significantly different from controls at 92-100 min. †Significantly different from controls at 80-90 min. ($p < 0.05$).

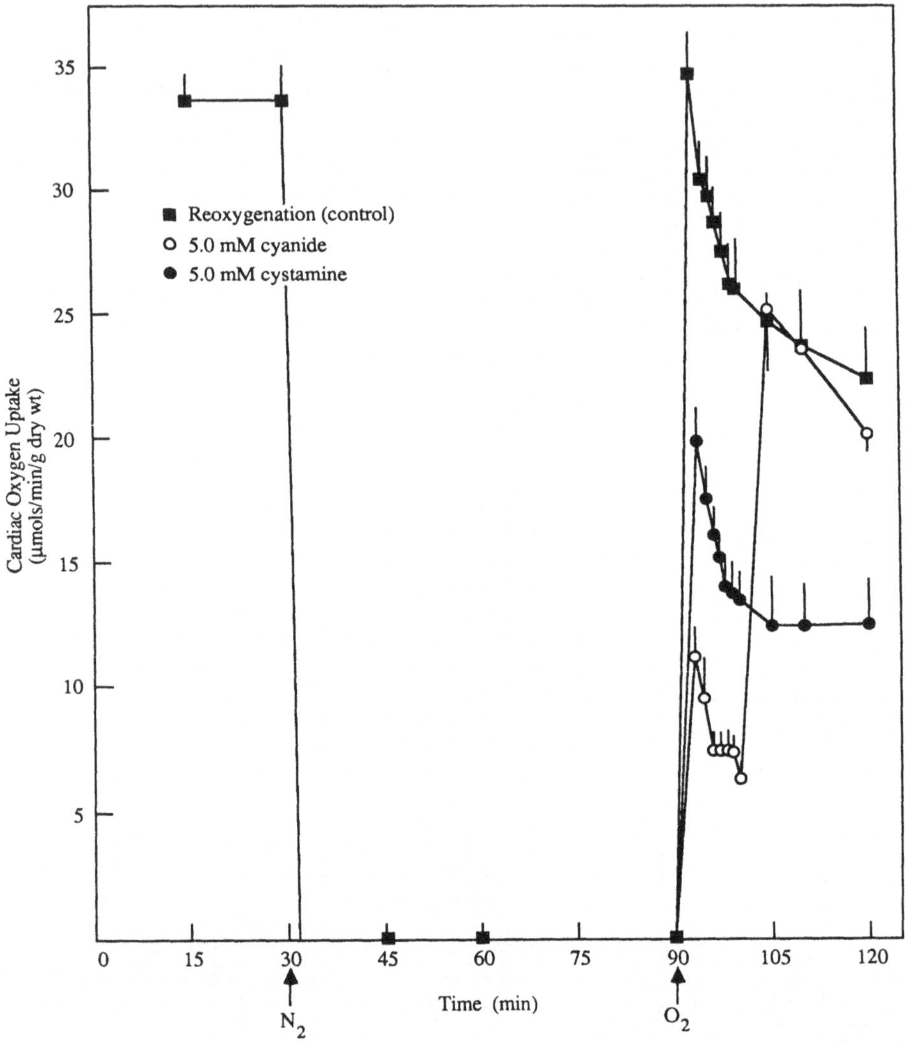

Figure 5: Cardiac oxygen uptake. All hearts were perfused with hypoxic medium from 30-90 min and reoxygenated from 90-120 min. Cyanide was infused from 85-100 and cystamine from 80-100 min. Prehypoxic oxygen uptake was the same in all hearts and only the data from controls are shown. Data are expressed as mean ± S.E. N = 3 for all points.

study, massive damage developed upon calcium-free perfusion; a "reverse" calcium paradox. Whether the basic mechanism leading to plasma membrane lysis is similar in all cases is not clear.

Clinical Implications

The localization of xanthine oxidase in the capillary endothelial cells has been well documented by immunologic techniques (Jarasch *et al.*, 1981; Jarasch *et al.*, 1986). Despite the loss of 20% of tissue LDH, the specific activity of xanthine oxidase was actually slightly higher in reoxygenated heart tissue. Since xanthine oxidase activity is localized in endothelial cells, this may be due to the loss of myocyte, but not endothelial, cell protein suggesting that the cells which contain xanthine oxidase are less susceptible to reoxygenation injury. Clincially, these results suggest that the beneficial effects seen with allopurinol in some models of reperfusion injury will be limited and are probably unrelated to any decreased cell breakdown. Furthermore, the massive release of LDH during hypoxia upon calcium-free perfusions indicates that myocardial contracture is not necessary for cellular breakdown. Finally, manipulating calcium concentrations in hypoxic or ischemic tissue may initiate cell lysis and could, therefore, be detrimental.

ACKNOWLEDGEMENTS

Thanks go to Dr. Helmut Sies for many fruitful discussions and in whose laboratory this work was performed. Thanks also to Dr. Toshihisa Ishikawa for helpful discussions, and to Florian Baltzer for his participation in some of the experiments. The author is the Gustavus Pfeiffer Centennial Fellow of Pharmacology at the College of Pharmacy, The University of Texas at Austin, and was supported by Research Career Development Award HL 01435 from the National Institutes of Health. This work was supported by Deutsche Forschungsgemeinschaft.

REFERENCES

Battelli, M.G., Della Corte, E. and Stirpe, F., 1972. Xanthine oxidase type D (dehydrogenase) in the intestine and other organs of the rat. Biochem. J. **126**: 747-749.

Bernier, M., Hearse, D.J. and Manning, A.S., 1986. Reperfusion-induced arrhythmias and oxygen-derived free radicals. Studies with "anti-free radical" interventions and a free radical-generating system in the isolated perfused rat heart. Circ. Res. **58**: 331-340.

Chambers, D.E., Parks, D.A., Patterson, G., Roy, R., McCord, J.M., Yoshida, S., Parmley, L.F. and Downey, J.M., 1985. Xanthine oxidase as a source of free radical damage in myocardial ischemia. J. Mol. Cell. Cardiol. **17**: 145-152.

Cheung, J.Y., Bonventre, J.V., Malis, C.D. and Leaf, A., 1986. Calcium and ischemic injury. N. Engl. J. Med. **314**: 1670-1676.

Della Corte, E. and Stirpe, F., 1972. The regulation of rat liver xanthine oxidase. Involvement of thiol groups in the conversion of the enzyme activity from dehydrogenase (type D) into oxidase (type O) and purification of the enzyme. Biochem. J., **126**: 739-745.

Ganote, C.E., Worstell, J. and Kaltenbach, J.P., 1976. Oxygen-induced enzyme release after irreversible myocardial injury. Effects of cyanide in perfused rat hearts. Am. J. Pathol., **84**: 327-350.

Ganote, C.E., McGarr, J., Liu, S.Y. and Kaltenbach, J.P., 1980. Oxygen-induced enzyme release. Assessment of mitochondrial function in anoxic myocardial injury and effects of the mitochondrial uncoupling agent 2,4-dinitrophenol (DNP). J. Mol. Cell. Cardiol. **12**: 387-408.

Gaudel, Y. and Duvelleroy, M.A., 1984. Role of oxygen radicals in cardiac injury due to reoxygenation. J. Mol. Cell. Cardiol. **16**: 459-470.

Granger, D,N., Rutili, G. and McCord, J.M., 1981. Superoxide radicals in feline intestinal ischemia. Gastroenterology, **81**: 22-29

Granger, D.N., Höllwarth, M.E. and Parks, D.A., 1986. Ischemia-reperfusion injury: role of oxygen-derived free radicals. Acta Physiol. Scand. **548**: (suppl.) 47-63.

Grisham, M.B., Russell, W.J., Roy, R.S. and McCord, J.M., 1986. Reoxygenation injury in the isolated perfused working rat heart: roles of xanthine oxidase and transferrin. In: G. Rotilio (Editor), Superoxide and Superoxide Dismutase in Chemistry, Biology and Medicine, Elsevier, New York, pp. 571-575.

Hearse, D.J., Humphrey, S.M. and Chain, E.B., 1973. Abrupt reoxygenation of the anoxic potassium-arrested perfused rat heart: a study of myocardial enzyme release. J. Mol. Cell. Cardiol., **5**: 395-407.

Hearse, D.J., Humphrey, S.M. and Bullock, G.R., 1978. The oxygen paradox and the calcium paradox: two facets of the same problem? J. Mol. Cell. Cardiol. **10**: 641-668.

Hearse, D.J., Manning, A.S., Downey, J.M. and Yellon, D.M., 1986. Xanthine oxidase: a critical mediator of myocardial injury during ischemia and reperfusion? Acta Physiol. Scand. **548**: (suppl.) 65-78.

Hess, M.L. and Manson, N.H., 1984. Molecular oxygen: friend or foe. The role of the oxygen free radical system in the calcium paradox, the oxygen paradox and ischemia/reperfusion injury. J. Mol. Cell. Cardiol., **16**: 969-985.

Ishikawa, T and Sies, H., 1984. Cardiac transport of glutathione disulfide and *S*- conjugate. Studies with isolated perfused rat heart during hydroperoxide metabolism. J. Biol. Chem. **259**: 3838-3843.

Itzhaki, R.F. and Gill, D.M., 1964. A micro-biuret method for estimating proteins. Anal. Biochem. **9**: 401-410.

Jarasch, E-D., Grund, C., Bruder, G., Heid, H.W., Keenan, T.W. and Franke, W.W., 1981. Localization of xanthine oxidase in mammary-gland epithelium and capillary endothelium. Cell **25**: 67-82.

Jarasch, E-D., Bruder, G. and Heid, H.W., 1986. Significance of xanthine oxidase in capillary endothelial cells. Acta Physiol. Scand. **548**: (suppl.) 39-46.

Jolly, S.R., Kane, W.J., Bailie, M.B., Abrams, G.D. and Lucchesi, B.R., 1984. Canine myocardial reperfusion injury. Its reduction by the combined administration of superoxide dismutase and catalase.Circ. Res. **54**: 277-285.

Kehrer, J.P. and Sies, H., 1987. Xanthine oxidase is not responsible for reoxygenation injury in isolated-perfused rat heart. Free Rad. Res. Commun. (in press).

Langendorff, O., 1895., Untersuchungen am überlebenden Säugertierherzen. Pflüger's Arch. Physiol., **61**: 291-332.

Lowry, O.H. and Passoneau, J.V., 1972. A collection of metabolite assays. In: O.H. Lowry and J.V. Passoneau (Editors), A Flexible System of Enzymatic Analysis, Academic Press, New York, pp. 146-163.

Lowry, O.H., Rosebrough, N.J., Farr, A.L. and Randall, R.J., 1951. Protein measurements in the folin phenol reagents. J. Biol. Chem. **193**: 265-275

Lucchesi, B.R. and Mullane, K.M., 1986. Leukocytes and ischemia-induced myocardial injury. Ann. Rev. Pharmacol. Toxicol. **26**: 201-224.

Myers, C.L., Weiss, S.J., Kirsh, M.M. and Shlafer, M., 1985. Involvement of hydrogen peroxide and hydroxyl radical in the "oxygen paradox": reduction of creatine kinase release by catalase, allopurinol or deferoxamine, but not by superoxide dismutase. J. Mol. Cell. Cardiol. **17**: 675-684.
Myers, C.L., Weiss, S.J., Kirsh, M.M., Shepard, B.M. and Shlafer, M., 1986. Effects of supplementing hypothermic crystalloid cardioplegic solution with catalase, superoxide dismutase, allopurinol, or deferoxamine on functional recovery of globally ischemic and reperfused isolated hearts. J. Thorac. Cardiovasc. Surg. **91**: 281-289.
Nayler, W.G. and Elz, J.S., 1986. Reperfusion injury: laboratory artifact or clinical dilemma? Circulation **74**: 215-221.
Nicotera, P., 1986. On the role of intracellular Ca^{2+} accumulation in chemical toxicity. Dissertation, Karolinska Institute, Stockholm, Sweden.
Oei, H.H.H., Zoganas, H.C., McCord, J.M. and Schaffer, S.W., 1986. Role of acetaldehyde and xanthine oxidase in ethanol-induced oxidative stress. Res. Commun. Chem. Pathol. Pharmacol. **51**: 195-203.
Otani, H., Engelman, R.M., Rousou, J.A., Breyer, R.H., Leneshow, S. and Das, D.K., 1986. Cardiac performance during reperfusion improved by pretreatment with oxygen free-radical scavengers. J. Thorac. Cardiovasc. Surg. **91**: 290-295.
Peterson, D.A., Asinger, R.W., Elsperger, K.J., Homans, D.C. and Eaton, J.W., 1985. Reactive oxygen species may cause myocardial reperfusion injury. Biochem. Biophys. Res. Commun. **127**: 87-93.
Peterson, D.A., Kelly, B. and Gerrard, J.M., 1986. Allopurinol can act as an electron transfer agen. Is this relevant during reperfusion injury? Biochem. Biophys. Res. Commun. **13**: 76-79.
Poole-Wilson, P.A., Harding, D.P., Bourdillon, P.D.V. and Tones, M.A., 1984. Caclium out of control. J. Mol. Cell. Cardiol. **16**: 175-187.
Reimer, K.A. and Jennings, R.B., 1985. Failure of the xanthine oxidase inhibitor allopurinol to limit infarct size after ischemia and reperfusion in dogs. Circulation **71**: 1069-1075.
Roy, R.S. and McCord, J.M., 1983. Superoxide and ischemia: conversion of xanthine dehydrogenase to xanthine oxidase. In: R. Greenwald and G. Cohen (Editors), Oxy Radicals and their Scavenger Systems. Volume II: Cellular and Medical Aspects, Elsevier, New York, pp. 145-153.
Shatney, C.H., MacCarter, D.J. and Lillehei, R.C., 1976. Effects of allopurinol, propranolol and methyl prednisolone on infarct size in experimental myocardial infarction. Am. J. Cardiol. **37**: 572-580.
Shlafer, M., Kane, P.F. and Kirsh, M.M., 1982. Superoxide dismutase plus catalase enhances the efficacy of hypothermic cardioplegia to protect the globally ischemic, reperfused heart. J. Thorac. Cardiovasc. Surg. **83**: 830-839.
Slater, T.F. and Eakins, M.N., 1975. Interactions of (+)-cyandianol-3 with free radical generating systems. In: A. Bertelli (Editor), New Trends in the Therapy of Liver Diseases, Karger: Basel, pp. 84-89.
Stirpe, F. and Della Corte, E., 1969. The regulation of rat liver xanthine oxidase. Conversion *in vitro* of the enzymatic activity from dehydrogenase (type D) to oxidae (type O). J. Biol. Chem. **244**: 3855-3863.
Thor, H., Hartzell, P., Svensson, S-Å., Orrenius, S., Mirabelli, F., Marinoni, V. and Bellomo, G., 1985. On the role of thiol groups in the inhibition of liver microsomal Ca^{2+} sequestration by toxic agents. Biochem. Pharmacol. **34**: 3717-3723.
Zivin, J.A. and Bartko, J.J., 1976. Statistics for disinterested scientists. Life Sci. **18**: 15-26.

OXIDATIVE STRESS IN THE MYOCARDIUM: RELATIONSHIP WITH EICOSANOID BIOSYNTHESIS AND TISSUE DAMAGE.

Fulvio Ursini[a b], Gualtiero Pelosi[b], Antonio Benassi[b] and Renata Barsacchi[b c]

Istituto di Chimica Biologica dell'Università di Padova[a]
Istituto di Fisiologia Clinica C.N.R. Pisa[b]
Dipartimento di Fisiologia e Biochimica dell'Università di Pisa[c]

ABSTRACT

The oxidative stress was evaluated in the perfused rat heart by monitoring chemiluminescence (CL) emission at the surface of the organ. While ischemia decreased photon emission, reoxygenation restored the CL at a level not significantly above the basal. Partial depletion of Vit.E stimulated CL emission during post-ischemic reperfusion. In order to get a better insight into the relationship between oxidative stress and heart function and tissue viability, we induced an oxidative stress by infusing glutathione depleting agents or organic hydroperoxides. In both cases an increase of CL paralleled the decrease of the heart function leading eventually to the "stone heart", a pathologic pattern associated to an impairment of calcium homeostasis. Dietary manipulations (substitution of sunflower oil for olive oil or vit.E depletion) enhanced the response to the hydroperoxide induced oxidative stress (CL emission and morphofunctional derangement). Oxidative stress also increased prostaglandins (PG) release. Aspirin prevented PG release but greatly stimulated CL emission, while both effects were inhibited by nor-dihydroguaiaretic acid. These results suggest that oxidative stress leads to an increased steady state concentration of electronically excited molecules, possibly enzimatically generated, and that the functional derangement may also be due, at least in part, to peroxidic compounds active on calcium fluxes.

INTRODUCTION

Myocardial ischemia produces a series of biochemical changes related both to the impaired removal and to the interrupted supply of metabolites. The decreased oxidative metabolism and therefore the reduced synthesis of ATP at the level of the cytochrome oxidase is claimed to drive the sequence of events leading eventually to cell death (Reimer et al.,1981).

Cellular deterioration during the ischemic period is obviously time dependent and the restoration of oxygen supply can prevent cellular damage (Bush et al.,1983). However, a critical time exists, beyond which the reflow has not a beneficial effect and can even exacerbate myocardial damage (Hearse,1984).

In recent years, experimental evidences have been accumulated that an increased generation of free radicals and therefore an oxidative stress during reperfusion are the molecular events possibly leading to post-ischemic reoxygenation damage (Chambers et al.1983). It has been shown that free radicals are generated during ischemia (Rao et al., 1983) and even more during reperfusion (Guarnieri et al.,1980), that lipid peroxidation products can be detected in ischemic and reoxygenated tissues (Meerson et al., 1982), that intracellular thiols are oxidized under these conditions (Bindoli et al., personal communication) and that different antioxidants or free radical scavengers protect against the reperfusion injury (Ganote et al., 1982. Shlafer et al., 1982. Woodward et al., 1985). This "oxidative stress", occurring during reoxygenation, has been related to the "reductive stress" that occurs during ischemia, when the amount of reduced electron carriers is increased, due to the lack of O_2 acting as the terminal electron acceptor. Reductive stress would lead to the generation of free radicals during ischemia and to the univalent reduction of O_2 during reperfusion (Meerson et al., 1982). A production of superoxide anion radicals has also been claimed to be related to the ischemia - dependent conversion of xanthine oxidase into xanthine dehydrogenase (Hearse et al.,1986). The free radicals or the oxy radicals generated under these conditions would produce lipid peroxidation of the membranes and in this sense it would also be important the release of ferritin iron induced by the "reductive stress" and by the increased fluxes of superoxide (Thomas et al., 1985. Biemont et al., 1984). The elucidation of the precise mechanisms supporting the biochemical events occurring during ischemia, and responsible for irreversible damage during reperfusion, would assist the planning of therapeutical approaches as well as the design of specific drugs for myocardial protection.

Moreover, although both an increased generation of prooxidizing species and a decrease of antioxidant defenses - therefore a cellular condition of oxidative stress - have been demonstrated during ischemia-reperfusion, there are no clear data on the relationship between oxidative stress and myocardial damage. This chapter reviews this area of research and deals particulary with our studies on the oxidative stress in the heart, how it can be monitored, which are the physiopathological consequences and the possible mechanisms, and how it can be modulated in vivo.

ULTRAWEAK CHEMILUMINESCENCE EMISSION

The measurement of low level chemiluminescence has been recently introduced to evaluate the formation of excited species and to monitor the occurrence of oxidative free radical reactions in isolated or exposed organs (Boveris et al.,1980). The non-invasive character of this approach as well as its high sensitivity makes the use of this technique extremely valuable for in vivo studies of oxidative stress. Although the chemical and physical background of the photon emission in complex biological samples is not completely understood, the available data support the concept that cellular damage is associated with an increased chemiluminescence emission. The research therefore is directed both to the analysis of pathological situations and to the recognition of the fine mechanisms in simplified model systems. An example of the former is the demonstration of an increased chemiluminescence from the liver of animals bearing tumors (Boveris et al., 1985).

The peroxidation of linoleic acid (Nakano et al.,1978) as well as the increased peroxidation rate induced by different agents such as iron or hydroperoxides or hyperoxia in subcellular fractions, tissue homogenates, isolated cells and perfused organs, is always accompained by chemiluminescence emission (Cadenas,1985). Singlet oxygen and/or excited carbonyl compounds derived from free radical interactions during lipid peroxidation, prostaglandin biosynthesis, or lipoxigenase-catalyzed reactions might contribute to the observed photoemission (Cadenas,1985; Schulte-Herbruggen et al., 1985; Marnett et al.,1974). However, the correlation between lipid peroxidation and photon emission is usually, and legitimately, inferred when the spectral analysis is humpered by the low amplitude of the recorded signal.

OXIDATIVE STRESS IN THE RAT HEART AND CHEMILUMINESCENCE

The rat hearts were perfused retrogradely (Langendorff perfusion) in a light-tight box and the light emitted at the surface of the organ was collected by a lucite rod and measured by an EMI 9814 photomultiplier with an applied potential of 1.6 kV, connected to a computer. The scheme of the apparatus and of the electronics is reported in Fig.1. The careful setting of the discriminator and of the threshold allowed the detection of the "spontaneous" photon emission (Bottigli et al. 1984). This emission was oxygen dependent, being decreased when the perfusion was stopped (Barsacchi et al. 1983). The addition to the perfusion medium of hydroperoxides produced an increase of photon emission intensity with a polyphasic time course. Alike the "spontaneous" chemiluminescence, the "hydroperoxide-induced" chemiluminescence was oxygen dependent. The relation between the initial rate of photon emission vs the hydroperoxide concentration shows that the phenomenon is saturable with a sigmoid kinetics (Fig 2 A). This saturation kinetics suggests the presence of cellular rate limiting factors involved in the formation of the first oxidizing species or in the propagation of the peroxidative chain reactions. The free radical and oxidative nature of this photon emission is supported by: i) its oxygen dependence, ii) its dramatic enhancement following vit.E depletion (see below), and iii) the inhibitory effect of polyphenolic antioxidants such as nor-dihydro guairetic acid.

Also the depletion of glutathione, induced by perfusing the heart either with substrates of glutathione transferases or with thiol oxidant diamide, produced an increase of chemiluminescence intensity (Barsacchi et al., 1984). The pattern of photon emission in this condition was simpler than that observed in the presence of hydroperoxides. Chemiluminescence emission increased progressively, with a slope proportional to the concentration of the agent used, and reached a maximum 70% higher than the basal level when the concentration of GSH in the heart was practically nil.

The oxidative stress induced in the heart by hydroperoxides or by glutathione depletion produced lipid peroxidation, as confirmed by a HPLC analysis of the conjugated diene containing phospholipids and by HPLC quantitation of the thiobarbituric acid reactive material.

Chemiluminescence detection has been used to get direct information on the sensitivity of the heart to an oxidative challenge. The diet composition is known to modify the cellular balance between prooxidant and antioxidant factors. Feeding the rats for three weeks vitamin E and Selenium deficient diets caused, during cumene hydroperoxide induced oxidative stress, a ten-fold increase in chemiluminescence rate (Fig 2B), associated to a more extensive tissue damage. However, even mild modifications of the diet, compatible with different human habits, were able to modify the susceptibility of the rat heart to an oxidative stress. We observed indeed that an increase of polyunsaturated fatty acids or a decrease of antioxidants, induced by the substitution of the alimentary oil, produced a significantly different chemiluminescence response following the usual oxidative challenge by cumene hydroperoxide. The pattern of fatty acid saturation and the content of vitamin E in the hearts of rats fed with diets containing olive oil or sunflower oil or pork fat are reported in Table I. As shown in Fig.3, the initial rate of chemiluminescence was dramatically lower when the diet contained olive oil, apparently due to the optimal ratio between autoxidable polyunsaturated fatty acids and antioxidants.

The changes in heart function and tissue viability following an oxidative stress show a typical pattern, independently of the inducing agent. There are first rhythm abnormalities and coronary vasodilation, followed by a reduction of R waves amplitude on the electrocardiogram and by coronary flow decrease, and, finally, electric and mechanical arrest, characterized by heart hypercontracture at gross examination. Observation of these hearts under light microscopy reveals extensive contraction band necrosis (coagulative myocytolysis), a feature described in human pathology and particularly in the "stone heart" (Baroldi et al., 1974), as well as in experimental studies on the reperfusion of the ischemic myocardium (Ganote,1983).

In conclusion, in the experimental models adopted, the rate of chemiluminescence initial rise appears to be proportional to the extent of tissue damage and, moreover, the same feature of myocardial injury is evidenced following an oxidative stress as well as during post-ischemic reperfusion.

The direct evaluation of the oxidative stress occurring during ischemia-reperfusion is a rather complicated task. In fact, although the monitoring of the ultraweak chemiluminescence allows a sensitive evaluation of an oxidative stress in an intact organ, the direct evidence of a substantially increased photon emission during the post-ischemic reperfusion is apparent only if the heart is, at least partially, vit.E depleted (Fig. 4).

MECHANISM OF THE OXIDATIVE STRESS DEPENDENT TISSUE DAMAGE

Contraction band necrosis is the specific morphological feature common to an experimentally induced oxidative stress and to the post-ischemic reoxygenation damage. Therefore, the understanding of the biochemical events promoted by the oxidative stress and leading to irreversible hypercontraction, would permit to identify some of the mechanisms of the functional impairment occurring on the heart during ischemia and at reperfusion. Since a sudden increase of cytosolic free calcium is apparently the determinant factor of cellular hypercontraction (Ganote, 1983), the major goal is to understand whether and why an oxidative stress can induce an impairment of calcium homeostasis.

The direct measurement of the cytosolic free calcium would be obviously the best analytical approach, but extremely complicated, as the heart is an excitable tissue, and therefore the experimental approaches are usually indirect. On the other hand, most of the experimental studies on this field have been carried out in liver cells, and only few reports in myocardial cells have been published. However, the observed analogies between the results obtained with both cell preparations seem to support the hypothesis of a common biochemical pathway leading to cellular damage as a consequence of an oxidative stress. In isolated cells of both heart (Noronha-Dutra et al., 1982) and liver (Thor et al., 1982) the chemically induced glutathione depletion increases lipid peroxidation rate and produces a severe blebbing of plasma membranes, which in hepatocytes has been demonstrated to be specifically due to an increase of free calcium in the cytoskeletal environment (Jewell et al.,1982).

The ATP dependent calcium uptake by liver microsomes (Jones et al.,1983) or by sarcoplasmic reticulum (Player et al., 1978) is inhibited by lipid peroxidation and an increased calcium release has been observed in liver mitochondria following the addition of organic hydroperoxides (Lotschen et al., 1980). Menadione, which generates active oxygen species by a redox cycling and oxidizes glutathione, inhibits the mitochondrial calcium uptake and the plasma membrane calcium ATPase (Bellomo et al., 1983). The phosphorilase A activity, which can be used as an indirect evidence of the rise of cytosolic calcium, is increased following a menadione induced oxidative stress both in hepatocytes (Bellomo et al., 1984) and in isolated myocytes (Maiorino and Chan, unpublished observation). In conclusion, the homeostasis of intracellular calcium seems to be affected by an oxidative stress by one or both of these two major mechanisms: the inhibition of calcium translocases (possibly mediated by an oxidation of thiols) or the increase of calcium permeability (possibly mediated by lipid peroxidation products). The evidence that a substantial amount of GSH is lost during reperfusion (personal communication from dr. Bindoli and dr. Cavallini) could be explained by both mechanisms.

The observation that lipid peroxidation can induce in bilayer membranes an increase in transmembrane calcium current suggested sophisticated studies which showed that the lipid peroxides fulfil all the structural and functional criteria to exhert a specific calcium ionophoric effect (Lebedev et al., 1983). However, the quantity of lipid peroxides which can be generated during post ischemic reperfusion, and the concentration of peroxides required to exhert an ionophoretic effect in vivo are still unsolved issues.

CHEMILUMINESCENCE, OXIDATIVE STRESS AND EICOSANOID BIOSYNTHESIS

It is well known that hydroperoxides stimulate the activity of prostaglandin endoperoxide synthetase, and to this activity seems to be partially related the suggested regulatory role of lipid peroxides in cell physiology, differentiation, ageing and pathology (Lands et al., 1984).

A typical example could be the spawning of the mollusks, an event ultimately calcium-dependent, which is stimulated by hydrogen peroxide and inhibited by catalase and aspirin (Morse et al., 1977). Moreover, some eicosanoids fulfil the chemical criteria to be considered active as calcium ionophors (Carsten et al., 1978).

On this ground, we devised to study the relationship between eicosanoid biosynthesis and oxidative stress in the heart. As suspected, the hydroperoxides and the glutathione depleting agents evoked, in the perfused heart, a release of eicosanoids evaluated as tromboxane B2 and 6ketoPGF1a (Barsacchi et al., 1986). This release closely paralleled the rate of chemiluminescence emission (Fig.5) and, like photon emission, was sensitive to dietary factors (Fig 6). Since the peroxidase activity of prostaglandin endoperoxide synthetase generates singlet oxygen (Cadenas, 1985), it was reasonable to suppose that the activation of this enzyme by the peroxides would lead both to an enhancement of cellular damage and of light emission in an aspirin-sensitive manner. However, the opposite was observed. Aspirin strongly stimulated the cumene hydroperoxide induced

TABLE I

Degree of unsaturation of fatty acids and vit.E content in the heart of rats fed with diets containing different fats

	Olive oil	Sunflower oil	Pork fat
PUFA	15.7 ± 1.1	46.8 ± 2.3	18.1 ± 0.9
MUFA	59.8 ± 3.2	21.8 ± 1.8	49.3 ± 2.7
SFA	24.5 ± 1.6	31.4 ± 1.9	32.6 ± 2.3
Vit.E	21.2 ± 1.2	17.0 ± 0.9	16.3 ± 0.8

Polyunsaturated (PUFA), monounsaturated (MUFA) and saturated (SFA) fatty acids myocardial composition is expressed as relative percentage of the total heart fatty acids; vit. E is expressed as µg/100 mg of dry weight. The mean values and standard deviations of five determinations are reported.

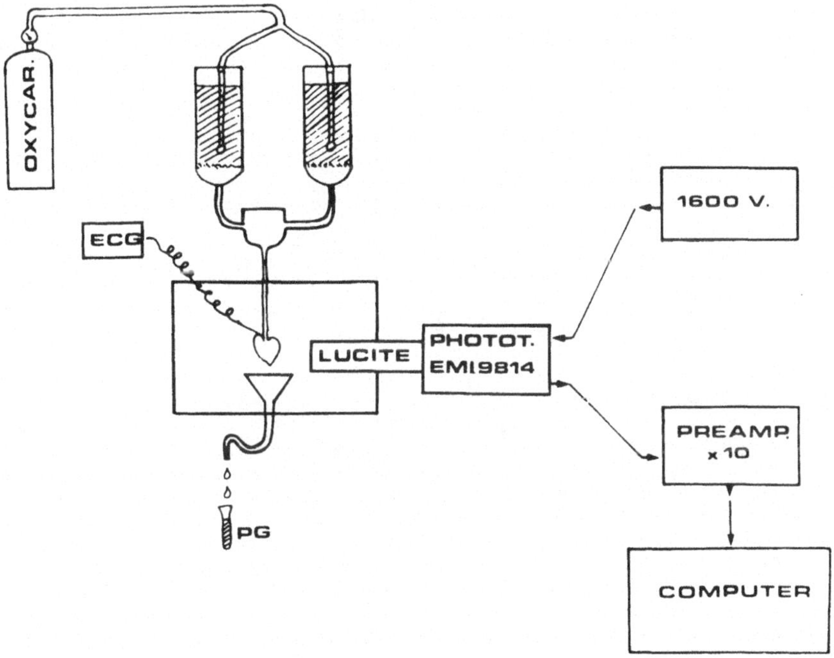

Fig.1. Scheme of the experimental equipment used to measure chemiluminescence emission from the surface of the isolated perfused rat heart.

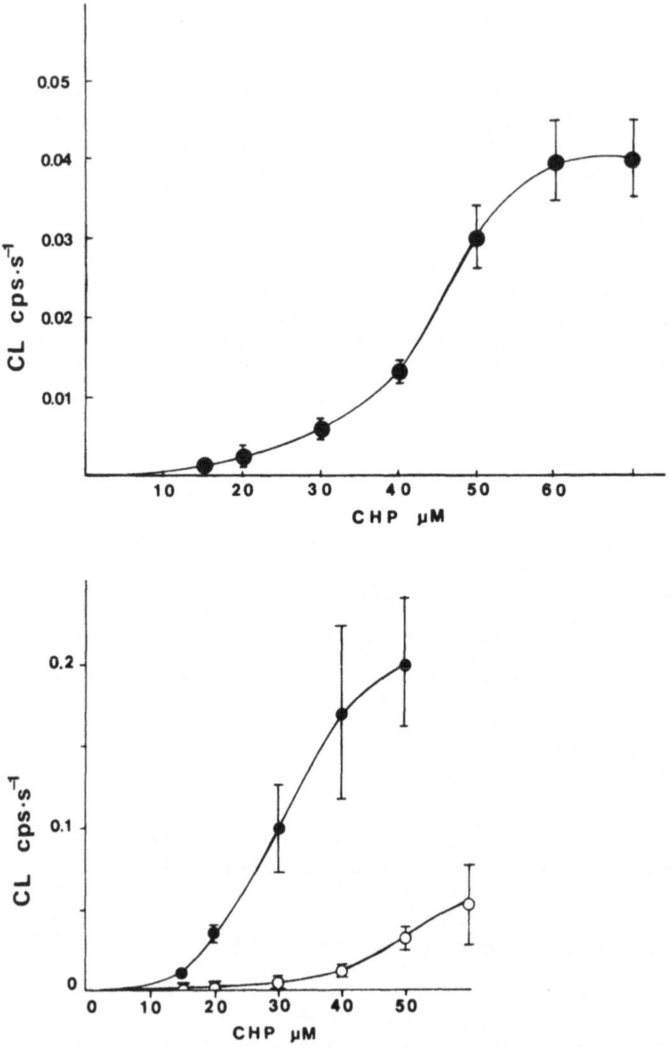

Fig. 2. Upper panel : relation between the initial rate of chemiluminescence emission and the cumene hydroperoxide concentration in the perfusate; lower panel : the same relation of upper panel is shown (open circles) together with the relation obtained from the hearts of rats fed with vitamin E and Selenium deficient diet (closed circles).

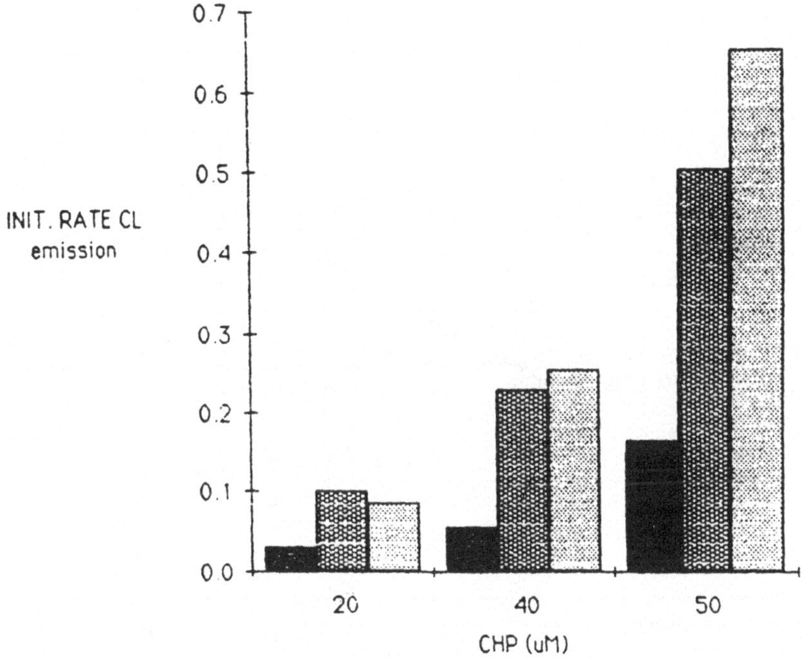

Fig. 3. Effect of different alimentary oils containing diets on the cumene hydroperoxide induced initial rate of chemiluminescence emission (black bars = olive oil, dark gray bars = sunflower oil, pale gray bars = pork fat).

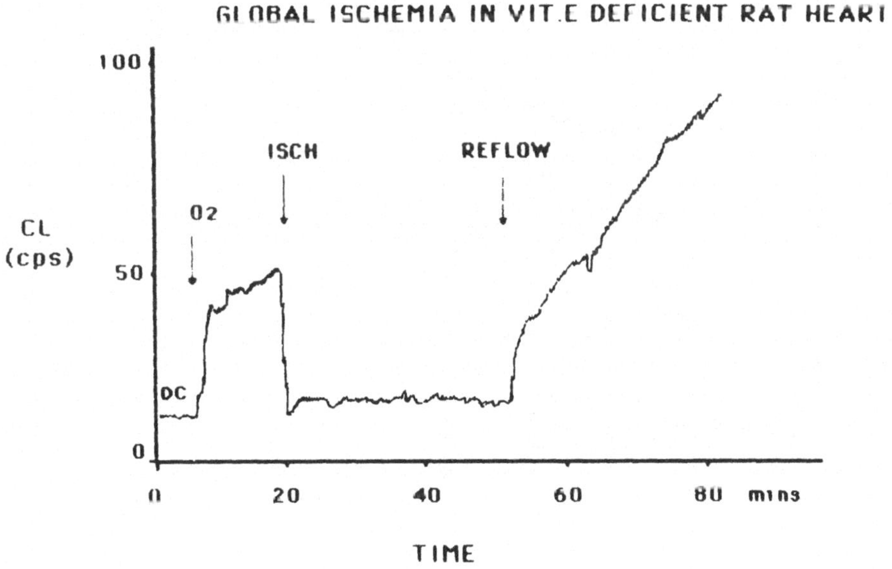

Fig. 4. Chemiluminescence tracing from the heart of a vit.E-Se deficient rat during global ischemia and at reperfusion.

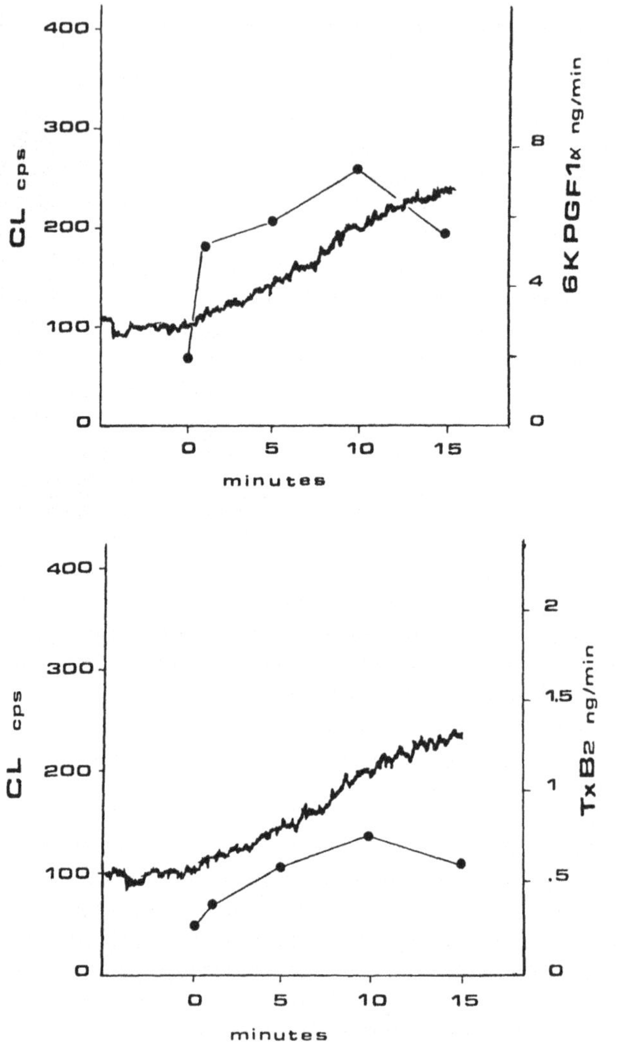

Fig. 5. Tromboxane B2 and 6ketoPG1a release and chemiluminescence tracing during the perfusion with 40μM cumene hydroperoxide.

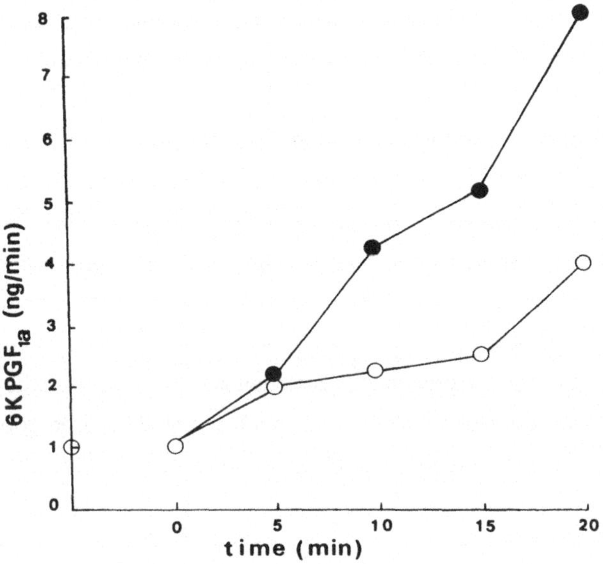

Fig. 6. Effect of different alimentary oils containing diets on cumene hydroperoxide (40 μM) induced eicosanoids release (open circles =olive oil; closed circles = sunflower oil).

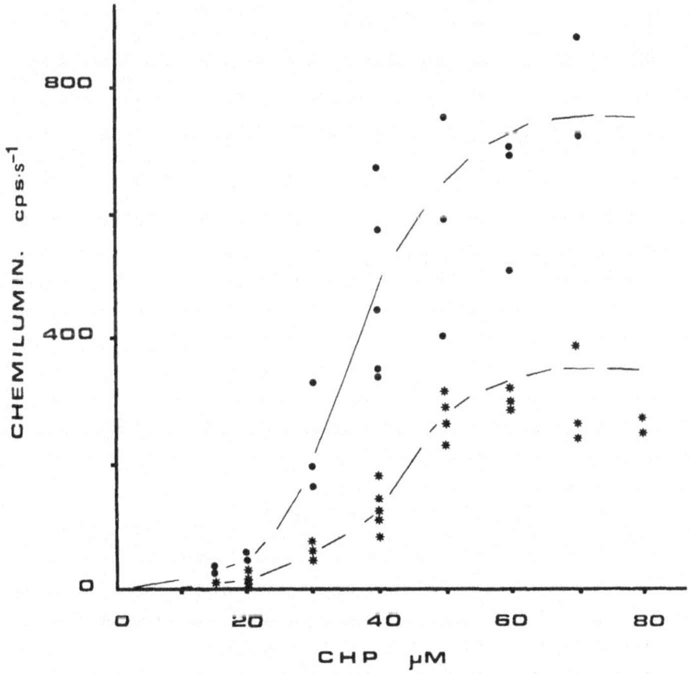

Fig. 7. Effect of 500μM aspirin on the relation between initial rate of chemiluminescence emission and cumene hydroperoxide concentration (asterisks = CHP, closed circles = CHP plus 500 μM aspirin).

light emission (Fig 7) and augmented myocardial damage, despite the inhibition of prostaglandins biosynthesis. One possible explanation is that the steady state concentration of hydroperoxides is increased, due to the aspirin induced inhibition of the peroxidase activity of the prostaglandin endoperoxide synthetase. However, we have to assume that a substantial amount of peroxides are metabolized by this activity, and this seems very unlikely because of the presence in the heart of other extremely active Se dependent and non Se dependent peroxidases. Another possibility is that some products of prostaglandin endoperoxide synthetase act as inhibitors on the generation of electronically excited species, and that these species play a role in modulating calcium fluxes. The possible candidates for this role are the products of lipoxigenase. The lipoxigenase reaction indeed is accompained by the generation of excited species (Schulte-Herbruggen et al., 1985), and leucotrienes have been recently identified as mediators of different types of shock (Lefer, 1985).

CONCLUSIONS

The use of chemiluminescence detection allows a sensitive and non invasive evaluation of oxidative stress in the heart. Chemiluminescence is always paralleled by cellular damage and calcium overflow is likely to be the ultimate functional event leading to cell death. Although a direct evidence is still lacking, post ischemic reperfusion produces an oxidative stress and the molecular mechanisms of the consequent cell damage, as envisaged from the analogy with model systems, seem to be related to an increased steady state concentration of hydroperoxides acting on calcium fluxes i) as ionophors, ii) by inhibiting calcium translocases, or iii) by stimulating the synthesis of specific molecules (lipoxigenase products?) active on calcium fluxes.

REFERENCES

Baroldi, G., Milam, J.D., Wukasch, D.C., Sandiford, F.M., Romagnoli, A. and Cooley, D.A., 1974. Myocardial cell damage in"stone heart". J. Molecul. Cell. Cardiol., 6: 395-399.

Barsacchi, R., Camici, P., Bottigli, U., Salvadori, P.A., Pelosi, G., Maiorino, M. and Ursini, F., 1983. Correlation between hydroperoxide-induced chemiluminescence of the heart and its function. Biochem. Biophys. Acta, 762: 241-247.

Barsacchi, R., Pelosi, G., Camici, P., Bonaldo, L., Maiorino, M. and Ursini, F., 1984. Glutathione depletion increases chemiluminescence emission and lipid peroxidation in the heart. Biochem. Biophys. Acta, 804: 356-360.

Barsacchi, R., Nanni, N., Pelosi, G., Camici, P. and Ursini, F., 1986. Relationship between oxidative stress eicosanoid biosynthesis and heart damage. In: Benzi, G., Packer, L. and Siliprandi, N. (Editors) Biochemical aspects of physical execise.

Elsevier, Amsterdam. pp.129-132.

Bellomo, G., Mirabelli, F., Richelmi, P. and Orrenius, S., 1983. Critical role of sulfhydryl group(s) in ATP-dependent calcium sequestration by the plasma membrane fraction from rat liver. FEBS Lett., 163: 136-139.

Bellomo, G., Thor, H. and Orrenius, S., 1984. Increase in cytocolic calcium concentration during t-butyl hydroperoxide metabolism by isolated hepatocytes involves NADPH oxidation and mobilization of intracellular calcium stores. FEBS Lett.,168: 38-42.

Biemont, P., VanEijk, H.G. and Koster, J.F.,1984. Iron mobilization from ferritin by superoxide derived from stimulated polymorphonuclear leucocytes. J. Clin. Invest., 73: 1576-1579.

Bottigli, U., Camici, P., Bellina, R., Salvadori, P., Mazzarisi, R.A., Barsacchi, R., Quaglia, M. and Ursini, F., 1984. Measurement of ultraweak chemiluminescence emitted from isolated and perfused rat hearts. Il Nuovo cimento- Europhysics Journal, 3d: 936-941.

Boveris, A., Cadenas, E., Reiter, R., Filipkowski, M., Nakase, Y. and Chance,B., 1980. Organ chemiluminescence: non-invasive assay for oxidative radical reactions. Proc. Natl. Acad. Sci. USA, 77: 347-351.

Boveris, A., Llesuy, S.F. and Fraga, C.G., 1985. Increased liver chemiluminescence in tumor-bearing mice. J.Free Rad. in Biol. and Med., 1: 131-138.

Bush L.R., Buja, L.M., Samowitz, W., Rude, R.E., Walthan, N., Tilton, G.P.,Willerson, J.T., 1983. Recovery of left ventricular segmental function after long-term reperfusion following temporary coronary occlusion in conscious dogs. Circulation Res., 53: 248-263.

Cadenas, E., 1985. Oxidative stress and formation of excited species. In Sies, H. (Editor), Oxidative stress. Academic Press, New York, pp.311-330.

Carsten, M.E. and Miller, J.D., 1978. Comparison of calcium association constants and ionophoretic properties of some prostaglandins and ionophores. Arch. Biochem. Biophys., 185: 282-287.

Chambers, D.E., Parks, D.A., Patterson, G., Yoshida, S., Burton, K., Parmley, L.F., McCord, J.M. and Downey, J.M., 1983. Role of oxygen-derived radicals in myocardial ischemia. Fed. Proc., 42: 1093.

Ganote, C.E., Sims, M., Kaltenbach, J.P., 1982. Dimethylsulfoxide (DMSO) inhibition of the oxygen-paradox in perfused rat hearts. Am.J.Pathol., 109: 270-276.

Ganote, C.E., 1983. Contraction band necrosis and irreversible myocardial injury. J. Mol. Cell. Cardiol., 15: 67-73.

Guarnieri, C., Flamigni, F. and Caldarera, C.M., 1980. Role of oxygen in the cellular damage induced by re-oxygenation of hypoxic heart. J. Mol. Cell. Cardiol., 12: 797-808.

Hearse, D.J., 1984. Reperfusion of the ischemic myocardium. Clin. Res. Rev., 4: 58-61.

Hearse, D.J., Manning, A.S., Downey, J.M. and Yellon, D.M., 1986. Oxygen-derived free radicals and myocardial injury: a critical role for xanthine oxidase?. In: Novelli, G. and Ursini, F.(Editors), Oxygen free radicals in shock. Karger, Basel, pp.149-164.

Jewell, S.A., Bellomo, G., Thor, H., Orrenius, S. and Smith, M.T., 1982. Bleb formation in hepatocytes during drug metabolism is caused by disturbances in thiol and calcium ion homeostasis. Science, 217: 1257-1259.

Jones, D.P., Thor, H., Smith, M.T., Jewell, S.A. and Orrenius, S., 1983. Inhibition of ATP-dependent microsomal calcium sequestration during oxidative stress and its prevention by glutathione. J. Biol. Chem., 258: 6390-6393.

Lands, W.E.M., Kulmacz, R.J. and Marshall, P.J., 1984. Lipid peroxide actions in the regulation of prostaglandin biosynthesis. In Pryor, W.A. (Editor), Free radicals in biology. Vol VI. Academic Press Inc. New York. pp.39-61.

Lotscher, H.R., Winterhalter, K., Carafoli, E. and Richter, C., 1980. Hydroperoxide induced loss of pyridine nucleotides and release of calcium from rat liver mitochondria. J.Biol.Chem., 255: 9325-9330.

Lebedev, A.V., Levitsky, D.O. and Loginov, V.A., 1983. Oxygen as an inductor of divalent cation permeability through biological and model lipid membranes. In Chazov, E.and Smirnov, V.(Eds) Advances in myocardiology, Vol III, Plenum Med.Book Co.New York. pp. 425-438.

Lefer, A.M., 1985. Eicosanoids as mediators of ischemia and shock. Feder. Proc., 44: 275-280.

Marnett, L.J., Wlodawer, P. and Samuelsson, B., 1974. Light emission during the reaction of prostaglandin synthetase Biochem. Biophys. Res. Commun., 60: 1286-1294.

Meerson, F.Z., Kagan, V.E., Kozlov, Yu.P., Belinka, L.M. and Arkhipenko, Yu.V., 1982. The role of lipid peroxidation in pathogenesis of ischemic damage and the antioxidant protection of the heart. Basic Res.Cardiol., 77: 465-485.

Morse, D.E., Duncan, H., Hooker, N. and Morse, A., 1977. Hydrogen peroxide induces spawning in molluscs, with activation of prostaglandin endoperoxide synthetase. Science, 196: 298-300.

Nakano, M. and Sugioka, K.,1978. Excitation of indole-3-acetic acid (an auxin) in a linoleate-lipoxigenase system. Biochem. Biophys.Acta, 529: 387-397.

Noronha-Dutra, A.A. and Steen, E.M., 1982. Lipid peroxidation as a mechanism of injury in cardiac myocytes. Lab. Invest., 47: 346-353.

Player, T.J. and Hultin, H.O., 1978. The effect of lipid peroxidation on the calcium-accumulating ability of the microsomal fraction isolated from chicken breast muscle. Biochem.J., 174: 17-22.

Rao, P.S., Cohen, M.V. and Mueller, H.S., 1983. Production of free radicals and lipid peroxides in early experimental myocardial ischemia. J. Mol. Cell. Cardiol., 15: 713-716.

Reimer, K.A., Hill, L.M., and Jennings, R.B., 1981. Prolonged depletion of ATP and of adenin nucleotide pool due to the delayed resynthesis of adenin nucleotides following reversible myocardial ischemic injury in dogs. J.Mol.Cell.Cardiol., 13:229-239.

Shlafer, M., Kane, P.F., Wiggins, V.Y. and Kirsh, M.M., 1982. Possible role for cytotoxic oxygen metabolites in the pathogenesis of cardiac ischemic injury. Circulation, 66 (suppl.I): I-85-92.

Russel, G.A., 1957. Deuterium-isotope effects in the autoxidation of aralkyl hydrocarbons. Mechanism of the interaction of peroxy radicals. J. Am. Chem. Soc., 79: 3871-3877.

Schulte-Herbruggen, T. and Cadenas, E., 1985. Electronically excited states generation during the lipoxygenase-catalyzed aerobic oxidation of arachidonate. Photobiochem. Photobiophys., 10: 35-51.

Thomas, C.E., Morehouse, L.A. and Aust, S.D., 1985. Ferritin and superoxide dependent lipid peroxidation. J. Biol. Chem., 260: 3275-3280.

Thor, H., Smith, M.T., Hartzell, P., Bellomo, G., Jewell, S.A. and Orrenius, S.,1982. The metabolism of menadione (2-methyl-1, 4-naphthoquinone) by isolated hepatocytes. J.Biol.Chem., 257: 12419-12425.

Woodward, B. and Zakaria, M.N.M., (1985). Effect of some free radical scavengers on reperfusion induced arrhythmias in the isolated rat heart. J. Mol. Cell. Cardiol., 17,485-493.

THE REACTION BETWEEN OXYMYOGLOBIN AND HYDROPEROXIDES
Formation of electronically excited states detected by low-level chemiluminescence

Diego Mira*, Ulf Brunk, Fulvio Ursini**, and Enrique Cadenas

Department of Pathology II, University Hospital,
University of Linköping, Linköping, Sweden
and
**Institute of Biological Chemistry, University of Padova
Padova, Italy

ABSTRACT

The O-O spliting of t-butyl hydroperoxide by oxymyoglobin is associated with hemoprotein destruction, and organic hydroperoxide- and oxygen consumption. In addition, electronically excited states -detected by low-level chemiluminescence- are formed in a side reaction. The excited states probably originate from the interaction of free radical products generated during the decomposition of t-butyl hydroperoxide by oxymyoglobin. This is indicated by the effect of the free radical scavenger, (+)-cyanidanol-3, which inhibits chemiluminescence, prevents hemoprotein destruction, and enhances t-butyl hydroperoxide and oxygen utilization.

The oxidative character of the reaction between organic hydroperoxide and oxymyoglobin is pointed out by its capacity to peroxidize polyunsaturated fatty acids. This process gives rise to a new chemiluminescence pathway -mainly that involving the mechanism(s) of lipid peroxidation- as shown by a shift toward shorter wavelengths in the spectral distribution of emission.

The excited states generated during the interaction between oxymyoglobin and organic hydroperoxide might contribute to the spectrum of oxidants mediating ischemia/reperfusion cardiac injury as well as in oxidative damage to red cells.

*On leave from Institute of Biological and Physical Chemistry, School of Pharmacy and Biochemistry, University of Buenos Aires.

INTRODUCTION

Hemoproteins are involved in many and important reactions of dioxygen and its reduction products. The spliting of the O-O bond of hydroperoxides catalyzed by various hemoproteins can be understood in terms of a metal- catalyzed Fenton reaction, a homolytic scission of the hydroperoxide, or a compound I intermediate similar to that of peroxidase or catalase. These three mechanisms predict peroxy radical formation, which, for the case of hematin/peroxide system has been identified by esr with spin trapping technique (Kalyanaraman, 1982). Other oxidizing species, such as alkoxy radicals and hematin-bound hydroxyl radical have been hypothesized to occur during this reaction. The interaction of these radical products has been implicated in the generation of electronically excited states detected by low-level photoemission (Cadenas et al., 1980a; Cadenas & Sies, 1982). Although the exact nature of the excited states was not assessed, they might contribute to the spectrum of strong oxidants generated upon the O-O spliting of hydroperoxides by hemoproteins. The interaction of hemoproteins with organic hydroperoxides usually is associated with changes in structure and function of the protein, probably involving the methene bridges of the porphyrin system and the aromatic amino acids, these leading to cross-linking and protein inactivation (Hemler & Lands, 1980; Rice et al., 1983).

The decomposition of organic hydroperoxides by hemoproteins is known to initiate peroxidation of polyunsaturated fatty acids (Tappel, 1955; Kashnitz & Hatefi, 1975; Kanner & Harel, 1985). The latter process seems to be triggered by the free radical products formed or by an active hemoprotein intermediate with a reactivity similar to hydroxyl free radical (Grisham, 1985).

The oxidative character of the hydroperoxide/hemoprotein interaction has been suggested to play a role in the free radical-mediated ischemia/ reperfusion cardiac injury (Grisham, 1985) as well as in red blood cell free radical damage.

We report here on the generation of electronically excited states associated with low-level chemiluminescence and as a consequence of the free radical interactions resulting from the spliting of the O-O bond of t-butyl hydroperoxide by oxymyoglobin. A cycling process is suggested in which the enzyme is partially destroyed due to the formation of free radicals upon hydroperoxide breakdown. The time course of photoemission is similar to that described during the organic peroxide-infused rat heart (Barsachi et al., 1983), thus suggesting that in the latter system a primary component to the photoemission might involve the direct interaction of myoglobin with the organic hydroperoxide. Moreover, further sources of electronically excited states are provided by the interaction of free radical products with polyunsaturated fatty acids leading to lipid peroxidation.

MATERIALS AND METHODS

Chemicals and biochemicals. t-Butyl hydroperoxide, (+)-cyanidanol-3, arachidonate, linoleate, linolenate, and myoglobin were from Sigma Chemical Co. (St. Louis, MO, USA). NADPH, glutathione reductase, glutathione peroxidase, and GSH were from Boehringer (Mannheim, FRG). Oxymyoglobin was prepared from horse heart myoglobin by titration with sodium dithionite in stoichiometric amounts; the formation of reduced myoglobin was monitored by the spectral changes at 416, 540, and 580 nm (Rothgeb & Gurb, 1978).

Spectrophotometric assays. t-Butyl hydroperoxide was measured according to the method of Heath & Tappel (1976) in which the remaining hydroperoxide is reduced by the glutathione peroxidase system, following NADPH oxidation at 340 nm (ϵ = 6.2 $mM^{-1}cm^{-1}$). Malondialdehyde formation was measured by the thiobarbituric acid-reactive material assay at 535 nm (ϵ = 156 $mM^{-1}cm^{-1}$). Spectral changes of oxy- and metmyoglobin were followed at the Soret band absorption region (ϵ_{406} = 123 $mM^{-1}cm^{-1}$ and ϵ_{414} = 130 $mM^{-1}cm^{-1}$, respectively) (Rothgeb & Gurb, 1978).

Oxygen uptake. O_2 consumption was followed with a miniature Clark- type electrode (Instech Lab., Philadelphia, PA, USA).

Low-level chemiluminescence. Photoemission was measured with a red-sensitive photomultiplier (type 9658AM, EMI Gencom, New York, NY, USA) as described previously (Cadenas & Sies, 1984). The photomultiplier efficiency was 2 x 10^{-3} photons/count, calculated after the luminol reaction.

Assay conditions. The standard reaction mixture consisted of 40 μM oxymyoglobin and 1 mM t-butyl hydroperoxide in 0.1 M potassium phosphate buffer, pH 7.4. Assays were carried out at 37°C.

RESULTS

The reaction between myoglobin and t-butyl hydroperoxide involves (a) main reaction pathways implying absorption spectra changes of the hemoprotein, t-butyl hydroperoxide- and O_2 consumption, and (b) side reaction pathways related to the generation of electronically excited states detected by low-level photoemission. The link between the main and side reaction pathways seems to be established by the formation of free radical products during the former reaction pathway; these free radical products would maintain the formation of photoemissive species. The oxidative potential of this reaction, resting on an intermediate formed during either the main or/and the side pathway, is indicated by the peroxidation of lipid targets, i.e., linoleic, linolenic, and arachidonic acid. This process is accompanied by an enhancement of photoemission intensity as well as changes in the spectral distribution of luminescence.

Main reaction pathways

The supplementation of oxymyoglobin with t-butyl hydroperoxide is accompanied by a decrease in the main absorption bands of the hemoprotein, this probably indicating heme destruction. Fig. 1 shows the continuous decrease of the Soret absorption band (414 nm) of oxymyoglobin following its supplementation with t-butyl hydroperoxide. Metmyoglobin

(Fe^{3+}) showed similar changes, which were preceded by a rapid shift of its Soret absorption band at 406 nm toward that of oxymyoglobin at 414 nm.

The consumption of t-butyl hydroperoxide and O_2 during the reaction of myoglobin with organic hydroperoxide show a biphasic time course pattern (Fig. 1): the first phase proceeds rapidly (68.4 and 72 μM . min^{-1}, respectively), reaching completion in about 1-2 min and accounting for the bulk of hydroperoxide and O_2 consumed during the reaction (over 60%), whereas the reactions contributing to the second phase proceed at about 10-fold slower rates (7.8 and 4.1 μM . min^{-1}, respectively). The close to the unit (0.95) ratio of the rate of t-butyl hydroperoxide consumption over the rate of O_2 consumption during the first phase might indicate a common -possibly myoglobin-mediated- pathway. The total amount of t-butyl hydroperoxide and O_2 consumed during the reaction (taken at 15 min) is 190 and 181 μM, respectively.

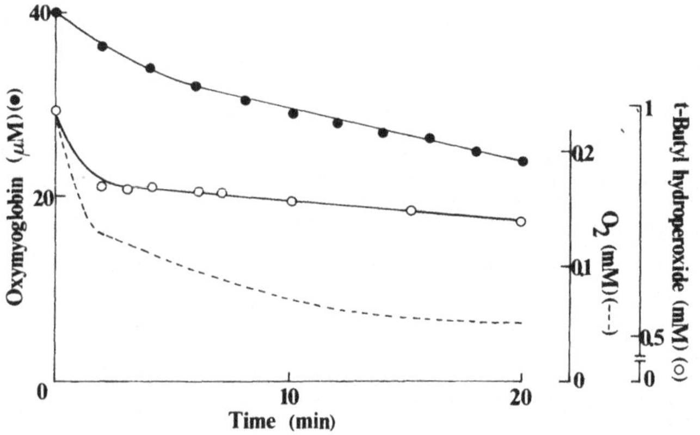

Fig.1. Time course of oxymyoglobin destruction and t-butyl hydroperoxide and oxygen consumption.Experimental conditions: 40 μM oxymyoglobin in 0.1 M potassium phosphate buffer, pH 7.4, was supplemented with 1 mM t-butyl hydroperoxide to start the reaction.

Side reaction pathways

The decomposition of t-butyl hydroperoxide by oxymyoglobin is accompanied by the generation of electronically excited states, similarly to what was described for H_2O_2- or t-butyl hydroperoxide-supplemented cytochrome c (Cadenas et al., 1980a,b) and cytochrome P_{450} (Cadenas & Sies, 1982). Fig. 2A shows the biphasic time course of photoemission arising from the decomposition of t-butyl hydroperoxide by oxymyoglobin. The first phase reaches its maximal intensity at 40s, whereas the second phase intensity augments slowly, reaching its maximum at about 15 min. The second phase is linearly dependent on oxymyoglobin and t-butyl hydroperoxide concentration, whereas the first phase shows two slopes (Fig. 2B,C). The relative chemiluminescence efficiencies of the first and second phase are 5×10^4 and 1×10^6 photons x s^{-1} . µM oxymyoglobin^{-1}, respectively. 77% of the emission is observed in the red region of the spectrum, beyond 610 nm (table I)

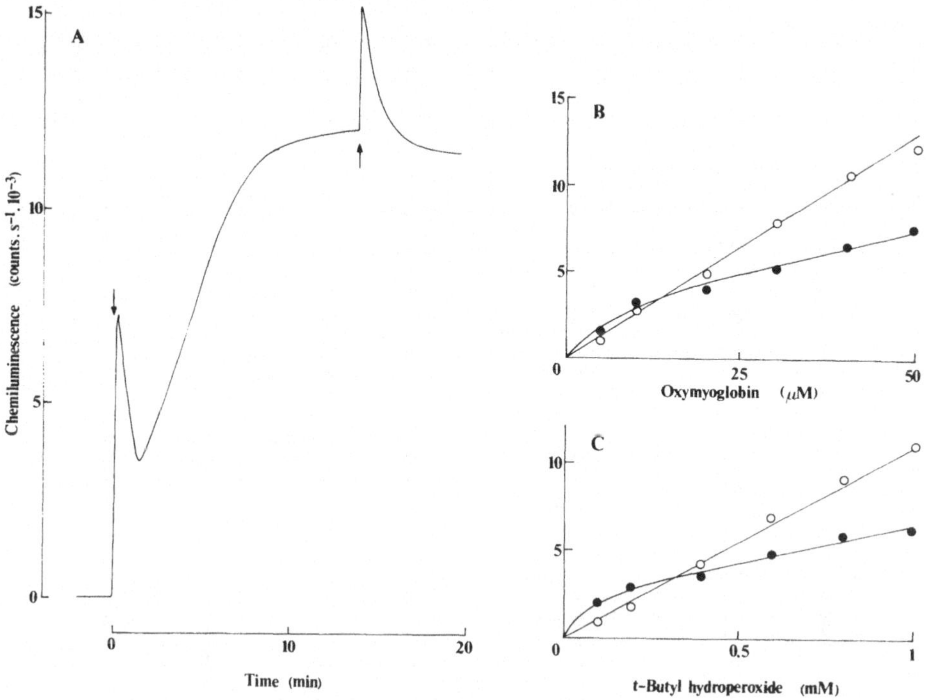

Fig. 2. Low level chemiluminescence from t-butyl hydroperoxide- supplemented oxymyoglobin. (A) Time course of photoemission. Assay conditions: 40 µM oxymyoglobin in 0.1 M potassium phosphate buffer, pH 7.4, was supplemented with 1 mM t-butyl hydroperoxide to start the reaction (downward arrow); upward arrow indicates a second addition of 20 µM oxymyoglobin to the ongoing photoemissive reaction. (B) and (C), dependence of first (●) and second (○) phase of chemiluminescence on oxymyoglobin and t-butyl hydroperoxide concentration, respectively.

The time course of O_2 uptake indicates that most of the O_2 is consumed during the development of the first phase, whereas the generation of excited states during the second phase is accompanied by a small consumption of O_2 (3×10^{-14} and 1×10^{-12} photons x s^{-1} x O_2 molecule consumed^{-1}, for phase I and II, respectively). Only about 20% of the t-butyl hydroperoxide is consumed during its reaction with oxymyoglobin (Fig. 1). Residual t-butyl hydroperoxide can react with subsequent additions of oxymyoglobin, triggering *de novo* a fast O_2 consumption and a first phase-like burst of photoemission (Fig. 2). This suggests that (a) the first component of O_2 consumption and the first phase of photoemission are mainly related to a hemoprotein-mediated activity; (b) that, though O_2 and t-butyl hydroperoxide are still available, the hemoprotein was rapidly inactivated at the onset of the reaction, and (c) the second phase of emission along with the slow-rate component of O_2 consumption seem to be principally related to a less-specific, probably of a free radical nature, pathway.

This last assumption is supported by the effect of (+)-cyanidanol-3 on myoglobin spectral changes, O_2 and t-butyl hydroperoxide consumption, as well as photoemission (Fig. 3).

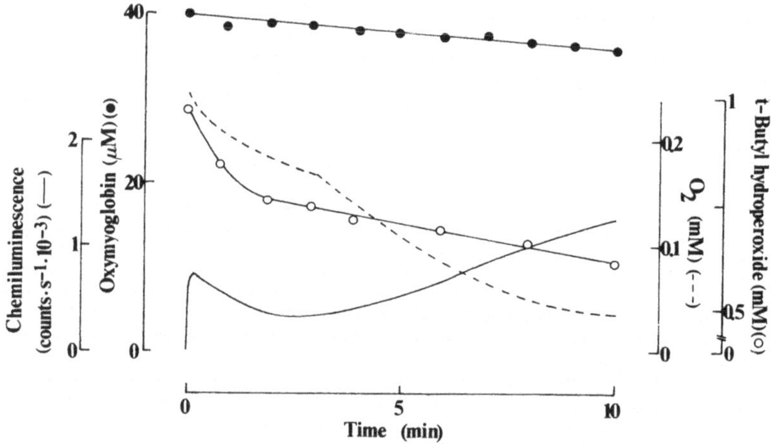

Fig. 3. Effect of (+)-cyanidanol-3 on the myoglobin-catalyzed decomposition of t-butyl hydroperoxide reaction. Assay conditions as in Fig.1 in the presence of 0.1 mM (+)-cyanidanol-3.

The higher O_2 and organic hydroperoxide consumption in the presence of the free radical quencher can be accounted for by a prevention of oxymyoglobin destruction, probably due to the formation of free radical products. In this regard, the decrease in absorption at 414 nm of myoglobin was averted in the presence of (+)- cyanidanol-3. These effects result also in a quenching of emission and further suggests the intermediacy of free radicals leading to the formation of electronically excited states.

Peroxidation of polyunsaturated fatty acids during t-butyl hydroperoxide decomposition by myoglobin

Addition of arachidonate to a mixture of oxymyoglobin and t-butyl hydroperoxide is associated with (a) increase of the rate of O_2 consumption and of total O_2 consumed; (b) accumulation of malondialdehyde, and (c) increase of chemiluminescence intensity at expense of the second phase. These observations are summarized in Fig. 4.

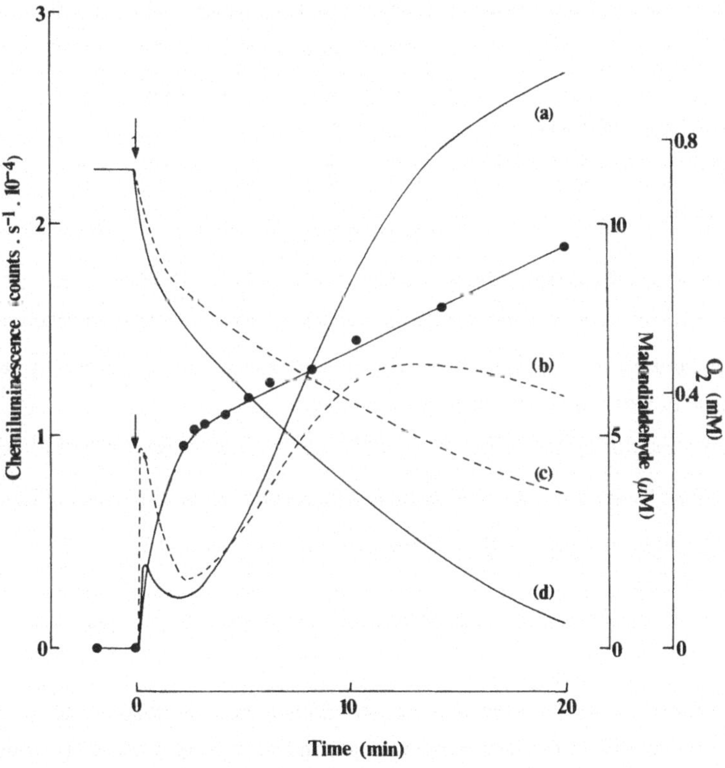

Fig. 4. Peroxidation of arachidonate by the oxymyoglobin / t-butyl hydroperoxide system. Enhancement of photoemission. Assay conditions as in Fig. 1. (●), malondialdehide; (a) and (b) photoemission in the presence and abscence of 1mM arachidonate; (c) and (d) O_2 uptake in the abscence and presence of 1 mM arachidonate.

The effects of polyunsaturated fatty acids on the first and second phase of photoemission are different. The intensity of the first phase, on the one hand, is decreased by the different polyunsaturated fatty acids, probably involving their chemical reaction with the excited state, without altering the process leading to its generation. The intensity of the second phase, on the other hand, is enhanced as a result of the presence of the polyunsaturated fatty acid, the extent of increase being proportionally related to the degree of unsaturation of the fatty acid: 20:4 >18:3>18:2 (not shown). A similar effect has been described for the soybean lipoxygenase-catalyzed oxidation of fatty acids (Schulte-Herbrüggen & Cadenas, 1985). The increase of intensity of the second phase of emission implies the contribution to photoemission of a different excited state, as indicated by spectral changes: whereas 77% of chemiluminescence was observed beyond 610 nm in the absence of arachidonate, only 24% was observed beyond this wavelength in the presence of the fatty acid (table I).

Table I. Effect of arachidonate on low-level chemiluminescence from t-butyl hydroperoxide supplemented oxymyoglobin. t-BuOOH, t-butyl hydroperoxide; 20:4, arachidonic acid.

	Chemiluminescence (%)	
	>350 nm	>610 nm
Oxymyoglobin + t-BuOOH	23	77
Oxymyoglobin + t-BuOOH + 20:4	76	24

DISCUSSION

The results described above indicate that the reaction between t-butyl hydroperoxide and oxymyoglobin involve hemoprotein destruction, organic hydroperoxide and O_2 consumption, and formation of electronically excited states, the latter probably supported by the occurrence of free radical intermediates in the system.

O_2 consumption during the myoglobin-catalyzed decomposition of t-butyl hydroperoxide can be explained by the formation of oxymyoglobin (Fe^{2+}), the O_2 bonding indicated as an iron (II) oxygenil or as an iron (III) superoxide complex (reaction 1).

$$Fe^{2+} + O_2 \longrightarrow [Fe^{2+}O_2 \longleftrightarrow Fe^{3+}O_2^{\cdot -}] \qquad [1]$$

This "active form" of the hemoprotein can catalyze the decomposition of hydroperoxide, yielding t-butyl peroxy and hydroperoxy radicals and myoglobin-iron (II) (reaction 2).

$$Fe^{3+}O_2^{\cdot -} + H_3C-\overset{CH_3}{\underset{CH_3}{C}}-OOH \longrightarrow Fe^{2+} + HO_2^{\cdot} + H_3C-\overset{CH_3}{\underset{CH_3}{C}}-OO^{\cdot} \qquad [2]$$

Convincing evidence that superoxide or perhydroxy radical are actually produced by reaction 2 is difficult to find. In our hands, the superoxide dismutase-sensitive reduction of cytochrome c, as well as the oxidation of epinephrine failed to provide clear evidence for the occurrence of $O_2^{\cdot -}$. The former method was handicaped by the destruction of cytochrome c by the organic hydroperoxide (Cadenas et al., 1980a,b), whereas the latter, epinephrine, was found to interfere with the photoemissive reaction.

Myoglobin-Fe^{2+}, generated in reaction 2, could participate in further reaction involving (a) its binding to O_2, as shown in reaction 1, thereby supporting O_2 consumption within a process of cycling characteristics, and/or (b) the decomposition of t-butyl hydroperoxide within the frame of a classical Haber-Weiss reaction (reactions 3a,3b).

$$Fe^{2+} + H_3C-\overset{CH_3}{\underset{CH_3}{C}}-OOH \longrightarrow Fe^{3+} + HO^- + H_3C-\overset{CH_3}{\underset{CH_3}{C}}-O^{\cdot} \qquad [3a]$$

$$Fe^{3+} + H_3C-\overset{CH_3}{\underset{CH_3}{C}}-OOH \longrightarrow Fe^{2+} + H^+ + H_3C-\overset{CH_3}{\underset{CH_3}{C}}-OO^{\cdot} \qquad [3b]$$

The occurrence of tertiary peroxy radicals in hemoprotein/organic hydroperoxide systems was identify by esr with spin trapping technique (Kalyanaraman, 1982). The termination reaction of tertiary peroxy radicals proceeds with O_2 evolution and formation of alkoxy radicals (reaction 4).

$$2\,H_3C-\overset{CH_3}{\underset{CH_3}{C}}-OO^{\cdot} \longrightarrow 2\,H_3C-\overset{CH_3}{\underset{CH_3}{C}}-O^{\cdot} + O_2 \qquad [4]$$

In addition to that of reaction 1, O_2 consumption could be supported by free radical interactions. The ß-scission of alkoxy radicals (reaction 5) (generated by either reactions 3a or 4) would yield a carbon-centered radical and acetone (Pryor, 1976). The former radical is quenched by molecular O_2 with near difussion-controlled rates (reaction 6).

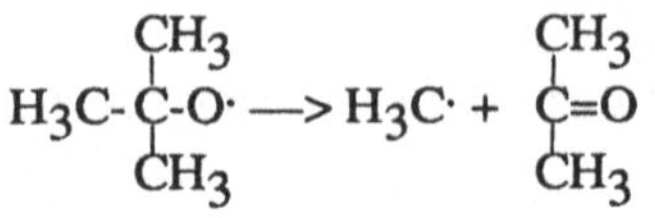

[5]

$$H_3C\cdot + O_2 \longrightarrow H_3COO\cdot \qquad [6]$$

In summary, the myoglobin-catalyzed decomposition of t-butyl hydroperoxide is accompanied by the formation of free radicals, such as tertiary peroxy and alkoxy radicals and probably carbon-centered radicals as well. The consequence of the formation of free radical intermediates might be expressed as a rapid inactivation of the hemoprotein as well as the formation of electronically excited states. The latter process might imply the termination reaction of t-butyl peroxy and t-butyl alkoxy radicals, with energy enough to yield an excited state product (Pryor, 1978) (reaction 7).

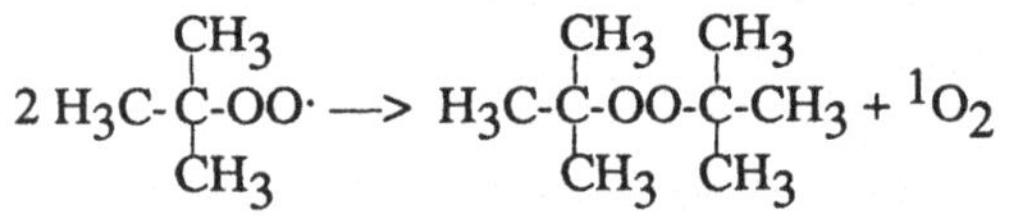

[7]

The weak intensity of photoemission does not allow a spectral analysis with high resolution; therefore, to ascribe the chemiluminescence observed to the relaxation of a sole excited state to the ground state is, at the present stage, merely speculative. We cannot exclude the possibility that reaction 5 could generate an excited acetone product, as expected from the free energy of the reaction. Excited acetone could contribute, upon relaxation, with emission in the blue region of the spectrum.

The molecular mechanism for the generation of excited states during the peroxidation of arachidonate by t-butyl hydroperoxide/oxymyoglobin system is obviously a distinct one to that of hydroperoxide/oxymyoglobin alone.

Two aspects should be considered in evaluating the formation of electronically excited states during the peroxidation of arachidonate by oxymyoglobin/organic hydroperoxide reactions. Firstly, the molecular mechanism leading to arachidonate peroxidation, process indicated by the increased O_2 uptake and malondialdehyde accumulation (Fig. 4). Secondly, the generation of excited states during the peroxidation process.

The former aspect would imply several reactive species as the initiators of arachidonate peroxidation. Initial H abstraction could be easily promoted by any of the reactive free radical intermediates formed in reactions 2-5, alkoxy radicals being by far more reactive than peroxy radicals (Pryor, 1978).

The latter aspect would imply any of the molecular mechanisms for lipid peroxidation-supported photoemission (Cadenas, 1984). The generation of triplet carbonyl compounds (with emission at 360-450 nm) during the termination reactions of fatty acid peroxy (LOO·) (Kellog, 1969) and alkoxy (LO·) (Hamberg, 1983) radicals (reactions 8,9) might account for the large shift of emission towards shorter wavelengths when arachidonate is peroxidized by myoglobin/organic hydroperoxide mixtures.

$$LOO\cdot + LOO\cdot \longrightarrow LOH + O_2 + LO^* \qquad [8]$$

$$LO\cdot + LO\cdot \longrightarrow LOH + LO^* \qquad [9]$$

The low-level chemiluminescence technique permits to assess noninvasively cellular oxidative conditions as indicated by studies with perfused-liver (Boveris et al., 1980), lung (Cadenas et al., 1980c) and heart (Barsachi et al., 1983). The biological relevance of electronically excited state formation during the O-O spliting of hydroperoxides by hemoproteins as well as during the peroxidation of fatty acids would rely on the reactivity of such excited states toward cellular constituents. Thus, electronically excited states might contribute to the oxidative damage of red cells as well as the free radical-mediated ischemia/ reperfusion injury of cardiac tissue (McCord, 1985).

Acknowledgements. Supported by grants 7697 and 4481 from the Swedish Medical Research Council.

REFERENCES

Barsacchi, R., Camici, P., Bottigli, U., Salvadori, P.A., Pelosi, G., Maiorino, M., and Ursini, F. (1983) *Biochim. Biophys. Acta* **762**, 241-247.
Boveris, A., Cadenas, E., Reiter, R., Filipkowski, M., Nakase, Y. and Chance, B. (1980) *Proc. Natl. Acad. Sci. USA* **77**, 347-351.
Cadenas, E. (1984) *Photochem. Photobiol.* **40**, 823-830.
Cadenas, E., Boveris, A. and Chance, B. (1980a) *Biochem. J.* **187**, 131-140.
Cadenas, E., Boveris, A. and Chance, B. (1980b) *FEBS Lett.* **112**, 285-288.
Cadenas, E., Arad, I.D., Boveris, A., Fisher, A.B. and Chance, B. (1980c) *FEBS Lett.* **111**, 413-418.
Cadenas, E. and Sies, H. (1982) *Eur. J. Biochem.* **124**, 349-356.
Cadenas, E. and Sies, H. (1984) *Methods Enzymol.* **105**, 221-231.
Grisham, M.B. (1985) *J. Free Radicals Biol. Med.* **1**, 227-232.
Hamberg, M. (1983) *Biochim. Biophys. Acta* **752**, 191-197.
Heath, R.L. and Tappel, A.L. (1976) *Anal. Biochem.* **76**, 184-191.
Hemler, M.E. and Lands, W.E.M. (1980) *J. Biol. Chem.* **255**, 6253-6261.
Kalyanaram, B., Mottley, K. and Mason, R.P. (1983) *J. Biol. Chem.* **258**, 3855-3858.
Kanner, J. and Harel, S. (1985) *Arch. Biochem. Biophys.* **237**, 314-321.
Kashnitz, R.M. and Hatefi, Y. (1975) *Arch. Biochem. Biophys.* **171**, 292-304.
Kellog, R.E. (1969) *J. Am. Chem. Soc.* **91**, 5433-5436.
McCord, J.M. (1985) *New England J. Med.* **312**, 159-163.
O'Brien, P.J. (1968) *Biochem. J.* **100**, 12.
Pryor, W.A. (1976) in *Free Radicals in Biology* (Pryor, W.A., ed.), vol. I, pp.1-36, Academic Press, New York.
Pryor, W.A. (1978) *Photochem. Photobiol.* **28**, 787-801.

Pryor, W.A. (1986) *Ann. Rev. Physiol.* **48**, 657-668.
Rice, R.H., Lee, Y.M. and Brown, W.D. (1983) *Arch. Biochem. Biophys.* **221**, 417-427.
Rothgeb, T.M. and Gurb, F.R. (1978) *Methods Enzymol.* **52**, 473-481.
Schulte-Herbrüggen and Cadenas, E. (1985) in *Free Radicals in Liver Injury* (Poli, G., Cheeseman, K.H., Dianzani, M.U. and Slater, T.F., eds.), pp. 91-98 , IRL Press,Oxford.
Tappel, A.L. (1955) *Arch. Biochem. Biophys.* **44**, 368-395.

THE ROLE OF IRON MOBILIZATION IN ISCHEMIC TISSUE DAMAGE

J.F. Koster, H. Stam and P. Biemond

Department of Biochemistry I, Medical Faculty, Erasmus University Rotterdam, Rotterdam, The Netherlands

Abstract

THE ROLE OF IRON MOBILIZATION IN ISCHEMIC TISSUE DAMAGE

It has been well established that the actual toxicity of free radical oxygen-species is dependent on the presence of catalytic amounts of free iron in the tissue. Accumulating evidence is present, indicating that for the myocardial tissue damage occurring during reperfusion after ischemic period, oxygen free radicals are partially responsible. It has been demonstrated that superoxide dismutase decreased the ischemic-induced tissue damage. Based on the hypothesis of McCord and coworkers, implying the conversion of heart tissue xanthine dehydrogenase (XDH) to xanthine oxidase (XO) during ischemia and subsequent superoxide (O_2^-) formation during the conversion of the ATP breakdown product(s) (hypo)xanthine to urate, we studied whether XO is able to mobilize free iron from the iron-binding protein ferritin and transferrin. It appeared that XO-mediated O_2^- formation is able to release free iron from the intracellular ferritin, but not from extracellular transferrin. Beside this O_2^--dependent iron release and O_2^--independent Fe mobilization could be demonstrated. The latter phenomenon indicates that during the anoxic/ischemic period iron is mobilized from the ferritin. During myocardial reperfusion when XHD is converted to XO and ATP breakdown happens, the previous released iron starts catalyzing the formation of the most potent oxygen free radical, $OH^\cdot$ (hydroxyl radical).

Introduction

Overwhelming evidence exist that free radicals are involved in the tissue damage occurring during reperfusion of ischemic tissue (Fridovich, 1979; Guarnieri et al., 1980; Meerson, et al., 1982). Most of these evidences are obtained indirectly from the effects of free radical scavengers and inhibitors of, for instance xanthine oxidase. In the well-known hypothesis of McCord and Roy (1982) the conversion of xanthine dehydrogenase to xanthine oxidase plays an important role. This conversion is assumed to occur during the ischemic period, in which also catabolism of ATP happens. This latter results in the formation of hypoxanthine, substrate for the xanthine dehydrogenase/oxidase. With the resupply of O_2 xanthine oxidase with hypoxanthine will give rise to the formation of O_2^- radicals. Although this hypothesis is rather attractive the well accepted relative inertness of O_2^- is overlooked. The toxicity of O_2^- is tremendously increased in the presence of transition metals, of which from physiological point of view iron is the most important. The presence of iron catalyses the formation of the highly agressive hydroxyl radical (OH˙). In the hypothesis of McCord and Roy (1982) it is not taken into account how the necessary iron becomes available. Intracellularly the most likely source will be ferritin. Practically all cells contain ferritin. Although under normal physiological conditions about 2000 Fe per mol protein are present, ferritin is able to store 4500 Fe per mol protein. Ferritin is considered to be the iron storage protein (Harrison et al., 1986) and during anemia liver ferritin decreases. The exact mechanism by which iron is stored in the ferritin and the mechanism by which iron is mobilized are both unknown.

MOBILIZATION OF IRON BY FREE RADICALS

As already stated ferritin is far most the most important iron storage protein. Although the mechanism by which the iron is mobilized unknown, it is well established that reducing equivalent are necessary. In a system of bleomycine dependent degradation of DNA and the xanthine + xanthine oxidase induced hydroxylation of salicylate the free radical damage was not increased by ferritin (Halliwel, 1978; Gutteridge et al., 1981). However, in many other test systems (Bannister et al., 1984; O'Connel et al., 1985, 1986; Gutteridge et al., 1983, Thomas et al., 1985; Carlin and Asford, 1985; Koster and Slee, 1986; Carlin and Djursater, 1984) ferritin stimulates the free radical damage, probably by the formation of hydroxyl radicals.

The necessity of one electron reduction for the mobilization of iron from ferritin and considering the fact that O_2^- is also an excellent reducing substance we studied the possibility if O_2^- might be able to release iron (Biemond et al., 1984).

IRON MOBILIZATION from HUMAN FERRITIN and TRANSFERRIN.

	Iron mobilized in 30 min (μM)	% Iron* mobilization
Human ferritin 0.25 mg/ml	3.6	100 %
+ SOD 33.3 μg/ml		46 %
Human transferrin 3 mg/ml iron saturation 60 %	< 0.1	

* compared to the complete system without additions

Table I

Table I shows that O_2^- generated by stimulated polymorphonuclear cells (PMN), are able to mobilize iron from ferritin. This mobilization is completely blocked by the addition of superoxide dismutase (SOD). Iron mobilization from transferrin, at least in this system, is negligible if it happens at all. Also O_2^- derived from the addition of solid KO_2 mobilizes iron from ferritin (Biemond et al., 1984).

For transferrin conflicting data are reported. Normally an inhibition of free radical damage is found, ascribed to the iron binding capacity of transferrin. However, an enhancement of free radical damage by transferrin is reported. It should be realized that in these systems, if the saturation is mentioned, mostly 100% saturated transferrin is used, a highly unphysiological condition (35%). After our initial report that O_2^- derived from stimulated PMN is able to mobilize iron from ferritin, the same results were shown for O_2^- derived from the xanthine + xanthine oxidase reaction (Thomas et al., 1985; Biemond et al., 1985).

In the reaction of xanthine + xanthine oxidase the iron mobilization from ferritin can be blocked partially with the addition of SOD (fig. 1).

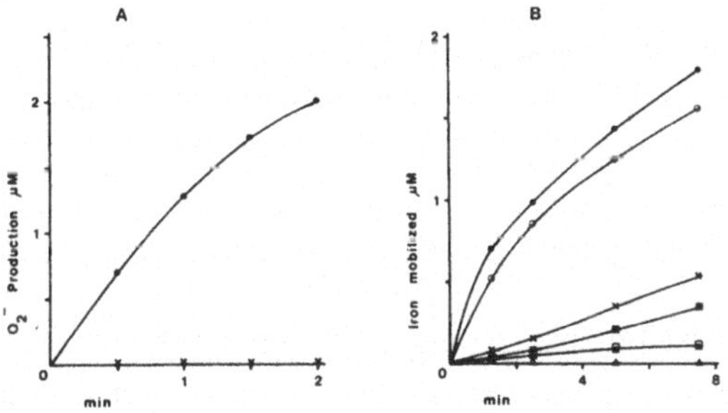

Fig. 1 The production of O_2^- (a) and iron mobilization from ferritin (b) by xanthine oxidase and xanthine ●, no addition; x, plus SOD, O, plus catalase, ■, plus SOD and catalase, ▲ without xanthine oxidase, □, without xanthine; △, without ferritin. (Biemond et al., 1986)

In the presence of SOD there is still about 30% of the total mobilizing capacity left (Biemond et al., 1986). This implicates that there is transfer of reducing equivalent from xanthine oxidase to ferritin by a unknown mechanism. Probably this reaction is the same as already observed by Mazur et al., (1955, 1958) in the fifties. These authors were unaware of O_2^-, but found an iron mobilization from ferritin by xanthine oxidase reaction under anaerobic conditions.

PHYSIOLOGICAL IMPLICATIONS OF THE O_2^- INDEPENDENT IRON MOBILIZATION FROM FERRITIN.

Ferritin is ubiquitous protein, present in alsmost any cell. Besides its storage role, it is probably also important for the cellular protection against free iron under normal physiological condition. However, under ischemic conditions tremendous amount of reducing equivalents are formed. Also under these conditions ATP will be broken down resulting in the formation of hypoxanthine, the substrate for xanthine dehydrogenase/oxidase. In the hypothesis of McCord and Roy (1982) the conversion of xanthine dehydrogenase to xanthine oxidase plays an important role. At the moment the occurrance of this conversion during ischemia is in debat (see this symposium). To our opinion this conversion is not obliged because the importance of xanthine dehydrogenase/oxidase is more important for the iron mobilization from the ferritin than actually the generation of oxygen radicals. Especially the O_2^- - independent mechanism is important, because due to this mechanism already iron can be mobilized under the ischemic conditions. This iron will be in the ferrous state and ready available to catalyse the formation of hydroxyl radicals, if the O_2 supply is restored. The O_2^- generation during reperfusion can be derived from the cyclooxygenase reaction, the impaired respiratory chain or other flavin protein.

INTERACTION BETWEEN ENDOTHELIAL CELLS AND CARDIOMYOCYTES

It is well established that after an ischemic period the actual damage occurs when the reperfusion is restored, the so-called O_2-paradox. Recently, it is claimed (Piper et al., 1985) that isolated cardiomyocytes do not exhibit the O_2-paradox phenomenon. This implicates that during the ischemic period in other cells of the heart tissue products are formed, which exert their actions on cardiomyocytes at the normal O_2·supply is restored. It is also important that xanthine oxidase is present in the endothelial cells and the cardiomyocytes are devoid of this activity. Therefore we considered the susceptibility of endothelial cells for the action of free radicals.

SUSCEPTIBILITY OF ENDOTHELIAL CELLS TOWARDS FREE RADICALS

Under normal conditions there is a balance between the formation and destruction of generated free radicals. This does not imply that all cells have the same capacity to cope with free radicals. Compared to liver, heart muscle has a much lower activity of SOD, catalase and glutathion peroxidase (Stam and Koster, 1985). Also various amounts of vitamine E are present. The variety in this protection capacity makes one cell type more susceptible than the other cell type for an increased generation of free radicals.

The following observations substantiate the possibility that coronary endothelial cells are more vulnerable to oxidative stress than the underlying cardiomyocytes:

a. Hardly any catalase activity is present in cultured endothelial cells. This is probably also valid for smooth muscle cells (Shingu et al., 1985).
b. Ferritin is present in cultural endothelial cells, in larger amount than in cardiomyocytes (Shingu et al., 1985).
c. Xanthine oxidase is virtually absent in cardiomyocytes, but together with cyclooxygenase activity, present in endothelial cells (Gerlach et al., 1985). Also the amount of ATP present in endothelial cells is higher than compared to the myocardium (Gerlach et al., 1985).
d. Endothelial cell membranes are enriched in polyunsaturated fatty acids (PUFA's) and synthesize polyene acids with 5 and 6 double bonds. These fatty acids are very prone to peroxidation.
e. Endothelial cells are exposed in vivo to higher oxygen tensions then the underlying smooth muscle cells and the deeper lying cardiomyocytes. Furthermore, oxygen is a rather lipophylic molecule and consequently a high "affinity" for biomembranes.
f. For the in vivo solution the endothelial layer is under a permanent pulsating, hydrostatic pressure, implicating that endothelial cells undergo a permanent mechanic stress.

Perfusion experiments with cumene hydroperoxide (Koster et al., 1985) clearly shows the susceptibility of the endothelial layer. With special perfusion technique which enables to collect separately the vascular bed fluid from the interstitial fluid. The interstitial fluid contains mainly metabolic products from the cardiomyocytes. During cumene hydroperoxide perfusion there is immediate rise of malondialdehyde in the vascular bed, while in the interstitial fluid malondialdehyde appears 15 min. later.

IRON MOBILIZATION, PEROXIDATION AND ISCHEMIA.

Ischemia does not imply the complete absence of O_2 supply. At a tissue pO_2 of 4 mm Hg, frequently observed during severe ischemia, free radical formation can take place (Hall, 1977). The free radical induced tissue damage is more likely to occur upon reintroduction of oxygen.

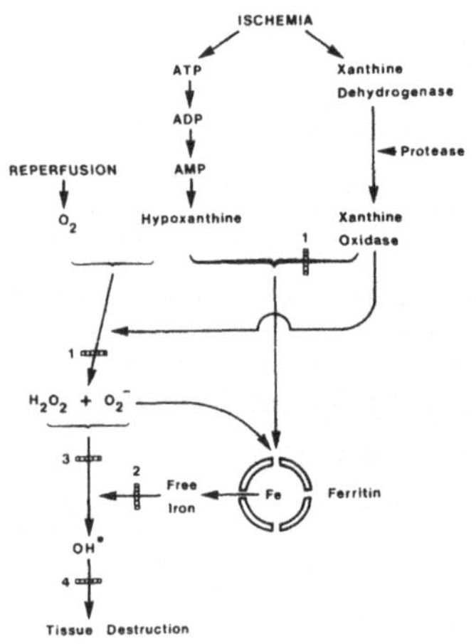

Fig. 2 Role of xanthine oxidase and iron mobilization from ferritin in tissue destruction in ischemia
1. allopurinol; 2. desferrioxamine; 3. SOD, catalase; 4. radical scavenger.

Fig. 2 shows the scheme proposed by McCord and Roy, (1982) but we have extended this scheme by putting in the role of iron. In concept of McCord and Roy, O_2^- is the culprit of the tissue damage, while in our proposal its more the mobilisation of iron together with the production of O_2^-, which create a situation to form hydroxyl radical. The iron is mobilized from ferritin already under ischemic condition by the O_2^- independent mechanism and at the time of restoration of the O_2 supply. This mobilization of iron explains the toxicity of O_2^-, which on itself is rather inert. Another difficulty with the original proposal of McCord and Roy, that it assumes that xanthine oxidase is present in the cardiomyocytes. As already mentioned this enzyme is localized in the endothelial cells. If xanthine oxidase is the main O_2^- source, the myocardial damage is done by the endothelial raised O_2^-. It is known that O_2^- itself can diffuse over rather large distances, but together with the mobilized iron, it is not likely that this occurs. The extent of reperfusion damage is dependent on the length of the ischemic period. It is possible that during this time there is diffusion of the mobilized iron. A free radical source can be fully reduced respiratory chain, which is impaired due to the ischemia. By reperfusion with oxygen O_2^- can be formed, probably on the ubiquinon site. This generated O_2^- can be converted to H_2O_2 by the mitochondrial superoxide dismutase and can leave the mitochondria. The H_2O_2 released from the mitochondria together with Fe^{++} mobilized from the ferritin can result in the formation of $OH^{\cdot}$ radicals. Furthermore a decreased cellular defence against free radicals during normal perfusion after ischemia is reported (Guarnieri et al., 1980; Julicher et al., 1984). Finally, for the in vivo situation the role of infiltration of granulocytes should not be under estimated. The stimulated granulocytes produce tremendous amount of O_2^- and Jolly et al. (1984) demonstrated that the tissue infiltration by granulocytes has its impact on the degree of reperfusion damage.

THERAPEUTIC POSSIBILITIES

In fig. 2 is indicated on which places in the scheme the cascade can be interrupted. These are inhibition of xanthine oxidase (1), desferrioxamine (2) to chelate the mobilized iron, the addition of SOD and catalase (3) and finally radical scavengers (4). All these four interventions have been applied (contribution of Hearse). The success of the therapy depends highly on the permeability characteristics of the various components. A promising possibility is desferrioxamine which is already clinically used in situation of iron-overloading.

REFERENCES

Bannister, J.V., Bannister, W.H. and Thornalley, P.J. (1984). The effect of ferritin iron loading on hydroxyl radical production. Live Chem. Rep. S2: 64-72.

Biemond, P., van Eijk, H.G., Swaak, A.J.G. and Koster, J.F. (1984). Iron mobilization from ferritin by superoxide derived from stimulated polymorphonuclear leucocytes. Possible mechanism in inflammation disease. J. Clin. Invest. 73: 1576-1579.

Biemond, P., Swaak, A.J.G., Beindorff, C.M. and Koster, J.F. (1986). Superoxide-dependent and independent mechanism of iron mobilization from ferritin by xanthine oxidase. Biochem. J. 239: 169-173
Carlin, J. and Djursater, R. (1984). Xanthine oxidase induced depolymerization of Hyalunoric acid in the presence of ferritin. FEBS Letters, 177: 27-30.
Carlin, G and Asford, K.E. (1985). Peroxidation of liposomes promoted by human polymorphonuclear cells leucocytes. J. Free Rad. Biol. Med. 1: 437-442.
Fridovich, I. (1979). Hypoxia and oxygen toxicity. Adv. Neurology 26: 255-259.
Gerlach, E., Nees, S. and Becker, B.F. (1985). The vascular endothelium: a servey of some newly evolving biochemical and physiological features. Basic Res. Cardiol. 80: 459-474.
Guarnieri, C., Flamigni, F. and Caldarara, C.M. (1980). Role of oxygen in the cellular damage induced by re-oxygenation of hypoxic heart. J. Mol. Cell. Cardiol., 12: 797-808.
Gutteridge, J.M.C., Rowley, D.A. and Halliwell, B. (1981). Superoxide-dependent formation of hydroxyl radicals in the presence of iron salts. Detection of "free" iron in biological systems by using bleomycine dependent degradation of DNA. Biochem. J. 199: 263-265.
Gutteridge, J.M.C., Halliwell, B., Treffry, A., Harrison, P.M. and Blake, D. (1983). Effect of ferritin-containing fractions with different iron loading on lipid peroxidation. Biochem. J. 209: 557-560.
Hall, E.T. (1977). The oxygen effect, in E.T. Hall (editor). pp. 48.
Halliwell, B. (1979). Superoxide-dependent formation of hydroxyl radicals in the presence of iron chelates. FEBS Letters, 92: 321-326.
Harrison, P.M. (1979). Ferritin: an iron storage protein. Semin. Hematol., 14: 55-70.
Jolly, S.R., Kane, W.J., Baillie, M.B., Abrams, G.D. and Lucchesi, B.R. (1984). Canine myocardial reperfusion injury. Its reduction by the combined administration of superoxide dismutase and catalase. Circ. Res. 54: 277-285.
Julicher, R.H.M., Tuburg, L.B.M., Sterrenberg, L., Bast, A., Koomen, J.M. and Noordhoek, J. (1984). Decreased defence against free radicals in rat heart during normal perfusion after hypoxic, ischemic and calcium-free perfusion. Life Sci. 35: 1281-1288.
Koster, J.F. and Slee, R.G. (1986). Ferritin, a physiological iron donor for microsomal lipid peroxidation. FEBS Letters, 199: 85-89.
Koster, J.F., Slee, R.G. and Stam, H. (1985). Studies on cumene hydroperoxide-induced lipid peroxidation in the isolated heart. J. Moll. Cell. Card. 17: 701-708.
Mazur, A., Baez, S., and Shorr, E., (1955). The mechanism of iron release from ferritin as related to its biological properties. J. Biol. Chem. 213: 147-160.
Mazur, A., Green, S., Saha, A. and Carleton, A. (1958). Mechanism of release of ferritin iron in vivo by xanthine oxidase. J. Clin. Invest. 37: 1809-1817.
McCord, J.M. and Roy, R.S. (1982). Pathophysiology of superoxide: Roles in inflammation and ischemia. Can. J. Physiol. 60: 1346-1352.
Meerson, F.Z., Kagan, V.E., Kozlov, Y.P., Belkina, L.M. and Arkhipanko, V. (1982). The role of lipid peroxidation in pathogenesis of ischemic damage and the antioxidant protection of the heart.

O'Connell, M.J., Ward, R.J., Baum, H. and Peters, T.J. (1985). The role of iron in ferritin and haemosiderin mediated lipid peroxidation of liposomes. Biochem. J., 229: 135-139.

O'Connell, M.J., Halliwell, B., Moorhouse, C.P., Aruoma, O.I., Baum, H. and Peters, T.J. (1986). Formation of hydroxyl radicals in the presence of ferritin and haemosiderin. Is haemosiderin formation a biological protective mechanism? Biochem. J., 234: 727-731.

Piper, H.M., Spahr, R., Hütter, J.F. and Spieckermann, P.G. (1985). The calcium and the oxygen paradox: non existent on the cellar level. Basic Res. Cardiol. 80; Suppl 2: 159-163.

Shingu, M., Yoshioka, M., Nobunoga, M and Yoshida, K. (1985). Human vascular smooth muscle cells and endothelial cells lack catalase activity and are susceptible to hydrogen peroxide. Inflammation, 9: 309-320.

Stam, H. and Koster, J.F. (1985). Fatty acid peroxidation is ischemia. In: Schrör (editor), Prostaglandines and other Eicosanoïds in the cardiovascular system, pp 131-148.

Thomas, C.E., Morehouse, L.A. and Aust, S.D. (1985). Ferritin and superoxide-dependent lipid peroxidation. J. Biol. Chem. 260: 3275-3280.

ROLE OF LIPID PEROXIDATION IN INCREASING CALCIUM PERMEABILITY OF MODEL AND NATURAL MEMBRANES.

D.O.Levitsky, A.V.Lebedev, A.V.Kuzmin and V.M.Brovkovich

USSR Cardiology Research Center of the Academy of Medical Sciences, 3rd Cherepkovskaya street, 15A, Moscow 121552 (USSR).

ABSTRACT

Artificial membranes formed from lipids containing products of peroxidation possess high calcium permeability. Ca^{2+} flux across the membrane was decreased in the presence of various antioxidants in the measuring cell. Initiation of lipid peroxidation of membranes of skeletal muscle sarcoplasmic reticulum was accompanied by a decrease in Ca^{2+} accumulation by the vesicles. The damage of the uptake system was prevented in the presence of antioxidants, their relative efficiency correlating with the ability to inhibit Fe^{2+}/ascorbate induced oxygen consumption by a lipid suspension. The decrease in the Ca^{2+}-pump activity of sarcoplasmic reticulum isolated from ischemic rat hearts was partially prevented by an antioxidant quercetin. It is shown that under oxygen atmosphere typical Ca^{2+} channels are formed in the artificial membranes. The data obtained indicate that one of the consequences of lipid peroxidation during myocardial ischemia could be an increase in Ca^{2+} permeability of heart membranes which is due to generation of substances possessing Ca^{2+}-ionophoric properties.

INTRODUCTION

Lipid peroxidation provokes the damage of cellular membranes (Kako, 1985, 1987). It has been demonstrated that during myocardial ischemia, and especially after reoxygenation of the heart, the concentration of lipid peroxides in the tissue increases (Gauduel and Duvelleroy, 1984, Guarnieri et al., 1980, Meerson et al., 1982, Rao et al., 1983, Shlafer et al., 1982). Reperfusion of ischemic myocardium results in marked damage of cell membranes (Gauduel and Duvelleroy, 1984) and influx of Ca^{2+} into the cells (Alto and Dhalla, 1979). Perfusion of the heart by a Ca^{2+}-free medium followed by the restoration of normal Ca^{2+} concentration in the perfusate also results in severe morphological and functional changes of cardiomyocytes and entry of Ca^{2+} into the cells (Ganote and Nayler, 1984, Zimmerman and Hulsmann, 1966, Zimmerman et al., 1967). This phenomenon, known as the calcium paradox (Zimmerman and Hulsmann, 1966), is also suggested to be a result of accumulation of free radicals in the myocardial tissue (Hess and Manson, 1984). The mechanisms of calcium and oxygen paradoxes are not yet clear. Nevertheless, these phenomena, representing "two facets of the same problem" (Hearse et al., 1978), are evidently related to a decrease of antioxidant capacity of the heart and an increase in concentration of oxygen radicals (Hess and Manson, 1984, Julicher et al., 1984a,b, Ursini et al., 1985).

In our previous studies we have shown that bilayer lipid membranes (BLM) formed from oxidized lipid possess increased cation permeability (Lebedev et al., 1982a,b). This fact by itself does not yet indicate that production of free radicals and lipid peroxides in living tissues causes an increase of cation passive transfer across lipid phase of cell membranes. The purpose of this study was to compare effects of prooxidant and antioxidant systems on transmembrane Ca^{2+} movements, using both a very simple model (BLM) and fragments derived from a major intracellular Ca^{2+}-pump system of muscle, sarcoplasmic reticulum. It is demonstrated that the effects of prooxidants and antioxidants on Ca^{2+} permeability of model and natural membranes are qualitatively similar.

MATERIALS AND METHODS

Bilayer lipid membranes were formed by the method described by Mueller et al. (1964) in a Teflon cell containing two symmetrical 2 ml compartments. Incubation medium contained either 0.04 mM EDTA, 25 mM histidine and 25 mM imidazole or 0.04 mM EDTA and 25 mM imidazole (pH 7.0-7.6). Membrane forming n-decane solutions contained phosphatidyl cholines (PC) and cholesterol (2:1 by weight). Electrical conductance of BLM was measured using Ag/AgCl electrodes connected with a functional generator Systron Donner 410 and a 10^9 Ohm resistance. Electrical transmembrane potential developed after formation of $CaCl_2$ gradient was measured by an electrometer Corning 125. Relative cation selectivity of the BLM was estimated using the values and the sign of the transmembrane potentials generated upon asymmetric additions of chlorides of calcium and other cations to the compartments of the cell.

Oxygen consumption by a suspension of egg phosphatidyl choline (Sigma) was induced by Fe^{2+}/ascorbate (1 µM and 50 µM, respectively) and measured with continuous stirring at room temperature using an a Clark electrode in an oxygen monitor YSI, model 53. Aliquots of the lipid suspension in alcohol (40 mg in 0.4 ml) were added to 4 ml of the incubation medium containing 25 mM histidine and 25 mM imidazole (pH 7.0).

Fragments of sarcoplasmic reticulum were isolated from rabbit skeletal muscle as described previously (Levitsky et al., 1976). Preincubation of SR suspension with $FeSO_4$ and ascorbic acid (1 μM and 50 μM, respectively) was performed for 30 min at 37°C in a medium containing 10% sucrose, 0.1 M KCl, 10 mM Tris-HCl and 0.5 mg SR protein/ml. The medium was also supplemented with antioxidants. Ca^{2+} uptake by SR vesicles was measured by a Ca^{2+}-selective electrode (Orion Research) in a solution containing 0.1 M KCl, 2 mM ATP, 3 mM $MgCl_2$, 5 mM sodium azide, 10 mM potassium oxalate, 10 mM creatine phosphate, 10 IU of creatine kinase/5 ml and 20 mM HEPES (pH 7.0, 25°C).

In the experiments on total ischemia, rat hearts were perfused and subsequently incubated at 37°C with 0.9 M NaCl in the presence and absence of the antioxidant. The hearts were homogenized using a Polytron homogenizer in ten volumes of the solution containing 0.1 M KCl, 5 mM sodium azide and 40 mM Tris-HCl (pH 7.4). The reaction medium for measuring Ca^{2+}-pump activity of cardiac muscle homogenates contained 0.1 M KCl, 5 mM ATP, 6 mM $MgCl_2$, 5 mM sodium azide, 15 mM potassium oxalate and 20 mM Tris-HCl buffer (pH 7.2, 37°C). The activity was expressed as umol Ca^{2+}/min/g weight heart.

RESULTS

Effects of prooxidant and antioxidant systems on Ca^{2+} fluxes across bilayer lipid membranes

Bilayer lipid membranes have been demonstrated to be an adequate model for testing ionophores of various nature. Insertion of a number of proteins or membrane fragments into BLM causes a marked increase in ionic conductance of the lipid bilayers (Shamoo and Goldstein, 1977, Smith et al., 1986). This is interpreted usually as an evidence of existance of selective ion channels or ionophores in the tested preparations.

As shown previously (Shamoo and Goldstein, 1977, Levitsky et al. 1984) large fragments and peptides of sarcoplasmic reticulum Ca^{2+}-ATPases increase permeability of BLM for calcium ions (cf. Fig. 1). In our studies, however, the effect of the fragments and peptides isolated from cardiac and skeletal muscles Ca^{2+}-ATPases on the conductance varied from one experiment to another. Moreover, in some cases the initial electrical conductance of bilayers formed from phosphatidyl choline and cholesterol was found to be so high that it hampered testing ionophoric substances. We proposed that lipid itself contains endogeneous compound(s) increasing ion permeability.

Depending on the source of commercial lipid used for formation of the BLM and conditions of the lipid storage, calcium ions increase more or less efficiently the electrical current through the membrane, the maximal effect being demonstrated if a freshly oxidized lipid suspension is employed (Fig. 2). A row of the cation selectivity estimated by transmembrane potentials generated upon additions of $CaCl_2$ and metal chlorides into opposite compartments of the measuring cell is the following: $Ca^{2+}>Mg^{2+}>Ba^{2+}>Sr^{2+}>>K^+>Rb^+>Cs^+>NH_4{}^+>Na^+>Li^+$.

The increase of bilayer conductance in the calcium containing medium was more pronounced in the presence of a prooxidant system, Fe^{2+}/ascorbate (Fig. 3). We suggested that the increased Ca^{2+} permeability is a consequence of the presence of endogeneous or generation of new lipid peroxides. To test the suggestion, experiments with different antioxidants were carried out.

The rise in conductance of BLM induced by Fe^{2+}/ascorbate is abolished by adding catalase into the measuring cell (Fig. 3). It is worthwhile mentioning that catalase, though arresting this process, as well as a free radical scavenger, superoxide dismutase (SOD), did not decrease the current through the membrane. A small effect on the current under these conditions was registered in the presence of quercetin (Fig. 3), an antioxidant of flavonoid nature (Cavallini et al., 1978).

Fig. 4 demonstrates effects of different antioxidants on the conductance of BLM formed from a lipid containing endogeneous oxidized products. SOD does not affect the increase of the current in the Ca^{2+}-containing medium. Addition of an antioxidant butylated hydroxytoluene (BHT) abolishes further rise of the conductance and only slightly decreases its level, another addition of the drug being ineffective. A sharp decline of the conductance takes place when quercetin is further added into the cell. Low level of conductance, which was close to the initial one, could not be changed by adding additional $CaCl_2$ or Fe^{2+}/ ascorbate into the medium (Fig. 4).

The data presented in Fig. 3 and Fig. 4 can be summarized as follows:

1) Catalase completely blocks accumulation of products of lipid peroxidation possessing Ca^{2+}-ionophoric properties. This enzyme, however, does not decrease the concentration of the active species;

2) Antioxidants BHT and quercetin, when added separately, do not decrease significantly the content of Ca^{2+} ionophores in the lipid. The

more pronounced effect on the conductance found in the presence of both of the compounds could reflect potentiation of scavenging of lipid peroxidation products by combinations of antioxidants (Kanematsu et al., 1983).

<u>Effects of antioxidants on lipid oxidation and Ca^{2+}-pump activity of sarcoplasmic reticulum</u>

The relative efficiency of different antioxidants was tested by their action on the velocity of oxygen consumption by phosphatidyl choline suspensions in the presence of Fe^{2+}/ ascorbate. BHT and quercetin at 5 μM concentration decreased markedly the lipid oxidation, the same concentration of α-tocopherol being ineffective (Table 1).

The same compounds were tested in the experiments with isolated SR vesicles treated with Fe^{2+}/ascorbate. 30 min incubation of the microsomes with the prooxidant system resulted in a two-fold decrease of the velocity of ATP-dependent Ca^{2+} uptake by the vesicles (Table 1). It was not due to the inhibition of catalytic activity of Ca^{2+}-ATPase (not shown) but resulted from an increase of the leakage of Ca^{2+} from the vesicles into the incubation medium. α-tocopherol in this system as well did not produce any effect. BHT and quercetin being added at 5 μM concentration prevented the Ca^{2+}-pump system from its deterioration by Fe^{2+}/ ascorbate.

Effects of SOD and catalase on oxidation of the lipid and the Ca^{2+}-pump activity were also compared (Table 1). Only catalase prevented (though partially) the damage of the Ca^{2+}-pump and oxidation of the lipid induced by Fe^{2+}/ascorbate. These results indicate that the agents decreasing the velocity of lipid oxidation protect also SR Ca^{2+}-pump.

The action of total ischemia of hearts on the activity of Ca^{2+}-pump system is illustrated by Fig. 5 A. After 30 min of the ischemia the velocity of Ca^{2+} uptake by SR in the homogenate decreases by 70%. Longer incubation of the hearts under ischemic conditions does not lead to an additional drop of the Ca^{2+}-pump activity.

To test if the decrease activity of SR under our experimental conditions is a consequence of lipid peroxidation, we pretreated the hearts with different concentrations of quercetin (Fig. 5 B). Addition of this compound into the preincubation medium at concentrations ranged from 10 to 100 μM resulted in an increase of the rate of Ca^{2+} uptake by SR from ischemic myocardium by 30-40%. α-tocopherol in the same concentration range did not influence the activity of the Ca^{2+}-pump from the ischemic myocardium. Pretreatment of the hearts with a higher dose of quercetin resulted in the inhibition of the pump system isolated from the heart. The latter phenomenon could be explained by a redistribution of quercetin inside the cell and its binding to SR; it has been shown that the flavonoid decreases Ca^{2+}-pump and Ca^{2+}-ATPase activities of skeletal muscle SR vesicles (Fewtrell and Gomperts, 1977; Shoshan and MacLennan, 1981). In separate experiments we demonstrated that this drug at 100 uM concentration induced a two-fold inhibition of the Ca^{2+}-pump activity of isolated fragments of cardiac SR if added directly into the incubation medium (not shown).

Ca^{2+} channels in bilayers generated by oxygen

As shown in Fig. 2, depending on the source and storing conditions of commercial lipid, calcium ions more or less efficiently increase conductance of BLM. Since the effect of Ca^{2+} was found to be more pronouced if BLM were prepared from freshly oxidized lipid than from highly oxidized ones, we suggested that ionophoric lipid peroxides were not stable and could be converted in time into inactive species.

Generation and decomposition of calcium ionophores in BLM upon changes of gas content above the incubation buffer is illustrated by the Fig. 6 and Fig. 7. Under nitrogen atmosphere and in the presence of low Ca^{2+} the current across the BLM is low at a transmembrane voltage of 30 mV (Fig. 6 A). It increases 5-fold at the voltage of 150 mV. When the nitrogen above the cell was substituted for air (Fig. 6 B), current noises appear, an average level of the current at 90 mV being 2 times higher than that under the nitrogen atmosphere (cf. curves f and c). Subsequent lowering of the voltage from 90 to 60 mV results in a decrease of the amplitute of current fluctuations and in the spontaneous cessations of the noises (Fig. 6 B, curve g).

When the gas content above the incubation medium was restored to the initial one (Fig. 6 C) the current fluctuations cease in a while even at the voltage as high as 120 mV. This indicates that ionoporic substances are accumulated in lipid upon its exposure to the air and they disappear under nitrogen atmosphere.

Under appropriate conditions, discrete jumps of the electrical current through the BLM can be recorded in Ca^{2+}-containing media (Fig. 7). At a low transmembrane voltage the noises of the current are small and deviations from the basal current level are rare (Fig. 7, curve a). Increase in the voltage makes the membrane excitable and the deviations of the current become more frequent (curve b). Occasionally, stable current values of higher amplitude are recorded. At last, further increase in the voltage leads to appearance of several excitable states of the membrane (curve c). The state of higher conductance of the BLM may last as long as tens of seconds. These data evidence that ionic channels are formed in the bilayer. It is not yet clear whether high transmembrane potential increases probability of channel formation or potentiates ion fluxes across preformed channels. Analysing the recordings presented in Fig. 7, one may suggest that more than one type of the channels operate in oxidized bilayers. An alternative suggestion is that clusters of channels of a single type are functioning in the BLM, their formation and disappearance occuring in a highly cooperative manner.

DISCUSSION

The data presented in this paper demonstrate that one of the effects of lipid peroxidation is accumulation of products possessing ionophoric properties. The oxidized membranes exibited a high cation selectivity. It is of importance that the permeability of the oxidized BLM for calcium is higher than that for other divalent and especially monovalent cations. It is well known that calcium transmembrane gradients across cellular membranes may be as high as four orders of magnitute. The dissipation of the gradients of this important second messenger would deteriorate major cellular function, including contractile function, and may kill the cell.

Another conclusion is that the initiation of the peroxidation results not only in an increase of cation permeability across artificial bilayer membranes but in a decrease of active accumulation of Ca^{2+} by SR vesicles. The latter phenomenon is due to an increase of passive efflux of Ca^{2+} from the vesicles. Our data indicate that cation channels are operating in membranes from oxidized lipid.

Experiments performed with antioxidants did not allow us to draw the final picture of the processes taking place in the lipid during its oxidation or to suggest the nature of a concrete ionophoric substance. However, these data indicate that those of the antioxidants which effectively decrease lipid oxidation, also diminish Ca^{2+} fluxes across oxidized BLM and are able to protect SR membrane against an increase of its passive permeability for calcium ions.

From the data presented we may conclude that $\cdot O_2$ does not participate in generation of ionophoric substances either in pure lipid or in SR membranes in the presence of Fe^{2+}/ascorbate. In this connection it is worthwhile to mention the data of Myers et al. (1985) showing that SOD does not affect the release of creatine kinase from the reoxygenated ischemic heart.

Unexpected results were obtained in the experiments with catalase. This enzyme not only protected the Ca^{2+} pump system of SR from the damage but also blocked the rise of Ca^{2+} conductance induced by Fe^{2+}/ascorbate. One may suggest that H_2O_2 and/or $OH^{\cdot}$ participate in generation of ionophoric peroxides under those conditions. The latter radical can be produced in the Fenton reaction (1) or in the reactions (2):

$$H_2O_2 + Fe^{2+} \longrightarrow Fe^{3+} + {}^{\cdot}OH + OH^- \quad (1)$$

$$ROOH + Fe^{2+} \longrightarrow Fe^{3+} + {}^{\cdot}OR + RO^- \quad (2),$$

where R corresponds to lipid. H_2O_2 could be present in trace amounts in the incubation media or originate from radical recombination:

$${}^{\cdot}OH + {}^{\cdot}OH \longrightarrow H_2O_2 \quad (3)$$

At last, a highly speculative explanation of the effect of catalase could be made if one suggests that the enzyme possesses peroxidase activity:

$$2ROOH \xrightarrow{\text{catalase}} 2ROH + O_2 \quad (4)$$

Moving from a simplest membrane system (BLM) to isolated membrane vesicles, we confirmed our original suggestion about a role of products of lipid peroxidation in an increase of Ca^{2+} permeability of cellular membranes. To find out if myocardial ischemia results in formation of "calcium ionophoric substances", we treated the ischemic heart with an antioxidant quercetin and studied Ca^{2+}-pump activity of the heart homogenates, rather than of isolated microsomal fractions. This approach allowed us to avoid an additional impairment of the calcium pump system during the isolation procedures and to investigate total Ca^{2+}-pump activity. Is is found that quercetin prevents partially the damage of the system of Ca^{2+} translocation. These data provide evidence that during myocardial ischemia substances are accumulated which play a role of calcium ionophores or calcium channel forming structures. Evidently additional mechanisms are operating in the ischemic heart, such as proteolysis and phospholipolysis, which aggravate the condition of the failing myocardium caused by free radicals and further impair function of Ca^{2+}-translocating systems.

Table 1. Effect of antioxidants on lipid oxidation and on the decrease of Ca^{2+}-pump activity of SR in the presence of the pro-oxidant system.

Additions	Relative velocity of oxygen consumption, %	Ca^{2+} uptake, µmol/min/mg protein
None	-	1.63±0.11
$FeSO_4$ and ascorbic acid	100	0.75±0.06
+ α-tocopherol	100	0.54±0.06
+ BHT	14.5	1.41±0.08
+ quercetin	12.1	1.72±0.03
+ catalase	53.5	1.38±0.08
+ SOD	72.5	0.60±0.14

The incubation media were supplemented as indicated with 1 µM $FeSO_4$, 50 µM ascorbic acid, 5 µM -tocopherol, BHT and quercetin, 320 IU catalase, 560 IU SOD.

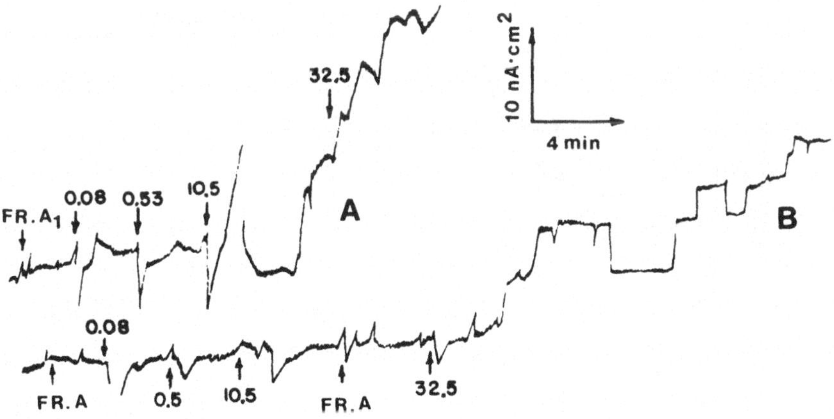

Fig. 1. Effect of fragments of Ca^{2+}-ATPase isolated from pigeon heart SR on electical current across BLM. A. The tryptic fragment of 55 kDa. B. The fragment of 35 kDa. Additions of $CaCl_2$ (in mM) are indicated. From Levitsky et al. (1984).

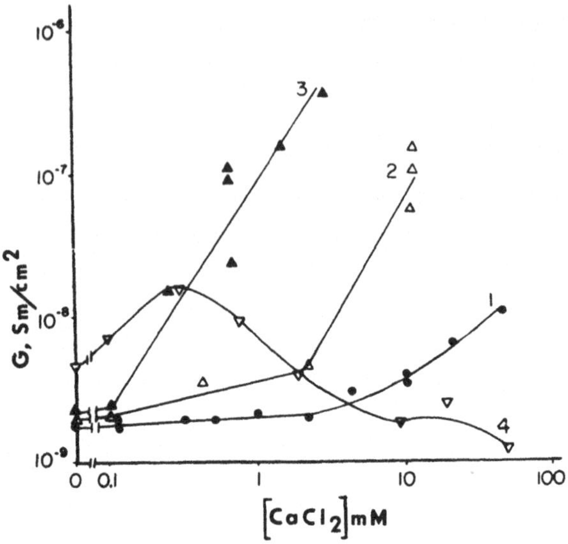

Fig. 2. Ca^{2+}-induced increase in conductance of BLM prepared from mixtures of cholesterol and synthetic dioleyl phosphatidyl choline (1); egg PC, 1 day after opening of the ampule, (2); egg PC stored at -20°C under air for a month (3) and stored in the dry state under air (4). From Lebedev et al. (1982a).

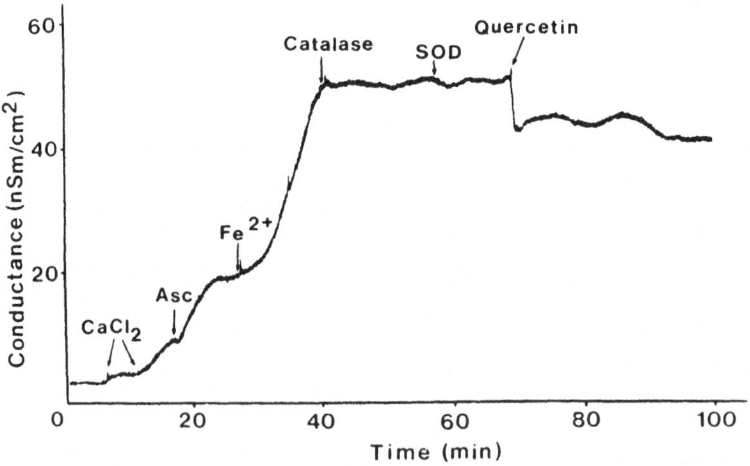

Fig. 3. Effects of Fe^{2+}-ascorbate, catalase, SOD and quercetin on BLM conductance. The BLM was prepared from a mixture of strongly oxidized egg PC and cholesterol. Additions: 1 mM $CaCl_2$ (twice), 50 μM ascorbic acid, 1 μM $FeSO_4$, 42 IU of catalase (Sigma), 40 IU of superoxide dismutase (Sigma), 40 μM quercetin.

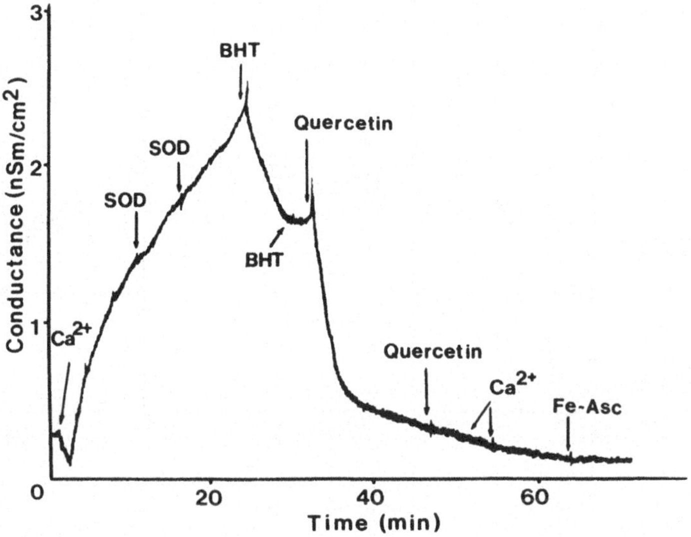

Fig. 4. Effect of antioxidants on the conductance of BLM prepared from egg PC and cholesterol and containing endogeneous calcium ionophores. Additions: 5 mM $CaCl_2$, 40 IU superoxide dismutase (twice), 40 μM BHT (twice), 40 μM quercetin, 5mM Ca^{2+} (twice), 1 μM $FeSO_4$ and 50 μM ascorbic acid.

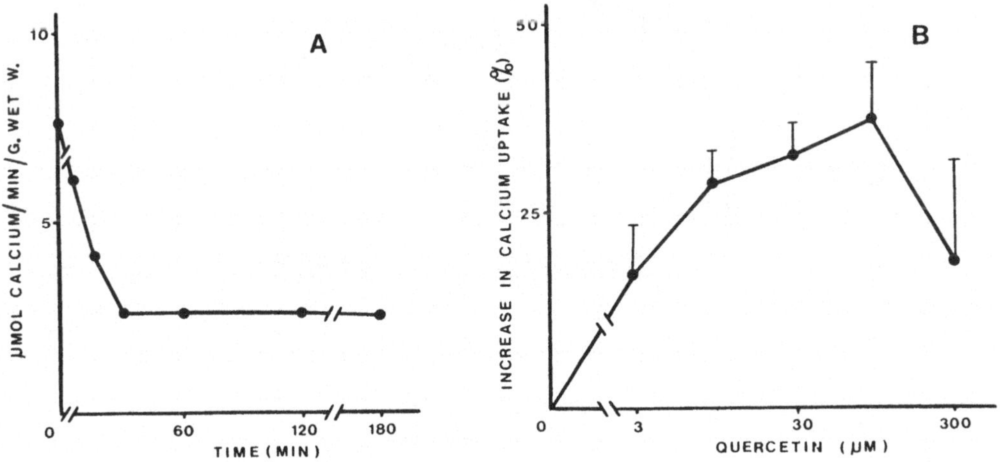

Fig. 5. Ca^{2+} uptake by sarcoplasmic reticulum from ischemic rat hearts. A. The uptake as a function of duration of global ischemia. B. Protection of the calcium pump system of SR isolated from rat hearts after 30 min ischemia by quercetin.

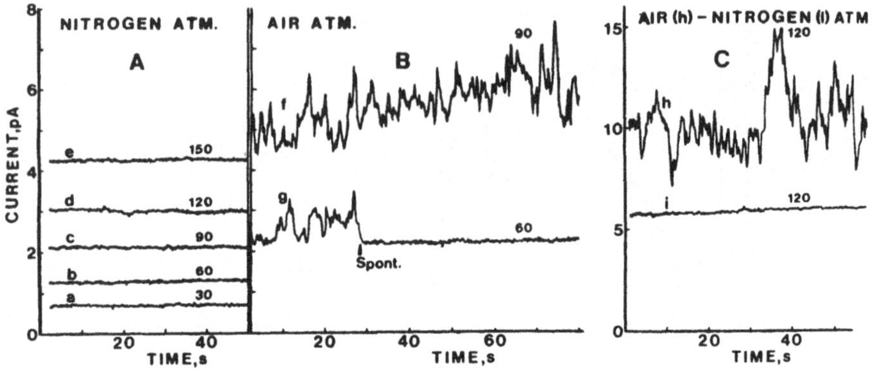

Fig. 6. Current noises in BLM dependent on the presence of oxygen and applied voltage. The recordings were obtained on the same membrane (in a sequence from a to i) formed from dioleyl PC and cholesterol. The medium contained 25 mM imidazole and 25 μM EDTA (pH 7.0 was adjusted by HCl). Values of the transmembrane voltage (in mV) are indicated above the curves.

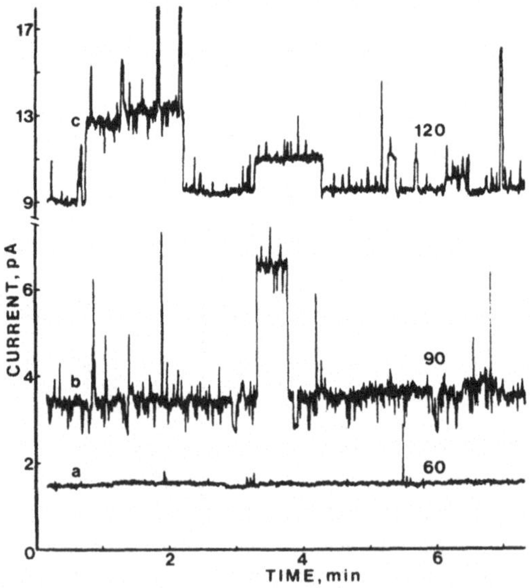

Fig. 7. Voltage-dependent jumps of the current through BLM formed from dioleyl PC and cholesterol. The medium contained 25 mM imidazole, 25 μM EDTA (pH 7.0 was adjusted by HCl) and 5 mM $CaCl_2$. Voltage values (60, 90, 120 mV) are indicated.

REFERENCES

Alto, L.E. and Dhalla, N.S., 1979. Myocardial cation contents during induction of calcium paradox. Am. J. Physiol., 237, H713-H719.

Cavallini, L., Bindoli, A. and Siliprandi N., 1978. Comparative evaluation of antiperoxidative action of silumarin and other flavonoids. Pharmacol. Research Commun., 10, 133-136.

Fewtrell, C.M.S. and Gomperts, B.D., 1977. Effect of flavon inhibitors of transport ATPases on histamin secretion from rat mast cells. Nature, 265, 635-636.

Ganote, C.E. and Nayler, W.G.,1985. Contracture and the calcium paradox. J. Mol. Cell. Cardiol., 17, 733-745.

Gauduel, Y. and Duvelleroy, M.A., 1984. Role of oxygen radicals in cardiac injury due to reoxygenation. J. Mol. Cell. Cardiol., 16, 459-470.

Guarnieri, C., Flamingi, F. and Gardarera, C.M., 1980. Role of oxygen in the cellular damage induced by re-oxygenation of hypoxic heart. J. Mol. Cell. Cardiol., 12, 797-808.

Hearse, D.J., Humphrey, S.M. and Bullock, G.R., 1978. The oxygen paradox and calcium paradox: two facets of the same problem? J. Mol. Cell. Cardiol.,10, 641-668.

Hess, M.L. and Manson, N.H., 1984. Molecular oxygen: friend and foe. The role of the oxygen free radical system in the calcium paradox, the oxygen paradox and ischemia/reperfusion injury. J. Mol. Cell. Cardiol., 16, 969-985.

Julicher, R.H.M., Sterrenberg, L., Koomen, J.M., Bast, A. and Noordhoek, J., 1984a. Evidence for lipid peroxidation during the calcium paradox in vitamin E deficient rat heart. Naunyn Schmiedebergs Arch. Pharmacol., 326, 87-89.

Julicher, R.H.M., Tijburg, L.B.M., Sterrenberg, L., Bast, A., Koomen, J.M. and Noordhoek, J., 1984b. Decreased defence against free radicals in rat heart during normal reperfusion, after hypoxic, ischemic and calcium free reperfusion. Life Sci., 35, 1281-1288.

Kako, K.J., 1985. Membrane damage caused by lipid peroxidation in myocardial ischemia. Jikei Med. J., 32, 609-639.

Kako, K.J., 1987. Free radical effect on membrane protein in myocardial ischemia/reperfusion injury. J. Mol. Cell. Cardiol., 19, 209-211.

Kanematsu, H., Aoyama, M., Maruyama, T., Niiya, I., Tsukamoto, M., Tokairin, S. and Matsumoto, T., 1983. Studies of antioxidant effect of tocopherols. III. Synergistic effect of monoacylglycerol citrate, malate, and succinate. Yukagaku, 32, 731-734.

Lebedev, A.V., Levitsky, D.O. and Loginov, V.A., 1982a. Oxygen as an inductor of divalent cation permeability through biological and model lipid membranes. In: E.Chazov, V.Smirnov, N.S.Dhalla (Editors), Advances in Myocardiology, vol., Plenum Medical Book Company, New York, London, pp. 425-438.

Lebedev, A.V., Levitsky, D.O., Loginov, V.A. and Smirnov, V.N., 1982b. The effect of primary products of lipid peroxidation on transmembrane transport of calcium ions. J. Mol. Cell. Cardiol., 14, 99-103.

Levitsky, D.O., Aliev, M.K., Kuzmin, A.V., Levchenko, T.S., Smirnov, V.N. and Chazov, E.I., 1976. Isolation of calcium pump system and purification of calcium ion-dependent ATPase from heart muscle. Biochim. Biophys. Acta, 443, 468-484.

Levitsky, D.O., Grishin, E.V., Biryukova, T.V., Lebedev, A.V. and Nikolaeva, L.N., 1984. Ca^{2+}-dependent ATPases of the sarcoplasmic reticulum of skeletal and heart muscles and their iontransporting fragments. J. Sov. Cardiovasc. Res., 4, 262-269.

Meerson, F.Z., Kagan, V.E., Kozlov, Yu.P., Belkina, L.M. and Arkhipenko, Yu.V., 1982. The role of lipid peroxidation in pathogenesis of ischemic damage and the anti-oxidant protection of the heart. Basic Res. Cardiol., 77, 465-485.

Mueller, P., Rudin, D. O., Tien, H. T. and Wescott, W. C., 1964. Formation and properties of bimolecular lipid membranes. In: Recent Progress in Surface Science, vol. 1, Acad. Press, New York, London, 379-393.

Myers, C.L., Weiss S.J., Kirsh M.M. and Shlafer, M., 1985. Involvement of hydrogen peroxide and hydroxyl radical in the "oxygen paradox": Reduction of creatine kinase release by catalase, allopurinol or deferoxamine, but not superoxide dismutase. J. Mol. Cell. Cardiol., 17, 675-684.

Rao, P.S., Cohen, M.V. and Mueller, H.S., 1983. Production of free radicals and lipid peroxides in early experimental myocardial ischemia. J. Mol. Cell. Cardiol., 15, 713-716.

Shamoo, A.E. and Goldstein, D.A., 1977. Isolation of ionophores from ion transport systems and their role in energy transduction. Biochim. Biophys. Acta, 472, 13-53.

Shlafer, M., Kane, P.F., Wigging, V.Y. and Kirsch, M.M., 1982. Possible role for cyto-toxic oxygen metabolites in the pathogenesis of cardiac ischemic injury. Circulation, 66, 85-92.

Shoshan, V. and MacLennan, D.H., 1981. Quercetin interaction with the (Ca^{2+}+Mg^{2+})-ATPase of sarcoplasmic reticulum. J. Biol. Chem., 256, 887-892.

Smith, J.S., Coronado, R. and Meissner, G., 1986. Single channel measurments of the calcium release channel from skeletal muscle sarcoplasmic reticulum. J. Gen. Physiol., 88, 573-588.

Ursini, F., Maiorino, M. and Gregolin, C., 1985. The selenoenzyme phospholipid hydroperoxide glutathion peroxidase. Biochim. Biophys. Acta, 839, 62-70.

Zimmerman, A.N.E., Daems, W., Hulsmann, W.C., Synder, J., Weisse, E. and Durer, D., 1967. Morphological changes of heart muscle caused by successive perfusion with calcium-free and calcium-containing solutions (calcium paradox). Cardiovasc. Res., 1, 201-209.

Zimmerman, A.N.E. and Hulsmann, W.C., 1966. Paradoxical influence of calcium ions on the permeability of cell membranes of isolated rat heart. Nature, 211, 646-647.

CYTOTOXIC MECHANSIMS FOR CHOLESTEROL OXIDATION PRODUCTS IN FIBROBLASTS AND ENDOTHELIAL CELLS.

Alex Sevanian

Institute for Toxicology and Department of Pathology, University of Southern California, 1985 Zonal ave. Los Angeles, CA

ABSTRACT

Several cholesterol oxides form during free radical oxidation of membrane lipids. These cholesterol oxides have been recovered from tissues and at least eight of these are products consistently detected after oxy-radical induced oxidation of membrane lipids. The proportions of these products can serve as a "fingerprint" of the oxidation process in membranes. Three common cholesterol oxides have been tested for their cytotoxic potency in cell culture systems. The isomeric cholesterol 5,6 epoxides, 7-keto-cholesterol and cholestane-3β,5α,6β-triol are potent cytotoxins with remarkable stability under conditionsof cell culture. All three compounds are toxic at concentrations half of that seen with bile acids such as lithocholic, cholic or deoxycholic acids. Their toxicity appears to be directed towards the cell membrane and includes marked perturbations of calcium homeostasis. The potency of each compound follows the order: pulmonary endothelial cells > lung fibroblasts (V79 cells) > hepatocytes. The cytotoxic potency of each cholesterol oxide is reduced more than 50% in calcium deficient media (<0.05 mM) indicating the involvement of calcium in cytotoxicity. The LD_{50} for cholestane triol (20 uM) approaches the toxicity of linoleic acid hydroperoxides (10 uM) in endothelial cells. Although endothelial cells represent the most sensitive cell type examined for virtually all cholesterol oxides, each cell type displays approximately equal sensitivity to linoleic acid hydroperoxides. In addition to their membrane toxicity, the cholesterol epoxides also produce DNA damage which correlates with extensive DNA binding. The epoxides are also weak mutagens as demonstrated in V79 cells. A unique aspect of cholesterol epoxide toxicity is the equal LD_{50}'s and IC_{50}'s.(ie. 50% inhibition of DNA synthesis) in both V79 and endothelial cells, suggesting that the two events may proceed via a common mechanism. Since cholesterol epoxides are major products derived from lipid peroxidation, rapidly accumulation on treatment of membranous cholesterol with linoleic and other organic hydroperoxides, it is concievable that a number of toxic effects of lipid peroxides may be attributable to the more long-lived cholesterol oxides which are produced.

INTRODUCTION

It is widely recognized that elevated serum cholesterol significantly increases human risk to coronary artery disease. The development of atherosclerosis can be summarized as a multistage process which begins with injury to the vascular intima followed by a series of events including the accumulation of platelets and macrophages, denudation of the endothelium at the site of initial injury, outgrowth of smooth muscle cells from the vascular media and accumulation of lipid laiden cells (foam cells) in the growing plaque. Cholesterol is a major lipid component of developing plaques and elevated serum cholesterol contributes to the multiplicity and growth of atherosclerotic plaques (Kritchevsky et al. 1979, Benditt 1977, Mahley 1980). There remains, however, considerable controversy over the manner by which cholesterol per se contributes to the development of atheromatous lesions. More recently, several investigators have presented evidence showing that the course of vascular injury and progression of the atheroma is influenced not so much by serum cholesterol as by cholesterol oxidation products which are more readily derived when serum cholesterol is markedly elevated (Brooks et al. 1983).

Several of the cholesterol oxidation products have been shown to accumulate during free radical-induced lipid peroxidation where cholesterol is a major component (Smith 1981, Mitton et al. 1971, Watabe and Sawahata 1979). Many of these cholesterol oxidation products are detected in human serum (Brooks et al. 1983), are significantly elevated in humans with hypercholesterolemia (Gray et al. 1971), and can be isolated from foods (Tsai et al. 1980) and tissues (Sevanian, et al. 1979, Pertrakis et al. 1981), often at high concentrations. The impact of these observations is strengthened by studies demonstrating considerable toxicity for a number of cholesterol oxides. Among the most commonly studied cholesterol oxides are cholesterol-5α,6α-epoxide, (αCE) cholesterol-5β,6β-epoxide (βCE), cholestan-3β,5α,6β-triol (CT), 7-keto cholesterol (7-keto) and cholesterol-7-hydroperoxide. The toxicity of each of these products has been examined in various in vitro preparations including, vascular explants (Imai et al. 1976), aortic smooth muscle cells (Peng et al. 1978) and fibroblasts (Sevanian and Peterson 1984). These cholesterol oxides produce marked injury, development of lesions, inhibition of cell growth and cell death in these tests systems at micromolar concentrations. These effects are not observed with cholesterol which is free of oxidation products. Observations such as these have led to the hypothesis that progression of vascular injury and development of atheromatous lesions includes the formation and accumulation of cytotoxic cholesterol oxides. The formation of these oxides is a free radical mediated event, however, the radical species and their origins have yet to be elucidated. Yagi has provided evidence that lipid hydroperoxides can precipitate atherosclerosis (presented in this monograph) providing further support for a free radical component associated with this disease process.

I present in this chapter a series of studies on the relationship between free radical generation and the formation of specific oxidation products derived from membranous cholesterol. The occurance of these cholesterol oxidation products in tissues will be reviewed from previous reports and cytotoxic properties described using two cell culture systems.

MATERIALS AND METHODS

Cholesterol oxidation studies

Cholesterol (free of oxidation products) was incorporated into small unilamellar liposomes by premixing with suspensions of bovine liver phosphatidylcholine (PC) and phosphatidylethanolamine (PE) in Tris/KCl buffer and sonication of the suspension as previously described (Sevanian and Kim 1985). The proportion of each lipid component was formulated to achieve a set ratio of cholesterol to phospholipid and corresponding level of unsaturation. The lipid composition of these liposomes is described in the following section. Radioactive cholesterol (4-^{14}C-cholesterol at 56 uCi/umol) was added during the preparation of liposomes at a level of 10^6 dpm/mg lipid. The resulting liposomes were immediately subjected to oxidation using the following conditions. 1) Incubation in the presence of 20 uM Fe^{+3}/120 uM ADP plus 4 units xanthine oxidase and 250 uM xanthine. This is referred to as the superoxide radical (O_2^-) generating system, however, considerable amounts of hydrogen peroxide (H_2O_2) are also formed (Nagano and Fridovich 1985). 2) Incubation in the presence of 200 uM cumene hydroperoxide (CuOOH) plus 50 uM hematin. This represents an organic peroxide-dependent oxidation system. 3) Irradiation with a ^{60}Co source under N_2O at a dose rate of 4.5 Gy/min for various time intervals. Liposomes were transferred to test tubes containing pH 7.0 water prior to irradiation and under these conditions the predominant radical species is hydroxyl radical (·OH). 4) Autoxidation of liposomes entailed incubating samples in buffer only for various intervals under air.

Following incubation the extent of lipid peroxidation was estimated by assaying aliquots of the samples for the levels of thiobarbituric acid reactive products (TBAR). The remaining samples were then extracted and the lipids recovered as previously described (Sevanian and Kim 1985). The lipid residue was applied to solid phase extraction columns for the fractionation of cholesterol and its oxidation products as well as phospholipids (Sevanian and Kim 1985). Using this procedure all radioactivity was found to be associated with the cholesterol and cholesterol oxide fraction. This fraction was then dissolved in 25 % isopropanol in hexane prior to high pressure liquid chromatography (HPLC). The methods and conditions for HPLC which permitted resolution of cholesterol and its various oxidation products have been previously reported (Sevanian and Peterson 1984, Sevanian and McLeod 1987). The HPLC eluent was simultaneously monitored for radioactivity and mass using a Ramona Instruments (IN/US) liquid scintillation flow detector, and differential refractometer (Erma Instruments), respectively. The identity of each component was verified using authentic standards and sample spiking during chromatography, and the levels of each product was calculated from its specific activity - based on the original specific activity of cholesterol.

For experiments involving the toxicity of lipid hydroperoxides, the following lipid hydroperoxides were prepared. Linoleic acid hydroperoxide was formed by autoxidation as previously described (Sevanian and Kim 1985). The product was found by HPLC to contain 60 % of the 13-hydroperoxide isomer, 35 % of the 9-hydroperoxide isomer with the remainder being other isomeric hydroperoxides. Cholesterol 7-hydroperoxide was prepared by isomerization of the cholesterol 5-hydroperoxide in chloroform, where cholesterol 5-hydroperoxide was formed by singlet oxygen-induced oxidation of cholesterol as described by Schenck et al. (1957). All products were stored in methylene chloride at $-80^{o}C$.

Endothelial and fibroblast cell cultures

Chinese hamster lung fibroblasts (V79 cells) are a continuous cell line which has been well characterized by our laboratory (Peterson et al. 1979). These cells were utilized either in log or stationary phase depending on the nature of the experiment. Cells in passage 12 - 16 were used in these studies. These cells have a 13-15 hr doubling time and remain differentiated and viable over 25 passages. The V79 cells were used for initial determinations of the cytotoxic levels of cholesterol oxides. They were also used to estimate the mutagenic potency of these compounds and the ability to inhibit DNA synthesis, as measured by the incorporation of ^{3}H-dThd into DNA (Sevanian and Peterson 1984). Bovine pulmonary endothelial cells were isolated from fresh beef hearts as described by Ryan et al (1978). Primary cultures of these cells were grown over three passages after which several clones were isolated. We utilized clone 6 for these studies.

Cytoxicity Studies

The toxicity of cholesterol and several of the major cholesterol oxidation products were measured in cultured cells using three criteria. 1) Suppression of clonal growth in which the growth of 600 cells seeded in 60 mm dishes is determined over 24 hr and compared to untreated cells (controls). 2) Inhibition of growth of 5×10^{3} cells treated for 72 hr with the test compounds. 3) Inhibition of ^{3}H-dThd uptake into DNA of cells following 24 hr treatment with the test compounds. In addition to the above, genotoxicity was assayed in V79 cells by measuring the numbers of 6-thioguanine-resistant colonies produced following 24 hr treatments with the test compounds as described previously (Sevanian and Peterson 1984).

The first three criteria above allowed for the estimation of the LD_{50} for each compound. Criteria 1 is a measure of irreversible toxicity (approximating cell death) in that the effect on cell survival is determined after the test compound is removed. A reduction in the surviving cells results in the growth of fewer colonies over the remaining 9 day period.

Effects of calcium on toxicity and measurements of calcium flux

Spinners minimal essential medium containing 10 % fetal calf serum was supplemented with 50 uM calcium. This preparation, representing a calcium deficient medium, was substituted for the standard Dulbeccos medium used in these studies. Endothelial cells were then treated with cholesterol oxides for 2 hr in the calcium deficient medium, the medium was removed and replaced with complete Dulbeccos medium. Effects of the cholesterol oxides on cell survival were compared to those produced by treatment in complete Dulbeccos medium using both the 72 hr growth, and 7 day clonal assays.

Uptake of calcium by endothelial cells was studied using $^{45}Ca^{+2}$ added to Dulbeccos medium. The medium contained 0.25 uCi of $^{45}Ca^{+2}$/ml and was added to confluent monolayers 1 hr after treatment with a given cholesterol oxide. The uptake of $^{45}Ca^{+2}$ in these experiments was assayed using cells grown in 25 mm multiwell chambers where each chamber represented a specific time point. The cells were washed with unlabeled medium, and harvested by trypsinization. The total cell suspension was collected and transferred to scintillation vials for measurement of radioactivity.

Efflux of calcium from endothelial cells was measured by initially loading cells with $^{45}Ca^{+2}$. Subconfluent endothelial cells grown on 60 mm dishes were incubated for 24-48 hr in 3 ml of complete medium containing 0.5 uCi $^{45}Ca^{+2}$. The cells reached confluency over this period and cell numbers did not increase more than 20 % if cells were incubated beyond this point. At this time the medium was removed and the cells washed 3 times with fresh unlabeled complete medium. Immediately afterwards 3 ml of media containing the desired quantity of test compound(s) was added and incubations begun. All petri dishes (for both calcium influx and efflux studies) were partially immersed into 37°C water baths during the periods of incubation. At selected time intervals 25 ul aliquots of the medium were removed, after gentle mixing of the dishes, and transferred to scintillation vials for measurement of radioactivity. The appearance of radioactivity in the medium vs time was used to estimate the rate of calcium efflux.

All results are shown as the mean and standard deviation computed from 3 - 5 independent experiments. Statistical comparisons were made utilizing linear regression analysis and the Students t-test.

RESULTS

The liposomes made in this study contained 20 mole % cholesterol. This proportion is similar to the amount of cholesterol found in the cell membrane of hepatocytes (Zambrano et al. 1978). **Table 1** shows the fatty acyl composition of the liposomes from which an unsaturation index can be calculated. The major fatty acids are palmitate, oleate, linoleate and arachidonate. Subjecting the liposomes to lipid peroxidation produced considerable oxidation of the unsaturated fatty acids as seen by the loss of polyunsaturated species (eg. arachidonic, docosahexaenoic and linoleic acids), the formation of TBAR and a concomitant loss of cholesterol. The relationships between loss of unsaturated fatty acids and TBAR formation have been described elsewhere (Jordan and Schenkman 1982), and in this paper we describe the pattern of cholesterol oxidation.

The profile of cholesterol oxidation products, and their relationship to the level of cholesterol oxidation and overall lipid peroxidation is presented in **Table 2**. The presence of cholesterol greatly limits the ability of the liposomal lipids to oxidize, however, the reduced level of lipid peroxidation is accompanied by a corresponding increase in cholesterol oxidation with the formation of 7 consistently recognized products. The isomeric 7-hydroperoxides were found as the early products under all conditions except γ-irradiation in the absence of oxygen. With continued oxidation the hydroperoxides ceased to accumulate and secondary products formed. Among the major products, we consistently encountered the diastereomeric cholesterol epoxides, 7-hydroxycholesterol (comprised of equal amounts of the α- and β-hydroperoxide isomers), and 7 keto.

Under conditions favoring initiation reactions, such as with γ-irradiation, where free radical reactions are induced by hydroxyl radical (Ansari and Smith 1979), the only appreciable products were the diastereomeric cholesterol epoxides (formed in approximately equal amounts). Under conditions where propagation reactions prevail, such as with cumene hydroperoxide induced lipid peroxidation, all products appeared in significant quantities. The major products were again cholesterol epoxides and derived CT along with 7-keto- and 7-hydroxycholesterol, derived from the hydroperoxide (Teng and Smith 1976). Prolonged oxidations yielded approximately twice as much βCE as αCE. Superoxide-dependent lipid peroxidation, derived from the xanthine oxidase/ADP-$Fe+^{2}$/xanthine reaction, produced a product profile intermediate between the initiation-type (autoxidation and γ-irradiation) and propagation-type (cumene hydroperoxide) reactions. With prolonged incubations this system yielded a product profile similar to that of cumene hydroperoxide-induced lipid peroxidation, albeit at an overall lower level of lipid peroxidation. It therefore appears that products characteristic of early "initiation" periods of lipid peroxidation (where oxyradicals may be largely responsible for lipid oxidation) are the cholesterol hydroperoxides, the derived 7-keto- and 7-hydroxycholesterols, as well as the isomeric cholesterol epoxides. As lipid peroxidation progresses, and where propagative chain reactions prevail, the major oxidation products are cholesterol β-epoxide, 7-keto and 7-hydroxy-cholesterols.

A hypothetical scheme for the peroxidation of cholesterol is proposed from these findings as shown in **Figure 1**. Oxy-radicals, such as hydroxyl radical, can abstract a hydrogen from the allylic carbon-7 of cholesterol, producing a radical which reacts with oxygen to form the isomeric cholesterol-7-hydroperoxides. These are early species encountered following initiation of lipid peroxidation. In unsaturated lipid systems (typical of cell membranes) the lipid peroxy-radicals may either react with cholesterol to abstract a hydrogen (where this is more likely to obtain from alkoxyl radicals derived from the fatty acid peroxides - RO˙), or add to the double bond of cholesterol (Sevanian et al 1979). Addition products such as these are thermally labile and can decompose to epoxides and other products. A similar mechanism may be involved in the addition of the cholesterol peroxy-radical to cholesterol, forming the epoxides (Smith and Kulig 1975), as depicted in the lower portion of figure 1. The predisposition to yield the βCE from reactions involving lipid peroxy-radicals may be due to the orientation of the β-surface of cholesterol's double bond toward the hydrophobic matrix of membranes (Vandenheuval 1963) wherein the unsaturated fatty acyl peroxides arise. Formation of the αCE may be favored by the orientation of the α-surface toward the membrane interface and attack by oxy-radicals or species of more hydrophilic character.

Based on the above results it appears that a number of cholesterol oxidation products accumulate during lipid peroxidation in membrane systems. Many of these oxidation products are consistently encountered, and their isolation from biological membranes (Mitropoulos and Balasubramaniam 1972) and tissues (Brooks et al. 1983, Sevanian et al. 1979, Petrakis et al. 1981, Lo and Black 1972) makes it reasonable to examine their biological and toxic properties further. These studies have begun with measurements of uptake and metabolism as well as the cytotoxic levels of the major cholesterol oxidation products in cultured cells.

We described previously the uptake and metabolism of the isomeric cholesterol epoxides in V79 cells (Sevanian and Peterson 1984). In the present report the uptake and metabolism of the epoxides is described using pulmonary endothelial cells. The endothelial cells used for these experiments were derived from clone 6 of primary cultures which had undergone two passages. This clone had a doubling time of 19 - 22 hrs over the course of 5 passages, and the doubling time then increased to 26 - 29 hrs over passages 6 - 10. By passage 11 the cells stopped dividing and the plating efficiency decreased to less than 10 %. Based on these attributes, and on the gradually diminishing plating efficiency for cells passaged more than 6 times, all studies were confined to cultures of passage 8 or less. A marker for the purity and state of differentiation of these endothelial cells is the production of angiotensin converting enzyme (ACE). This activity was routinely monitored in all cultures and typical activities are shown in **Table 3**. This table compares the ACE activities for cells from primary cultures at different passages (PEC), for the clone 6 cells (PEC clone 6) and for V79 cells. The advantages of the clone are apparent by its longer viability and the persistence of ACE activity. The PEC cultures have lost more than 60 % of this activity by passage 6, much of which was due to overgrowth by fibroblasts and smooth muscle cells which show comparatively little if any ACE activity. It appears, therefore, that the diminished viability of these cells and the loss of ACE activity coincide.

The addition of 10 uM cholesterol α- or β-epoxides to endothelial cells resulted in a rapid uptake and gradual metabolism of both compounds as described in **Figure 2**. Uptake during the first 6 hrs was much greater than over the remaining 18 hrs of analysis suggesting that incorporation was saturable. This property is remarkably similar to the findings with V79 cells (Sevanian and Peterson 1984). In addition, the metabolism of the epoxides to CT was similar for endothelial and V79 cells. The β-isomer was incorporated at a somewhat faster rate (statistically insignificant, $p>0.05$) and metabolized to CT more readily than the α-isomer. Taking the differences in uptake into consideration, the rates of metabolism of both isomers are also not significantly different.

Cytotoxicity measurements were performed using the major cholesterol oxidation products described above. **Table 4** presents a comparison of the toxicities of these cholesterol oxides towards endothelial cells, V79 cells and rat hepatocytes. All compounds tested produced a linear increase in toxicity with increasing dose. The results shown in table 4 utilized the method of measuring inhibition of the surviving fraction of cells treated with a given compound (suppression of clonal growth) for endothelial and V79 cells, and typan blue exclusion for hepatocytes. All values were corrected by the surviving fraction for untreated cells. For comparison, linoleic acid hydroperoxide, cholic and lithocholic acids were also examined. The results for these assays were in good agreement with the other measures of cytotoxicity described in the methods section. Hepatocytes were uniformly the least sensitive to all the compounds tested, whereas endothelial cells were most sensitive. Linoleic acid hydroperoxide was the most toxic among these compounds, and produced a uniform level of toxicity among all three cell types. CT was the most potent cytotoxic compound among the oxidized steroids with somewhat lower cytotoxic potencies observed for bCE, 7-keto and 3,5-cholestadiene-7-one. βCE was approximately twice as toxic as the corresponding α-isomer, suggesting that the basis for its greater cytotoxic potency may be a feature applicable to cells in general. It is also interesting to note that these cholesterol oxidation products are (with the exception of 7-hydroxycholesterol) approximately twice as toxic as the bile acids, cholic and lithocholic acids. The general resistance of hepatocytes to the cholesterol oxides may be related to their resistance to bile acid toxicity, since these cells are adapted for production, storage and release of large quantities of bile acids.

Recently, we reported that the genotoxic and cytotoxic potencies of the diastereomeric cholesterol epoxides are very similar (Peterson et al. 1987). It was hypothesized that the expression of genotoxicity and cytotoxicity may have a common origin, and that injury to the cell membrane may be a mechanism linking these two forms of toxicity. Several parameters of membrane injury are routinely used for membrane toxicity studies. We selected the commonly used measurements of disruption of ionic homeostasis as a measure of membrane damage, and effects on calcium fluxes was specifically studied. As a preliminary study the effects of extracellular calcium on cholesterol oxide toxicity was examined. It has been suggested that the loss of the membrane calcium barrier, and accumulation of intracellular calcium, is a mechanism by which many compounds produce cell death (Schanne et al. 1979). This hypothesis is supported by several experiments showing that injury by membrane toxicants is reversible provided that calcium in not permitted to accumulate in the affected cells. This possibility was tested using endothelial cells and the results are shown in **Table 5**. The toxicity of each of the cholesterol oxides tested in this manner was reduced by approximately 50 % when cells were treated in calcium deficient medium. These experiments were limited to the use of 50 uM calcium since total absence of calcium in the medium reduced the viability and recovery of these cells to unacceptable levels (< 20 %). Nevertheless, the results suggest that a significant component of the toxicity of these compounds involves the increased influx of extracellular calcium.

The effect of the cholesterol oxides on calcium transport was examined further by measurements of $^{45}Ca^{+2}$ influx and exchange-efflux using endothelial cells. **Table 6** shows the results for three of the cholesterol oxides, lithocholic acid and verapamil on calcium influx measured over a 2 hr period. A bimodal pattern of calcium uptake was observed during the initial 3 min (early phase) followed by a more rapid and linear uptake (late phase) which continued up to and beyond 2 hrs. Since both phases were linear with respect to time, the rates were computed on the basis of the slope for calcium uptake and are expressed as cpm $^{45}Ca^{+2}$/min/cell. Verapamil (30 uM) alone produced a 30 % inhibition of the early phase of calcium influx but had no effect on late phase uptake. Verapamil is known to inhibit primarily rapid voltage-gated calcium channels (Fleckenstein 1977). αCE (30 uM), βCE (25 uM), and CT (20 uM) significantly inhibited the early phase of calcium influx, and verapamil did not alter this effect. The inhibitory effect of αCE was found to continue during the late phase of calcium influx, while the β-isomer produced no prolonged inhibition. It also appears that in the presence of βCE, verapamil produced a mild but significant inhibition of late phase calcium influx. In the presence of CT, by contrast, verapamil increased the rate of late phase calcium influx. The effect of lithocholic acid (30 uM) resembled that of CT both in terms of early phase inhibition of calcium influx and the stimulation of calcium influx when both lithocholic acid and verapamil were added.

The effects of these compounds on calcium efflux are shown in **Table 7** and the results are expressed in the same manner as in table 6. Under the condition used in this study, we found a very rapid early phase for calcium efflux lasting approximately 2 min. This was followed by a prolonged late phase which remained linear up to the point where the experiment was terminated (2 hrs). It should be noted that the rate of calcium influx (table 6) and calcium efflux during the late phases are similar, suggesting that what is being measured is the rate of exchange-efflux under relatively steady-state conditions. All the compounds tested inhibited the rate of calcium efflux to varying degrees. The most potent inhibition was produced by αCE which was confined to the early phase only. Unlike the influx experiments the presence of αCE allowed for the inhibitory effect of verapamil to be expressed during the late phase of efflux. A similar effect was seen for βCE although this compound was considerably less potent an inhibitor than αCE and was ineffective during the late phase of calcium efflux. The effects of CT and lithocholic acid were again similar in several respects, producing an early phase inhibition which was reversed by verapamil.

By comparing the data in Tables 6 and 7 it is evident that the net effect of these cholesterol oxides is to produce an influx of calcium which appears to be sustained, particularly with CT and βCE, for extended periods. This net influx occurs by concurrent increase in influx and decrease in efflux rates. The results for measurements of calcium influx, therefore, agree with the findings showing decreased sensitivity to the cholesterol oxides in calcium deficient media. It also appears that these compounds are producing a generalized perturbation of calcium transport which only in part affects verapamil sensitive channels. The existance of two temporally distinct components for calcium influx and efflux may be an artifact of media change, and despite the fact that all changes utilized isotonic media, a gradient appears to have been induced for calcium and perhaps other constituents. This can be viewed as a favorable coincidence since it permits a secondary measure of the membranes ability to respond to rapid osmotic or pressure gradients, providing another measure of the membrane effects of cholesterol oxides.

CONCLUSIONS

Several oxidation products of cholesterol are commonly encountered following the free radical dependent oxidation of membrane lipids. It is, therefore, reasonable to expect that lipid peroxidation in cholesterol rich systems can produce appreciable quantities of cholesterol oxides. A situation such as this may exist in blood vessels where inflammatory cells, their derived oxyradicals and lipid rich deposits coexist. Accumulation of cholesterol oxides may contribute to lesion progression at the vascular media since many of the cholesterol oxides are toxic to endothelial cells at concentrations similar to the levels produced following peroxidation of membranous cholesterol. These levels are similar to those encountered in blood and tissues subjected to oxidative stress and obtainable via a "normal" human diet. A further aspect related to the progression of atheromatous plaques is the potential for genotoxicity along with the proliferation of transformed cell populations, a property noted for the commonly encountered cholesterol epoxides. Despite their remarkable toxicity, the cholesterol oxides as a group are relatively stable compounds with potentially long biological lifetimes. This is not the case for other lipid peroxidation products, such as the fatty acid hydroperoxides. Injury to the vascular barrier may progress via the accumulation of cholesterol oxides in cell membranes and attendant perturbations in membrane functions. We have found that one important property, the regulation of calcium transport is affected by the accumulation of small quantities of cholesterol oxides. Since the effects of these compounds may be additive, as they tend to accumulate as a group of products, considerable membrane perturbations may follow the formation of small amounts of specific cholesterol oxide.

TABLE I

Fatty Acyl Composition of Liposome Phospholipids

Fatty acid[‡]		% total fatty acids
palmitic	(16:0)	18.6 ± 0.22
palmitoleic	(16:1)	1.4 ± 0.04
stearic	(18:0)	29.5 ± 0.56
oleic	(18:1)	19.1 ± 0.17
linoleic, ω-6	(18:2)	6.6 ± 0.10
linolenic, ω-3	(18:3)	0.8 ± 0.05
eicosatrienoic, ω-9	(20:3)	4.2 ± 0.14
arachidonic, ω-6	(20:4)	10.3 ± 0.26
eicosapentaenoic, ω-3	(20:5)	1.5 ± 0.04
docosatetraenoic, ω-6	(22:4)	1.9 ± 0.02
docosahexaenoic, ω-3	(22:6)	0.9 ± 0.08
others		5.5 ± 0.19

‡ Fatty acids were analyzed as the fatty acid methyl esters derived from acidic methanolysis of phospholipids extracted from liposomal suspensions.

ACKNOWLEDGEMENTS

I wish to express my gratitude to Ms. Laurie McLeod and Mrs. Hazel Peterson for their excellent technical assistance in every aspect of this study. This project was supported by grant ES03466 from the National Institutes of Health.

TABLE 2

Major Oxidation Products of Cholesterol in Phospholipid Liposomes (1:4 molar ratio of cholesterol to phospholipid)

PRODUCTS (in micrograms)

conditions	αCE	βCE	7-OOH	7-keto	3,7diol	3,5diene	CT	umole* TBAR
Control								
0 min	0.08 ±0.01	0.10 ±0.03	0.03 -	0.04 ±0.01	0.08 ±0.02	0.02 -	nil	1.09 ±0.47
Autox.								
10 min	0.25 ±0.05	0.25 ±0.03	0.05 ±0.01	0.05 ±0.01	0.28 ±0.09	ND	ND	8.50 ±1.38
30 min	0.26 ±0.07	0.27 ±0.06	0.05 ±0.01	0.15 ±0.05	0.33 ±0.05	0.04 ±0.01	ND	11.70 ±2.12
60 min	0.28 ±0.04	0.28 ±0.06	0.06 ±0.02	0.18 ±0.04	0.29 ±0.07	0.06 ±0.02	0.10 ±0.07	17.47 ±5.79
ADP-Fe^{+3} + XO+								
10 min	0.26 ±0.04	0.26 ±0.03	0.20 ±0.08	0.19 ±0.02	0.25 ±0.06	ND	ND	18.17 ±1.03
30 min	0.27 ±0.09	0.36 ±0.09	0.19 ±0.06	0.19 ±0.05	0.34 ±0.03	0.13 ±0.04	0.09 ±0.02	39.62 ±9.42
60 min	0.31 ±0.09	0.57 ±0.13	0.23 ±0.02	0.34 ±0.07	0.35 ±0.12	0.10 ±0.04	0.09 ±0.01	45.03 ±12.96
CuOOH + hematin+								
10 min	0.16 ±0.02	0.26 ±0.03	0.18 ±0.07	0.25 ±0.03	0.40 ±0.06	0.04 ±0.01	ND	25.16 ±6.01
30 min	0.27 ±0.08	0.59 ±0.14	0.23 ±0.05	0.72 ±0.16	0.73 ±0.15	0.08 ±0.02	0.24 ±0.06	59.69 ±8.02
60 min	0.44 ±0.11	0.79 ±0.19	0.22 ±0.05	0.94 ±0.26	0.88 ±0.16	0.16 ±0.02	0.46 ±0.04	76.96 ±16.97
$^{60}Co/N_2O$								
30 min	0.074 ±0.008	0.152 ±0.025	0.029 ±0.007	0.153 ±0.003	0.069 ±0.008	0.081 ±0 014	ND	0.40 ±0.10
60 min	0.085 ±0.005	0.126 ±0.014	0.024 ±0.007	0.148 ±0.010	0.065 ±0.005	0.084 ±0.015	ND	0.50 ±0.11
90 min	0.110 ±0.018	0.160 ±0.025	0.028 ±0.005	0.137 ±0.025	0.064 ±0.010	0.108 ±0.055	ND	0.49 ±0.15

ND - not determined
\+ - see text for experimental details.
* - The levels of TBAR are expressed as equivalents of malonaldehyde and are calculated from the optical densities measured at 532 nm using a molar extinction coefficient of 1.56×10^4.

TABLE 3

ANGIOTENSIN CONVERTING ENZYME ACTIVITY AND PLATING EFFICIENCY OF PEC (UNITS/10^6 CELLS)

Passage no.						
PEC		PEC clone 6				V79
2	6	2	6	8	10	12
0.129 ±0.009	0.043 ±0.006	0.111 ±0.008	0.106 ±0.005	0.094 ±0.005	0.075 ±0.008	0.025 ±0.005

TABLE 4

CYTOTOXICITY OF LINOLEIC ACID HYDROPEROXIDE, CHOLESTEROL OXIDES AND BILE ACIDS IN CELL CULTURES

	LD_{50} (uM)		
compound	endothelial	hepatocytes	fibroblasts
linoleic acid hydroperoxide	10	18	14
cholesterol α-epoxide	45	75	56
cholesterol β-epoxide	18	65	30
cholestane triol	20	60	25
7-ketocholesterol	20	65	30
3,5-cholestadiene-7-one	25	60	-
7α-hydroxycholesterol	56	210	65
cholic acid	55	110	50
lithocholic acid	58	130	-

TABLE 5

EFFECT OF CALCIUM DEFICIENT MEDIA ON CHOLESTEROL OXIDE TOXICITY IN ENDOTHELIAL CELLS
(surviving fraction of control (1.00) cells exposed for 72 hrs)

CONDITIONS	DOSE (uM) 10	20	40	60
cholesterol α-epoxide				
normal Calcium	1.05	1.13	1.12	0.67
low Calcium	1.00	1.25	1.02	1.01
cholesterol β-epoxide				
normal Calcium	0.93	0.77	0.66	0.43
low Calcium	1.15	1.17	1.03	0.91
cholestane triol				
normal Calcium	1.14	0.80	0.45	0.05
low Calcium	1.05	0.79	0.76	0.15
7-ketocholesterol				
normal Calcium	1.03	1.21	0.78	0.12
low Calcium	0.96	1.11	1.07	0.22

Table 6

CALCIUM INFLUX INTO ENDOTHELIAL CELLS
(CPM $^{45}CA^{+2}/10^6$ CELLS/MIN)

CONDITION	EARLY PHASE	LATE PHASE
CONTROL	470 ± 34	873 ± 30
CONTROL + VERAP.	314 ± 56	862 ± 52
CHOLEST. α-EPOX.	246 ± 37	660 ± 34
CHOLEST. α-EPOX. + VERAP.	314 ± 36	683 ± 27
CHOLEST. β-EPOX	258 ± 27	862 ± 70
CHOLEST. β-EPOX. + VERAP.	246 ± 29	728 ± 33
CHOLESTANE TRIOL	302 ± 52	930 ± 26
CHOLESTANE TRIOL + VERAP.	368 ± 51	1008 ± 101
LITHOCHOLIC ACID	302 ± 40	1052 ± 44
LITHOCHOLIC ACID + VERAP.	730 ± 93	1120 ± 39

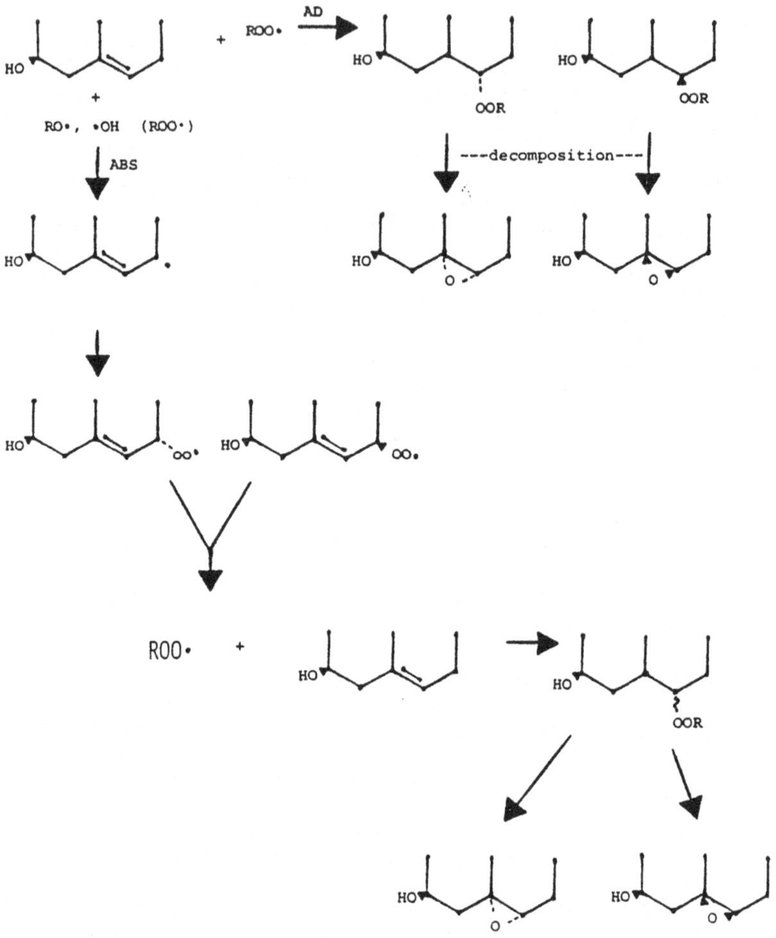

Figure 1. A scheme depicting possible mechanisms for the autoxidation of cholesterol and formation of the diastereomeric epoxides. Carbons 2 - 8 and 17 are shown for portions of sterol rings A and B. Alternate pathways for peroxide radical abstraction (ABS) or addition (AD) indicate the route to formation of the isomeric cholesterol-7-peroxy radicals. These may yield the cholesterol-7-hydroperoxides (not shown), or peroxide adducts which attack either axially or equitorially carbon 6 of the sterol. ROO$^{\cdot}$ represents either the cholesterol peroxy-radical(s) or other lipid peroxides which again attack carbon 6 of the sterol to form an unstable addition product.

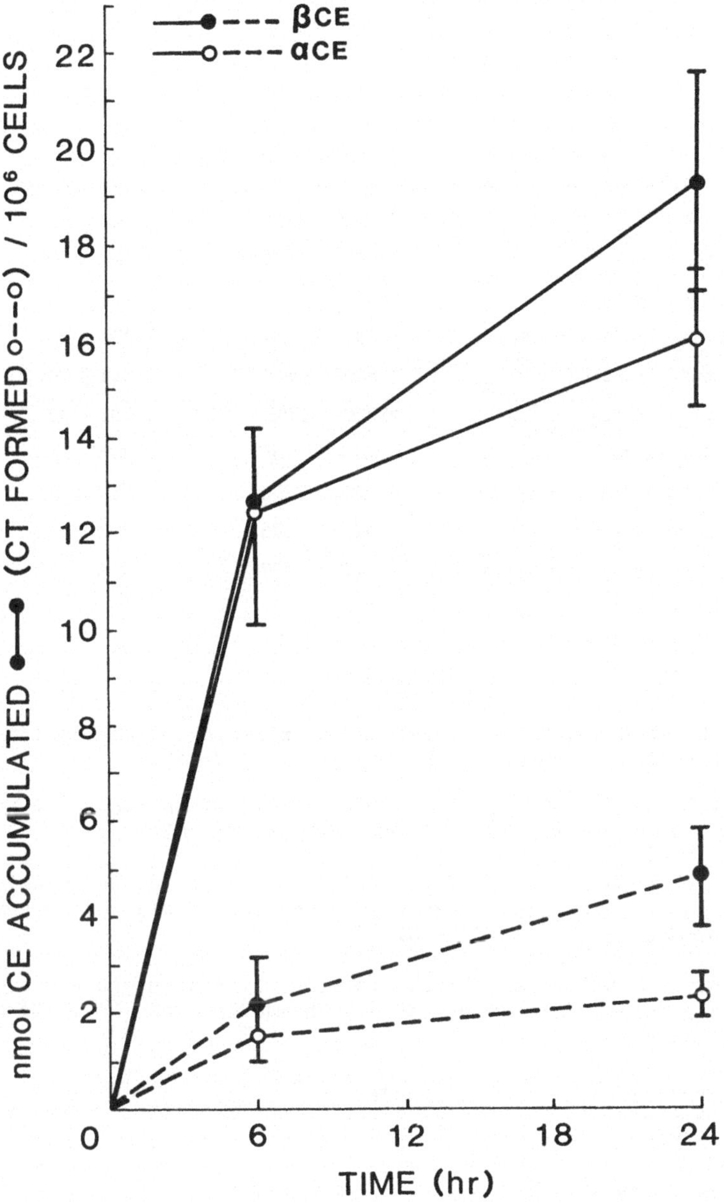

Figure 2. The uptake and conversion of the diastereomeric cholesterol epoxides by endothelial cells is indicated over a 24 hr interval. Values shown are the mean and standard deviation determined from two experiments. Cells were incubated with 10 uM of each compound containing 0.4 uCi/sample. See text for details.

Table 7

EFFLUX AND EXCHANGE-EFFLUX OF CALCIUM IN ENDOTHELIAL CELLS

CONDITION	(CPM $^{45}CA^{+2}/10^{6}$ CELLS/MIN) EARLY PHASE	LATE PHASE
CONTROL	45840 ± 4259	400 ± 58
CONTROL + VERAP.	49680 ± 3908	444 ± 64
CHOLEST. α-EPOX.	16320 ± 303	432 ± 57
CHOLEST. α-EPOX. + VERAP.	16800 ± 929	270 ± 17
CHOLEST. β-EPOX.	36980 ± 1442	414 ± 37
CHOLEST. β-EPOX. + VERAP.	42720 ± 1753	192 ± 14
CHOLESTANE TRIOL	25020 ± 909	125 ± 21
CHOLESTANE TRIOL + VERAP.	42240 ± 2700	127 ± 29
LITHOCHOLIC ACID	31320 ± 2105	148 ± 13
LITHOCHOLIC ACID + VERAP.	78000 ± 4398	299 ± 37

REFERENCES

Ansari, G.A.S., and Smith, L.L., 1976. The oxidation of cholesterol by hydroxyl radical. Photochem. Photobiol. 30:147-150.

Benditt, E.P., 1977. Implications of the monoclonal character of human atherosclerotic plaques. Am J. Pathol. 86:693-702.

Brooks, C.J.W., McKenna, R.M., Cole, W.J., McLachlan, J. and Lawrie, T.D.V., 1983. Profile analysis of oxygenated sterols in plasma and serum. Biochem. Soc. Trans. 11:700-701.

Fleckenstein, A., 1977. Specific pharmacology of calcium in myocardium, cardiac pacemakers and vascular smooth muscle. Ann. Rev. Pharmacol. Toxicol. 17:149-161.

Gray, M.F., Lawrie, T.D.V. and Brooks, C.J.W., 1971. Isolation and identification of cholesterol α-oxide and other minor sterols in human serum. Lipids. 6:836-843.

Imai, H., Werthessen, N.T., Taylor, B. and Lee, K.T., 1976. Angiotoxicity and atherosclerosis due to contaminants of USP-grade cholesterol. Arch. Pathol. Lab. Med. 100:565-571.

Jordan, R.A. and Schenkman, J.B., 1982. Relationship between malondialdehyde production and arachidonate consumption during NADPH-supported microsomal lipid peroxidation. Biochem. Pharmacol. 31:1393-1400.

Kritchevsky, D., Tepper, S.A., Klurfeld, D.M. and Story, J.A., 1979. Influence of cholesterol from various sources on experimental atherosclerosis in rabbits. Nutrition Rpts. Intl. 20:663-667.

Lo, W-B. and Black, H.S., 1972. Formation of cholesterol-derived photoproducts in human skin. J. Invest. Dermatol. 58:278-283.

Mahley, R.W., 1980. Cholesterol feeding: Effects on lipoprotein structure and metabolism. In: Atherosclerosis V. (A.M. Gotto, L.C. Smith and B. Allen, eds.) Springer Verlag, New York, pp. 641-652.

Mitropoulos, K.A. and Balasubramaniam, S., 1972. Cholesterol 7 α-hydroxylase in rat liver microsomal preparations. Eur. J. Biochem. 128:1-9.

Mitton, J.R., Scholan, N.A. and Boyd, G.S., 1971. The oxidation of cholesterol in rat liver sub-cellular particles. Eur. J. Biochem. 120:569-579.

Nagano, T. and Fridovich, I., 1985. Superoxide radical from xanthine oxidase acting upon lumazine. J. Free Rad. Biol. Med. 1:39-42.

Peng, S-K., Taylor, B., Tham, P., Werthessen, N.T. and Mikkelson, B., 1978. Effect of auto-oxidation products from cholesterol on aortic smooth muscle cells. Arch. Pathol. Lab. Med. 102:57-61.

Peterson, A.R., Peterson, H. and Heidelberger, C., 1979. Oncogenesis, mutagenesis, DNA damage and cytotoxicity in cultured mammalian cells with alkylating agents. Cancer Res. 39:131-138.

Peterson, A.R., Peterson, H., Spears, C.P., Trosko, J.E. and Sevanian, A., 1987. Mutagenic Characterization of cholesterol epoxides in Chinese hamster V79 cells. Mutation Res. (In press)

Petrakis, N.L., Gruenke, L.D. and Craig, J.C., 1981. Cholesterol and cholesterol epoxides in nipple aspirates of human breast fluid. Cancer Res. 41:2563-2565.

Ryan, U.S., Clements, E., Habliston, D. and Ryan, J.W., 1978. Isolation and culture of pulmonary artery endothelial cells. Tissue & Cell 10:535-554.

Schanne, F., Kane, A.B., Young, E.E. and Farber, J.L., 1979. Calcium dependence of toxic cell death: A final common pathway. Science 206:700-702.

Schenck, G.O., Gollnick, K. and Neumuller, O.A., 1957. Photosensitized oxidation of cholesterol. Liebig's Annalen 63:46-50.

Sevanian, A. and McLeod, L.L., 1987. Cholesterol oxidation in phospholipid membrane bilayers. Lipids (In press).

Sevanian, A., Mead, J.F. and Stein, R.A., 1979. Epoxides as products of lipid autoxidation in rat lungs. Lipids 14:634-643.

Sevanian, A. and Kim, E., 1985. Phospholipase A_2-dependent release of fatty acids from peroxidized membranes. J. Free Rad. Biol. Med. 1:263-271.

Sevanian, A. and Peterson, A.R., 1984. Cholesterol epoxide is a direct-acting mutagen. Proc. Natl. Acad. Sci. 81:4198-4202.

Smith, L.L., 1981. In: Cholesterol Autoxidation. Plenum Press, New York, pp. 49-69.

Smith, L.L. and Kulig, M.J., 1975. Sterol metabolism: On the derivation of carcinogenic sterols from cholesterol. Cancer Biochem. Biophys. 1:79-84.

Teng, J.I. and Smith, L.L., 1976. Sterol metabolism: The oxidation of cholesterol by dioxygenases. Bioorg. Chem. 5:99-119.

Tsai, L.S., Ijichi, K., Hudson, C.A. and Meehan, J.J., 1980. A method for the quantitative estimation of cholesterol α-oxide in eggs. Lipids 15:124-128.

Vandenheuval, F.A., 1963. Study of the biological structure at the molecular level with stereomodel projections I. The lipids of the myelin sheath of nerve. J. Amer. Oil Chem Soc. 40:455-471.

Watabe, T. and Sawahata, T., 1979. Biotransformation of cholesterol to cholestane-3β,5α,6β-triol via cholesterol α-epoxide in bovine adrenal cortex. J. Biol. Chem. 254:3854-3860.

Zambrano F., Fleisher, S. and Fleisher, B., 1978. Lipid composition of the golgi apparatus of rat kidney and liver in comparison with other sub-cellular organelles. Biochim. Biophys. Acta 380:357-369.

POSSIBLE IMPORTANCE OF PROTEOLYTIC SYSTEMS AS SECONDARY ANTIOXIDANT DEFENSES DURING ISCHEMIA-REPERFUSION INJURY

Kelvin J. A. Davies, Yin Zhang, and Olivier Marcillat

Institute for Toxicology & Department of Biochemistry

The University of Southern California, HSC-PSC 614-616

1985 Zonal Avenue, Los Angeles, California 90033, U.S.A.

Oxygen radicals, and other activated oxygen species, have been suggested as damaging agents during myocardial ischemia-reperfusion injury. Much attention has already been focused on lipid (per)oxidation, but here we show that proteins are also subject to oxidative damage. We have isolated novel proteolytic systems from the cytoplasm of cardiac cells, and from the cardiac mitochondrial matrix. These proteolytic systems are able to selectively recognize and degrade proteins which have undergone oxidative damage. The novel proteolytic systems exhibit no stimulation of activity with ATP, magnesium, or calcium, which are commonly found to enhance protein degradation in many cells. In contrast, the transition metal chelator EDTA strongly inhibits proteolysis, suggesting the involvement of metallo-proteases. It is suggested that these novel proteolytic systems may act to selectively degrade oxidatively damaged proteins <u>in vivo</u>, thus preventing more serious cross-linking reactions and providing amino acids for protein synthesis. Such proteolytic systems could be considered to form part of a series of "Secondary Antioxidant Defenses" which remove or repair oxidatively damaged cell components. The possible importance of such "Secondary Antioxidant Defenses" in ischemia-reperfusion injury is discussed.

INTRODUCTION

In recent years, tissue damage by oxygen radicals has become recognized as a major form of oxygen toxicity. In the past few years, the paradox that oxygen radical damage may be increased during or after the oxygen deprivation (and diminished blood flow) of ischemia, has received widespread attention (1,2). Ischemia-reperfusion injury to the heart has been a major focus of interest due to the large number of deaths attributable to coronary artery diseases and myocardial infarction. Despite such enthusiastic attention, the mechanisms by which oxygen radicals may be involved in ischemia-reperfusion injury remain largely unproven. As demonstrated by the papers presented at this conference, we have a great deal more to learn about the basic science of oxygen-radical toxicity.

The intent of this paper is to suggest a possible protective role for intracellular proteolytic systems in the process of ischemia-reperfusion injury. Particular attention will be paid to cardiac injury, since this is the theme of the conference, but most of the discussion could just as well be applied to ischemia-reperfusion injury in any organ. A proteolytic system consists of proteinases, proteases, and peptidases, and can catalyze the complete degradation of proteins to free amino acids. Proteinases recognize intact protein substrates and execute one or more initial cleavages. The large peptides produced by proteinases are substrates for proteases which further degrade them to small peptides. Peptidases conduct the final peptide bond cleavages to produce free amino acids.

Lipid peroxidation is a well established example of free radical toxicity, as is oxidative damage to RNA, DNA, and even carbohydrates. In contrast, the reactions of proteins with various radicals/oxidants have not been so extensively studied and it is sometimes assumed that proteins are not particularly susceptible to free radical damage. This assumption has been invalidated in recent years, and it is now clear that amino acids, peptides, and proteins are, indeed, vulnerable to attack by a variety of free radicals and related oxidants (3-21). Although mechanisms of damage may vary widely, it appears that oxidative processes are the common pathway for toxic reactions between free radicals and proteins. We have, therefore, used the term "oxidatively damaged proteins" to cover a wide variety of possibilities.

Antioxidant enzymes and compounds may protect proteins as efficiently as they guard lipids, nucleic acids, and carbohydrates. Nevertheless, research as shown that protein damage still occurs. Oxidation of particularly sensitive mino acid residues, aggregation or cross-linking, fragmentation, and loss of nzymatic or other functional properties are but a few of the documented xamples (3-21). At best, oxidatively damaged proteins would represent a pool useless cellular debris. More serious metabolic and immunological problems ould be created by large accumulations of protein aggregates, toxic fragments, deranged enzymes.

Since oxidatively damaged proteins serve no useful roles, one might predict hat cells would possess mechanisms for their removal. Proteolytic degradation ould be the most obvious means by which this might be achieved, with the bvious advantage that undamaged amino acids might be re-utilized. All cells re thought to contain both soluble (22-30) and membrane-bound (31,32) roteolytic enzymes, and most eukaryots also possess lysosomes which can injest nd degrade proteins (27). Many proteolytic enzymes are involved in the normal urnover of proteins, while others carry out a wide series of proteolytic ctivations. In recent years it has become increasingly apparent that several onsense or missense mutations, as well as products of certain post-ranslational modifications are also recognized and degraded by proteolytic nzymes (22-32). Thus, there is ample precedent for the intracellular egradation of damaged or abnormal proteins.

The studies of Stadtman, Levine, Rivett et al. (14,15,33-39), Dean, Wolff, al. (40,41), Rapoport et al. (42-45), Mattoo et al. (46), Kyle et al. (47), nd Fagan et.al. (48), as well as the investigations from our own laboratory 8-21,49-54), all indicate that several cell types (and subcellular rganelles) can conduct the recognition and selective degradation of xidatively damaged proteins. In our own work (18-21,49-54) proteolytic ystems are envisioned as secondary defenses which act to prevent the ccumulation of oxidatively damaged proteins, and to degrade potentially toxic protein fragments. Thus, proteolytic systems may have an important role in overall antioxidant defenses. Proteolytic systems could be of great importance when primary antioxidants, such as superoxide dismutase(55), glutathione peroxidase (56), vitamin E (57,58), uric acid (59-61), etc., are insufficient to cope with a major oxidative stress. Even the normal levels of oxidants which cells produce or encounter may necessitate constant protein turnover, since no antioxidant is likely to be 100% effective in preventing protein damage. In this paper we present evidence that the cytoplasm of mammalian heart muscle cells, and the matrix of cardiac mitochondria, contain soluble proteolytic systems which can preferentially recognize and degrade oxidatively damaged proteins. The possible protective role which these secondary antioxidant defense systems may play, in ischemia-reperfusion injury, is discussed.

MATERIALS & METHODS

Preparation of Cardiac Cytoplasm and Mitochondrial Matrix - Beef hearts were cleaned of fat and connective tissue, and cut into one inch cubes. The tissue was then passed through an electric meat grinder, rinsed with isolation buffer (0.25M sucrose, 1.0mM EDTA, 10.0mM HEPES, pH 7.4), and drained. Three hundred grams of ground heart was next homogenized, in 1.5L of isolation buffer using an electric blender at maximal speed for 30 seconds. The pH was maintained at 7.4 by addition of 6N KOH. The homogenate was centrifuged at 1,400 x g (10min) and the supernatant was filtered through gauze and then centrifuged at 7,500 x g (10min). The pellet from this first 7,500 x g centrifugation (a crude mitochondrial pellet) was used for preparation of the mitochondrial matrix (*vide infra*). The supernatant from the 7,500 x g centrifugation (a crude cytoplasmic preparation) was next centrifuged at 100,000 x g to remove any remaining mitochondria, and other cellular organelle

The 100,000 x g supernatant was then studied as representative of the cardiac cell cytoplasm.

The crude (7,500 x g) mitochondrial pellet was "washed" by another centrifugation at 7,500 x g in 100ml of 50mM sodium phosphate buffer (pH 7.4). The pellet was resuspended in 15ml of phosphate buffer containing 5mM $MnCl_2$, 10mM $MgCl_2$, and 1mM sodium succinate, and sonnicated (4 x 40 second bursts) under an atmosphere of argon. Sonicated mitochondria were centrifuged at 7,500 x g to remove any unbroken organelles, and the membranes (pellet) were removed by centrifugation at 100,000 x g. The remaining supernatant was taken to represent the mitochondrial matrix fraction.

Exposure of Proteins to Active Oxygen Species - Bovine serum albumin (BSA), hemoglobin (Hb), and superoxide dismutase (SOD) were obtained from Sigma Chemical Co. The proteins were reductively methylated, with ^{3}H-formaldehyde and sodium borohydride, and then extensively dialyzed as previously described (18-21,49-54). BSA and Hb were exposed to the hydroxyl radical (•OH) by ^{60}Co radiation under an atmosphere of N_2O (18-21,51,54); the exposure was 10nmol •OH/nmol protein. SOD was inactivated by exposure to 30mM H_2O_2 during 30min incubation at room temperature. The proteins were dialyzed before measurements of proteolytic susceptibility were made.

Measurements of Proteolysis - ^{3}H-labeled proteins were incubated with aliquots of cardiac cytoplasm or mitochondrial matrix, at 37°C for 1hr. All incubations involved 0.01ml of ^{3}H-protein substrate (3.3mg/ml), 0.06ml cytoplasm or mitochondrial matrix fraction (0.72mg protein), and 0.06ml of 75mM Tris buffer (pH 8.0). Incubations were terminated by the addition of .85ml of 12% trichloroacetic acid (to precipitate intact protein), and 0.06ml of 3% BSA (as carrier). Protein degradation was measured as the percent of initial acid-precipitable counts which were converted to (low molecular weight) acid-soluble forms, using liquid scintillation techniques.

RESULTS

The cytoplasm of cardiac cells was found to contain proteolytic enzymes which could degrade normal proteins (BSA, Hb, SOD) at a low rate. When these same proteins were oxidatively damaged by exposure to •OH or H_2O_2, their rates of degradation increased six to ten fold (Fig. 1). Thus, cardiac cells contain soluble proteolytic systems which can recognize, and preferentialy degrade, oxidatively damaged proteins.

The experiments of Fig. 1 were conducted in the absence of ATP, Mg^{2+}, and Ca^{2+}. These agents have been found to stimulate the degradation of several proteins in red blood cells and bacteria (22-32). When ATP-Mg^{2+} or Ca^{2+} were added to cardiac cytosol, we observed no increase in the degradation of •OH-treated BSA (Fig. 2). These results indicate that the degradation of oxidatively damaged proteins in the heart cytoplasm is conducted by ATP-independent, and Ca^{2+}-independent proteolytic systems. Leupeptin is a well known inhibitor of lysosomal, and Ca^{2+} activated thiol proteases (27,28). As shown in Fig. 2, leupeptin had no effect on the degradation of •OH-modified BSA, indicating that lysosomal contamination and Ca^{2+} activated thiol proteases cannot explain our results.

In contrast to the negative results above, the transition metal chelator EDTA caused approximately a 90% inhibition of the degradation of •OH-modified BSA (Fig. 2). This result may indicate the involvement of a metallo-enzyme (or enzymes) in proteolysis. We have previously observed inhibition by several metal chelators when studying the degradation of oxidatively damaged proteins in red blood cell, and bacterial extracts (18-21,50-54). Thus, metallo-proteases, with activity against oxidized proteins, may be of widespread biological inportance.

The soluble matrix fraction of cardiac mitochondria was also tested for the presence of proteolytic enzymes with activity against oxidatively damaged proteins. As shown in Fig. 3, the degradation of oxidatively damaged (•OH or H_2O_2) BSA, Hb, and SOD was seven to ten fold greater than the degradation of untreated proteins. As with heart cytoplasm (Fig. 1) no ATP-Mg^{2+} or Ca^{2+} were added to the mitochondrial matrix. The results of Fig. 3, therefore, indicate the presence of a soluble, ATP- and Ca^{2+}-independent, proteolytic system in mitochondria, which can preferentially degrade oxidatively damaged proteins.

It should be emphasized that the experiments of Figs. 1, 2,and 3 involved exposure of BSA, Hb, and SOD to •OH or H_2O_2 in the absence of cardiac material; the modified proteins were then added to heart cytoplasm or mitochondrial matrix fractions. At no time were cytoplasm or matrix fractions directly exposed to •OH or H_2O_2. Thus, the experiments of Figs. 1-3 represent true measures of the proteolytic susceptibility of BSA, Hb, and SOD in both the native state, and the oxidatively damaged state.

DISCUSSION

We propose that cardiac cytoplasm, and the cardiac mitochondrial matrix, contain soluble proteolytic systems which can conduct the selective recognition and degradation of oxidatively damaged proteins. We further propose that these proteolytic systems are ATP-independent and Ca^{2+}-independent, and may include metallo-proteases. The experimental results presented in this paper appear (to us) to be entirely consistent with such proposals.

We have previously reported the existence of similar, ATP- and Ca^{2+}-independent, soluble proteolytic systems in erythrocytes, reticulocytes, and E. coli (18-21,49-54). These proteolytic systems all appear to contain metallo-proteases and serine proteases, and are typically inhibited by hemin (18-21,49-54). In addition, we have observed increased rates of mitochondrial protein degradation following exposure to oxygen radicals (50,51,54). Other investigators have also reported oxidant-induced proteolysis in bacteria, mitochondria, chloroplasts, and red cells (33-48). Based on such findings, we (18-21,49-54) and others (39,41) have suggested that the selective proteolytic degradation of oxidatively damaged proteins may be a widespread biological phenomenon.

Since oxidatively damaged proteins appear to be preferential substrates for degradation (by soluble proteolytic enzymes) it is important to define the form(s) of damage which is/are recognized. At present, the most plausible explanation available is that oxygen radicals (and other oxidants) can cause protein denaturation, and can increase protein hydrophobicity. These (related) changes in conformation and charge may provide a simple and universal signal for proteolytic degradation (18-21,39,49-54). Additionally, certain oxygen radicals (in the presence of molecular oxygen) can cause direct fragmentation of proteins, and such protein fragments may be excellent substrates for proteolytic degradation (18-21,41,51,54).

Although the association between ischemia-reperfusion injury and oxygen radical production/damage in the heart remains somewhat circumstantial, the probability of a causal relationship appears to be quite good (1,2). If oxygen radicals are, indeed, generated following cardiac ischemia or a myocardial infarction, we suggest that cardiac proteins should be considered as potential targets for damage. We further suggest that the role of soluble (ATP- and Ca^{2+}-independent) proteolytic systems may be to selectively remove such damaged proteins.

Clearly, if an ischemia-reperfusion injury were so great that large areas of cardiac tissue died, there would be little "physiological" advantage in selective degradation. Furthermore, extensive protein damage would be likely to involve proteolytic enzymes, which may be as susceptible as other proteins to oxidative modification. Thus, we propose that the main role of these proteolytic systems may be to act in the early stages of ischemia-reperfusion njury. The degradation of oxidized proteins would provide amino acids (those hich are not modified) for protein synthesis. Early degradation of xidatively damaged proteins, which may contain carbon-centered radicals, may rovide an important protection against cross-linking reactions which serve to ropagate damage (18-21,51,54). Degradation of potentially toxic protein ragments (formed by direct scission reactions following protein peroxidation) ay also protect against the propagation of damage (18-21,41,51,54).

Our studies (and speculations) about proteolytic systems, and recent nvestigations of the repair of oxidatively damaged lipids (62,63) and nucleic cids (64), suggest that we should expand our view of antioxidant defenses. ntioxidants are classically considered to be those enzymes or compounds which rectly react with free radicals or oxidants to prevent initiation or ropagation rections; such enzymes and compounds may be considered to be "Primary Antioxidant Defenses". Superoxide dismutase(55), glutathione peroxidase (56 tamin E (57,58), uric acid (59-61), and others would all fit in the "Primary ntioxidant" class. In contrast, enzymes which remove and/or repair oxidative amage may be considered to be part of "Secondary Antioxidant Defenses". oteolytic systems, phospholipase A_2, and DNA repair systems, are suggested examples of "Secondary Antioxidant Defenses". These ideas are presented in formalized manner in Table 1.

It will be noted that the "Secondary Antioxidant Defense" category of able 1 contains several question marks. These serve both to indicate missing formation and to delineate those areas whch will require intensive study in e future. For the present, Table 1 can be considered only as a proposal ich may help to point out possible relationships between various components antioxidant defenses, and which (it is hoped) may suggest further periments. Of particular interest is the question of inducibility of nzymatic) "Secondary Antioxidant Defenses". Evidence has already been presented to suggest that DNA repair systems may be induced by exposure to oxidants (64) and similar studies with proteolytic systems are now in progress in our laboratory.

TABLE 1

Proposed System of Primary and Secondary Antioxidant Defenses

Primary Defenses

1. Antioxidant Enzymes - SOD, glutathione peroxidase, etc.
2. Antioxidant Compounds - vitamin E, uric acid, β-carotene, etc.

Secondary Defenses

1. Proteolytic Systems - proteinases, proteases, peptidases, ?
2. Lipolytic Enzymes - phospholipase A_2, ?
3. DNA Repair Systems - ?

In summary, we have presented data which indicate the presence of novel proteolytic systems in the cytoplasm of cardiac cells and in the matrix of cardiac mitochondria. These soluble proteolytic systems appear to recognize, and preferentialy degrade, oxidatively damaged proteins. The proteolytic systems are not stimulated by ATP-Mg^{2+} or by Ca^{2+}, but are strongly inhibited by the metal chelator EDTA; suggesting the involvement of metallo-proteases. We speculate that these proteolytic systems may act as "Secondary Antioxidant Defenses" during ischemia-reperfusion injury, by selectively removing oxidized proteins and preventing more serious cross-linking reactions. We hope that these proposals will stimulate further inquiry in the area of protein oxidation and proteolysis during cardiac ischemia.

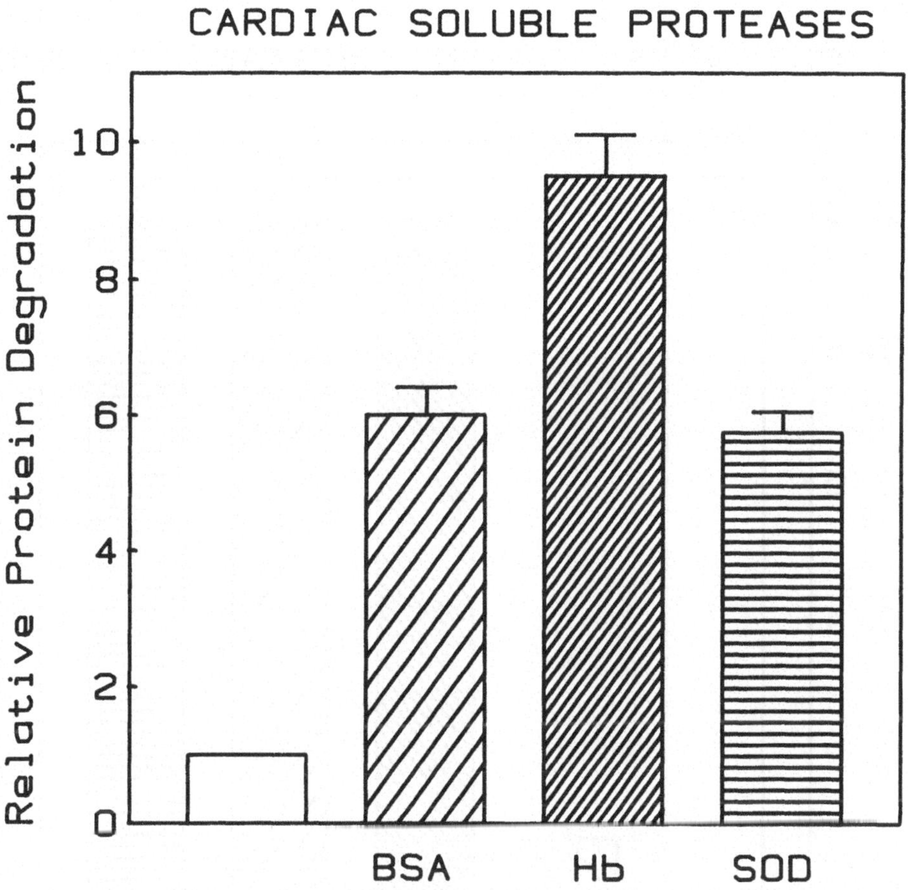

g. 1 Degradation of Untreated and Oxidatively Damaged Proteins in a Cardiac Cytoplasmic Fraction. BSA and Hb were oxidatively modified by exposure to •OH, whereas SOD was inactivated with H_2O_2. The degradation of untreated, and oxidatively damaged proteins was then assessed during incubation with a cardiac cell cytoplasmic fraction. The degradation of untreated proteins (column one, unlabeled) has been artificially set at a value of 1. The relative degradation of oxidatively damaged BSA, SOD, and Hb is expressed as multiples of the degradation rate for untreated samples. The values are means ± SE's of three independent determinations. All procedures are detailed in the Materials & Methods section.

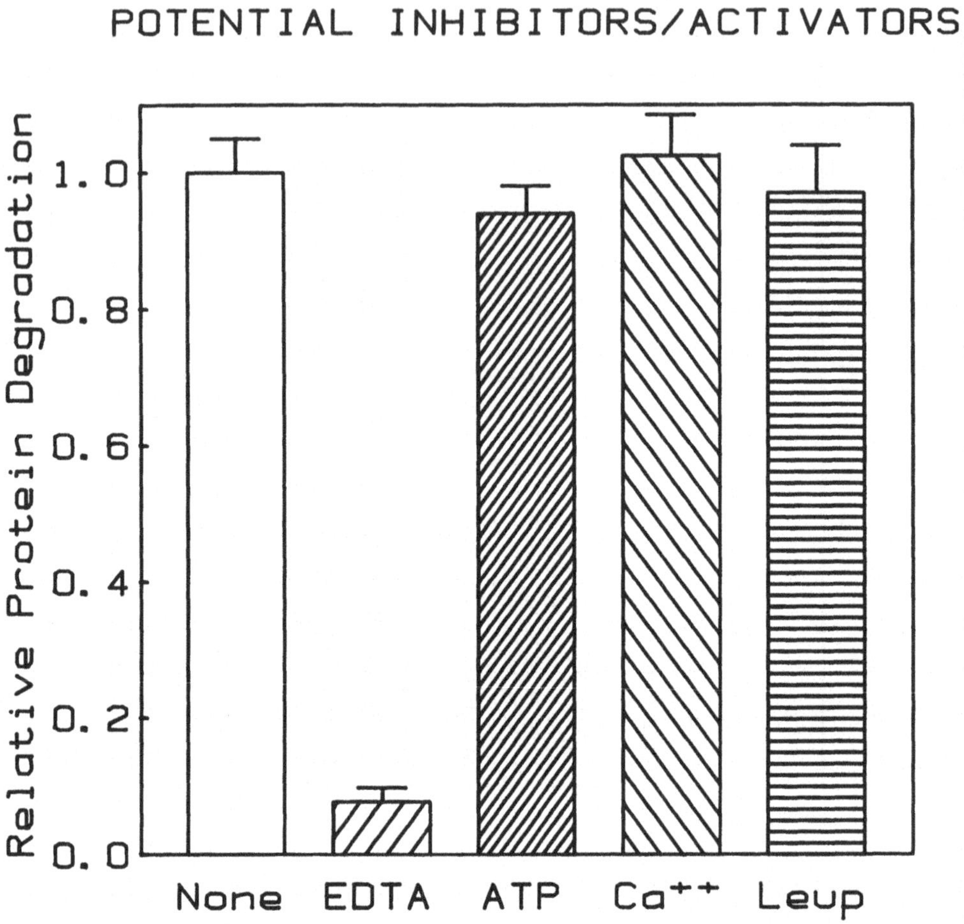

Fig. 2 Effects of Various Agents on the Degradation of Oxidatively Damaged BSA by the Cardiac Cell Cytoplasmic Fraction. The degradation of •OH-treated BSA was measured as described in Fig. 1. The value for this degradation rate, without additions ("None"), has been artificially set at 1.0, and the relative effects of various agents are shown as fractions. Where used, EDTA (10.0mM), ATP (5.0mM in the presence of 5.0mM Mg^{2+}), Ca^{2+} (1.0mM), or leupeptin (10.0µg/ml) were added to the cytoplasmic fraction prior to incubation with •OH-modified BSA. The data are means ± SE's of three independent determinations.

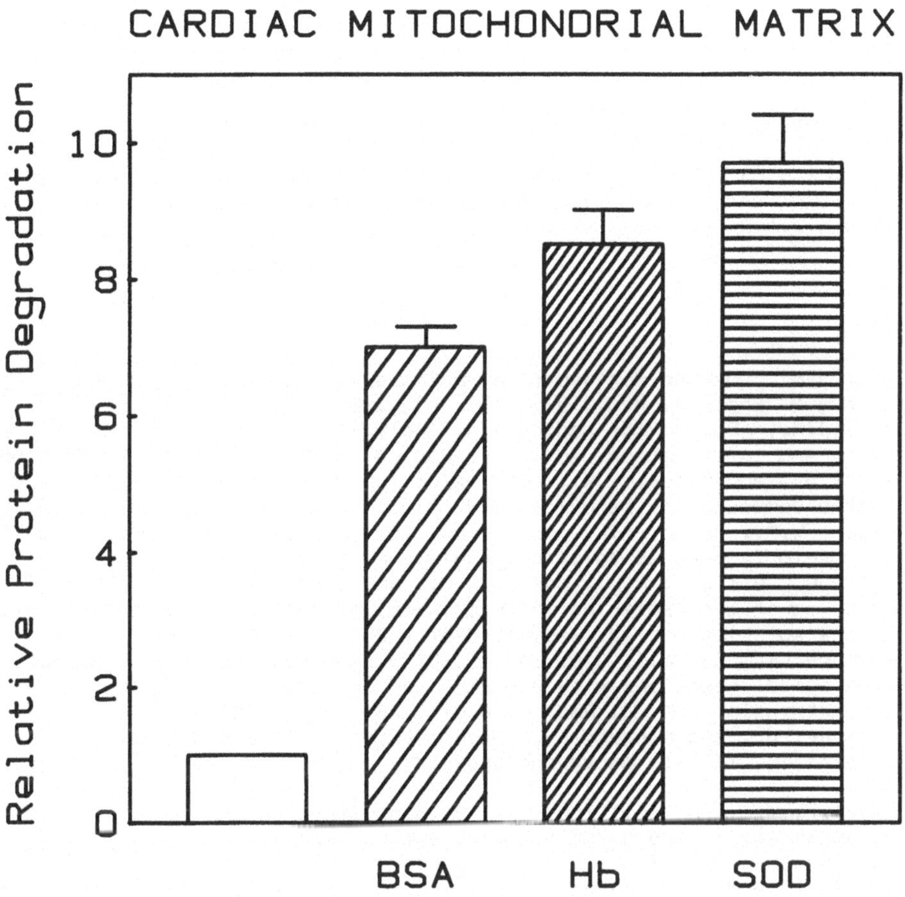

Fig. 3 Degradation of Untreated and Oxidatively Damaged Proteins in a Cardiac Mitochondrial Matrix Fraction. BSA and Hb were oxidatively modified by exposure to •OH, whereas SOD was inactivated with H_2O_2. The degradation of untreated, and oxidatively damaged proteins was then assessed during incubation with a cardiac mitochondrial matrix fraction. The degradation of untreated proteins (column one, unlabeled) has been artificially set at a value of 1. The relative degradation of oxidatively damaged BSA, SOD, and Hb is expressed as multiples of the degradation rate for untreated samples. The values are means ± SE's of three independent determinations. All procedures are detailed in the Materials & Methods section.

ACKNOWLEDGEMENTS

We wish to express our thanks to the organizers of this conference for providing us with the opportunity to participate. This research was supported by grant numbers ES 03598 and ES 03785 from The National Institutes of Health (U.S.A.) to K.J.A.D.

REFERENCES

1. McCord, J.M., Oxygen-derived free radicals in post-ischemic tissue injury, N. Engl. J. Med., 312, 159-163, 1985.
2. McCord, J.M., Superoxide radical: A likely link between reperfusion injury and inflammation, Adv. Free Radical Biol. Med., 2, 325-345, 1986.
3. Gross, A.J., and Sizer, I.W., The oxidation of tyramine, tyrosine, and related compounds by peroxidase, J. Biol. Chem., 234, 1611-1614, 1959.
4. Garrison, W.M., Jayko, M.E., and Bennett, W., Radiation-induced oxidation of protein in aqueous solution, Radiation Research, 16, 483-502, 1962.
5. Adams, G.E., Willson, R.L., Bisby, R.H., and Cundall, R.B., On the mechanism of the radiation-induced inactivation of ribonuclease in dilute aqueous solution Int. J. Radiat. Biol., 20, 405-415, 1971.
6. Baverstock, K., Cundall, R.B., Adams, G.E., and Redpath, J.L., Selective free radical reactions with proteins and enzymes: the inactivation of α-chymotrypsin, Int. J. Radiat. Biol., 26, 39-46, 1974.
7. Schuessler, H., and Herget, A., Oxygen effect in the radiolysis of proteins: I. lactate dehydrogenase, Int. J. Radiat. Biol., 37, 71-80, 1980.
8. Schuessler, H., and Schilling, K., Oxygen effect in the radiolysis of proteins; II. bovine serum albumin, Int. J. Radiat. Biol., 45, 267-281, 1984.
9. Butler, J., Land, E.J., Prutz, W.A., and Swallow, A.J., Charge transfer between tryptophan and tyrosine in proteins, Biochim. Biophys. Acta, 705, 150-162, 1982.
10. Boguta, G., and Dancewicz, A.M., Radiolytic and enzymatic dimerization of tyrosyl residues in insulin, ribonuclease, papain, and collagen, Int. J. Radiat. Biol., 43, 249-265, 1983.
11. Garner, W.H., Garner, M.H., and Spector, A., H_2O_2-induced uncoupling of bovine lens Na+,K+-ATPase. Proc. Natl. Acad. Sci. USA, 80, 2044-2048, 1983.
12. Shinar, E., Navok, T., and Chevion, M., The analogous mechanisms of enzymatic inactivation induced by ascorbate and superoxide in the presence of copper, J. Biol. Chem., 258, 14778-14783, 1983.
13. Wickens, D.G., Norden, A.G., Lunec, J., and Dormandy, T.L., Fluorescence changes in human gamma-globulin induced by free radical activity, Biochim. Biophys. Acta, 742, 607-616, 1983.
14. Levine, R.L., Oxidative inactivation of glutamine synthetase: I. inactivation is due to loss of one histidine residue, J. Biol. Chem., 258, 11823-11827, 1983.
15. Nakamura, K., and Stadtman, E.R., Oxidative inactivation of glutamine synthetase subunits, Proc. Natl. Acad. Sci. USA, 81, 2011-2015, 1984.
16. Gajewski, E., Dizdaroglu, M., Krutzsch, H., and Simic, M.G., OH radical-

induced crosslinks of methionine peptides, Int. J. Radiat. Biol., 46, 47-55, 1984.

.7. Zs.-Nagy, I., and Floyd, R.A., Hydroxyl free radical reactions with amino acids and proteins studied by electron spin resonance spectroscopy and spin trapping, Biochim. Biophys. Acta, 790, 238-250, 1984.

18. Davies, K.J.A., Protein damage and degradation by oxygen radicals: I. general aspects, J. Biol. Chem., 1987 (in press).

19. Davies, K.J.A., Delsignore, M.E., and Lin, S.W. Protein damage and degradation by oxygen radicals: II. primary structure, J. Biol. Chem., 1987 (in press).

0. Davies, K.J.A., and Delsignore, M.E., Protein damage and degradation by oxygen radicals: III. secondary and tertiary structure, J. Biol. Chem., 1987 (in press).

1. Davies, K.J.A., Lin, S.W., and Pacifici, R., Protein damage and degradation by oxygen radicals: IV. degradation of denatured protein, J. Biol. Chem., 1987 (in press).

2. Goldberg, A.L., and Dice, F.J., Intracellular protein degradation in mammalian and bacterial cells, Ann. Rev. Biochem., 43, 835-869, 1974.

3. Goldberg, A.L., and St. John, A.C., Intracellular protein degradation in mammalian and bacterial cells: Part 2, Ann. Rev. Biochem., 45, 747-803, 1976.

4. Goldberg, A.L., Voellmy, R., and Sreedhara Swamy, K.H., Studies of the pathway for protein degradation in Escherichia coli and mammalian cells, in Biological Functions of Proteinases, Holzer, H., and Tschesche, H., eds., Springer-Verlag, Berlin, 1979, 35-48.

5. Goldberg, A.L., Strnad, N.P., and Sreehara Swamy, K.H., Studies of the ATP dependence of protein degradation in cells and cell extracts, in Protein Degradation in Health and Disease, Ciba Foundation Symposium 75, Exerpta Medica/Elsevier, North Holland, 1980, 227-251.

6. Hershko, A., Ciechanover, A., Heller, H., Haas, A.L., and Rose, I.A., Proposed role of ATP in protein breakdown: Conjugation of proteins with multiple chains of the polypeptide of ATP-dependent proteolysis, Proc. Natl. Acad. Sci. USA, 77, 1783-1786, 1980.

7. Hershko, A., and Ciechanover, A., Mechanisms of intracellular protein breakdown, Ann. Rev. Biochem., 51, 335-364, 1982.

8. Pontremoli, S., Melloni, E., Salamino, F., Sparatore, B., Michetti, M., Benatti, U., Morelli, A., and De Flora, A., Identification of proteolytic activities in the cytosolic compartment of mature human erythrocytes, Eur. J. Biochem., 110, 421-430, 1980.

9. Mc Kay, M.J., Daniels, R.S., and Hipkiss, A.R., Breakdown of aberrant protein in rabbit reticulocytes decreases with cell age. Biochem. J., 188, 279-283, 1980.

0. McKay, M.J., and Hipkiss, A.R., ATP-independent proteolysis of globin cyanogen bromide peptides in rabbit reticulocyte cell-free extracts, Eur. J. Biochem., 125, 567-573, 1982.

1. Pontremoli, S., Salamino, F., Sparatore, B., Melloni, E., Morelli, A., Benatti, U., and De Flora, A., Isolation and partial characterization of three acidic proteinases in erythrocyte membranes, Biochem. J., 181, 559-568, 1979.

2. Melloni, E., Sparatore, B., Salamino, F., Michetti, M., and Pontremoli, S., Proteolysis of human reticulocyte membrane proteins: Evidence for a physiological role of the acid endopeptidases, Arch. Biochem. Biophys, 218, 579-584, 1982.

3. Levine, R.L., Oliver, C.N., Fulks, R.M., and Stadtman, E.R., Turnover of bacterial glutamine synthetase: Oxidative inactivation precedes

proteolysis, Proc. Natl. Acad. Sci. USA, 78, 2120-2124, 1981.
34. Fucci, L., Oliver, C.N., Coon, M.J., and Stadtman, E.R., Inactivation of key metabolic enzymes by mixed-function oxidation reactions: Possible implication in protein turnover and ageing, Proc. Natl. Acad. Sci. USA, 80, 1521-1525, 1983.
35. Levine, R.L., Oxidative modification of glutamine synthetase: II. Characterization of the ascorbate model system, J. Biol. Chem., 258, 11828-11833, 1983.
36. Rivett, A.J., Preferential degradation of the oxidatively modified form of glutamine synthetase by intracellular mammalian proteases, J. Biol. Chem., 260, 300-305, 1985.
37. Stadtman, E.R., and Wittenberger, M.E., Inactivation of Escherichia coli glutamine synthetase by xanthine oxidase, nicotinate hydroxylase, horseradish peroxidase, or glucose oxidase: Effects of ferredoxin, putidaredoxin, and menadione, Arch. Biochem. Biophys., 239, 379-387, 1985
38. Farber, J.M., and Levine,R.L., Oxidative modification of the glutamine synthetase of E. coli enhances its susceptibility to proteolysis, Fed. Proc., 41, 865, 1982.
39. Stadtman, E.R., Oxidation of proteins by mixed-function oxidation systems: Implication in protein turnover, ageing and neutrophil function, Trends Biol. Sci. (TIBS), 11, 11-12, 1986.
40. Dean, R.T., and Pollak, J.K., Endogenous free radical generation may influence proteolysis in mitochondria, Biochem. Biophys. Res. Commun., 126, 1082-1089, 1985.
41. Wolff, S.P., Garner, A., and Dean, R.T., Free radicals, lipids, and protein degradation, Trends Biol. Sci. (TIBS), 11, 27-31, 1986.
42. Rapoport, S., Schewe, T., Wiesner, R., Halangk, W., Ludwig, P., Janicke-Hohne, M., Tannert, Chr., Hiebsch, Ch., and Klatt, D., Lipoxygenase of Reticulocytes. Purification, characterization and biological dynamics of the lipoxygenase; its identity with respect to respiratory inhibitors of the reticulocyte, Eur. J. Biochem., 96, 545-561, 1979.
43. Rapoport, S., Muller, M., Dumdey, R., and Rathmann, J., Nitrogen economy and the metabolism of serine and glycine in reticulocytes of rabbits, Eur. J. Biochem, 108, 449-455, 1980.
44. Muller, M., Dubiel, W., Rathmann, J., and Rapoport, S., Determination and characteristics of energy-dependent proteolysis in rabbit reticulocytes, Eur. J. Biochem., 109, 405-410, 1980.
45. Dubiel, W., Muller, M., and Rapoport, S., ATP-dependent proteolysis of reticulocyte mitochondria is preceded by the attack of lipoxygenase, Biochem. Internat., 3, 165-171, 1981.
46. Mattoo, A.K., Hoffman-Falk, H., Marder, J.B., and Edelman, M., Regulation of protein metabolism: Coupling of photosynthetic electron transport to i vivo degradation of the rapidly metabolized 32-kilodalton protein of the chloroplast membrane, Proc. Natl. Acad. Sci. USA, 81, 1380-1386, 1984.
47. Kyle, D.J., Ohad, I., and Arntzen, C.J., Membrane protein damage and repair: Selective loss of a quinone-protein function in chloroplast membranes, Proc. Natl. Acad. Sci. USA, 81, 4070-4075, 1984.
48. Fagan, J.M., Waxman, L., and Goldberg, A.L., Red blood cells contain a pathway for the degradation of oxidant-damaged hemoglobin that does not require ATP or ubiquitin, J. Biol. Chem., 261, 5705-5713, 1986.
49. Davies, K.J.A., Free radicals and protein degradation in human red blood cells, in Cellular and Metabolic Aspects of Aging: The Red Cell as a Model, Eaton, J.W., Konzen, D.K., and White, J.G., eds., pp. 15-27, Alan R. Liss, New York, 1985.
50. Davies, K.J.A., The role of intracellular proteolytic systems in

antioxidant defenses, in Superoxide and Superoxide Dismutase in Chemistry, Biology, and Medicine, Rotilio, G., ed., pp. 443-450, Elsevier, Amsterdam, 1986.

51. Davies, K.J.A., Proteolytic systems may function as secondary antioxidant defenses: An hypothesis, J. Free Radicals Biol. Med., 2, 155-173, 1986.

52. Davies, K.J.A., and Goldberg, A.L., Oxygen radicals stimulate proteolysis and lipid peroxidation by independent mechanisms in erythrocytes, J. Biol. Chem., 1987 (in press).

53. Davies, K.J.A., and Goldberg, A.L., Proteins damaged by oxygen radicals are rapidly degraded in extracts of red blood cells, J. Biol. Chem., 1987 (in press).

54. Davies, K.J.A., Proteolytic systems as secondary antioxidant defenses: Concepts, methods, and evidence, in Cellular Antioxidant Defense Mechanisms, Chow,C.K., ed., CRC Press, Boca Raton, 1987 (in press).

55. Fridovich, I., Oxygen radicals, hydrogen peroxide, and oxygen toxicity, in Free Radicals in Biology, Pryor, W.A., ed., Vol. 1, pp.239-277, Academic Press, New York, 1976.

56. Cohen, G., and Hochstein, P., Glutathione peroxidase: The primary agent for the elimination of hydrogen peroxide in erythrocytes, Biochemistry, 2, 1420-1428, 1963.

57. Quintanilha, A.T., Packer, L., Davies, J.M.S., Racanelli, T.L., and Davies, K.J.A., Membrane effects of vitamin E deficiency: Bioenergetic and surface charge density studies of skeletal muscle and liver mitochondria, Ann. NY Acad. Sci., 393, 32-47, 1982.

58. Davies, K.J.A., Quintanilha, A.T., Brooks, G.A., and Packer, L., Free radicals and tissue damage produced by exercise, Biochem. Biophys. Res. Commun., 107, 1198-1205, 1982.

59. Ames, B.N., Cathcart, E., Schwiers, E., and Hochstein, P., Uric acid provides an antioxidant defense in humans against oxidant-and radical-caused aging and cancer: A hypothesis, Proc. Natl. Acad. Sci. USA, 78, 6858-6862, 1981.

60. Sevanian, A., Davies, K.J.A., and Hochstein, P., Conservation of vitamin C by uric acid in blood, J. Free Radicals Biol. Med., 1, 117-124, 1985.

61. Davies, K.J.A., Sevanian, A., Muakkassah-Kelly, S.F., and Hochstein, P., Uric acid-iron complexes: A new aspect of the antioxidant functions of uric acid, Biochem. J., 235, 747-754, 1986.

62. Sevanian, A., Muakkassah-Kelly, S.F., and Montestruque, S., Influence of Phospholipase A_2 and Glutathione Peroxidase on the Elimination of Membrane Lipid Peroxides, Arch. Biochem. Biophys., 223, 441-452, 1983.

63. Sevanian, A., and Kim, E., Phospholipase A_2 Dependent Release of Fatty Acids from Peroxidized Membranes, J. Free Radicals Biol. Med., 1, 263-271, 1985.

64. Demple, B., and Halbrook, J., Inducible repair of oxidative DNA damage in E. coli, Nature, 304, 466-468, 1983.

ABBREVIATIONS USED

Bovine serum albumin (BSA), superoxide dismutase (SOD), hemoglobin (Hb), hydroxyl radical (•OH)

INHIBITION BY SOME SYNTHETIC ANTIOXIDANTS OF THE AGONIST-INDUCED ACTIVATION OF ASPIRINATED PLATELETS AND OF THE DEPOLARIZATION-INDUCED RELEASE OF NEUROTRANSMITTER FROM BRAIN SYNAPTOSOMES.

Adolfo Alexandre, M. Gabriella Doni°, Franco Zoccarato and Renzo Deana

Institute of Biological Chemistry, C.N.R. Unit for the Study of the Physiology of Mitochondria, °Institute of Human Physiology, University of Padova, 35131 Padova, Italy.

Abstract.

We present observations on the action of some synthetic antioxidants on the functions of human platelets and guinea pig cerebral cortical synaptosomes.

The effects of BHT (2,3-tert-butyl-4-methoxyphenol), BHA (2,6-di-tert-butyl-4-methilphenol), NDGA (nordihydroguaiaretic acid) and of the one-electron donor I,I'-dimethylferrocene were studied in aspirinated human platelets challenged with physiological stimuli such as thrombin, platelet activating factor and vasopressin. The responses to such stimuli, namely the increase in cytosolic Ca^{++}, shape change, aggregation and secretion of intracellular granules were all strongly inhibited by these agents. The inhibitory effect could be observed also on the agonist-promoted cytosolic Ca^{++} increase originating from intracellular stores in experiments performed in the presence of EGTA. It is known that the activation of protein kinase C (i.e. with phorbol ester) promotes platelet aggregation and the secretion of cytosolic granules in the absence of cytosolic Ca^{++} increases. Also this effect has been shown to be antioxidant sensitive.

Agonist-promoted activation of aspirinated platelets does not involve the action of metabolites of the cycloxygenase or of the lipoxygenase pathways. It is therefore suggested that other still unknown free radical-dependent processes are involved in the mechanism of platelet activation.

The effect of BHT has been tested on the depolarization-induced cytosolic Ca^{++} increase and exocytosis of the neurotransmitter glutamate from guinea pig cerebral cortex synaptosomes. Also these processes appear to be significantly affected by this phenolic antioxidant.

Introduction

Much research has been devoted to platelet physiology in the last several years, owing to their central role in the process of clot formation and to their involvement in the onset of many pathological processes.

Different stimuli operate a receptor-mediated activation of blood platelets, the common outcome of the process being the formation of aggregates. Several well characterized events occur quite rapidly upon interaction of platelets with activating agents (such as thrombin, collagen, platelet activating factor, vasopressin, ADP etc.) including a sudden increase of the cytosolic Ca^{2+} concentration, a platelet shape change, exocytosis of secretory granules and aggregation (Rink and Hallam, 1984). The rise of the cytosolic Ca^{2+} is partly due to calcium influx from the extracellular space and partly to a release from intracellular stores, represented by the dense tubular system, which derives from the endoplasmic reticulum of the magacariocytes (Hallam et al., 1984 a; Hallam et al., 1984 b).

Much progress has been done in recent years in the understanding of the biochemical events leading to platelet activation (Berridge and Irvine, 1984; Brass and Joseph, 1985). Upon binding to specific receptors on the plasma membrane, agonists activate (probably via the intervention of a GTP-binding protein) a phosphodiesterase which specifically splits polyphosphoinositide (mainly phosphatidyl inositol-4,5-diphosphate) generating the two second messengers 1,2 diacylglycerol and inositol 1,4,5 Trisphosphate (IP_3), activators of a Ca-phospholipid dependent protein kinase (protein kinase C) and of Ca^{2+} release from the intracellular endoplasmic reticulum respectively (Brass and Joseph, 1985; Nishizuka, 1984; Israels, 1985; Aduniah and Dean, 1985). The increased cytosolic Ca^{2+} and the protein kinase C induced phosphorylation of some target proteins jointly cooperate, via the triggering of some still unidentified biochemical events, to the induction of platelet aggregation and the release of secretory granules. Platelet aggregation and exocytosis can be induced also at resting, or even below-resting cytosolic Ca^{2+} concentrations, provided that protein kinase C is maximally activated. This can be obtained by addition of sufficient amounts of the relatively permeable diglyceride 1-oleyl-2-acetyl glycerol, or with tumor promoters such as the active phorbol esters. It has been established that the biochemical effects of phorbol esters are largely to be ascribed to their extremely high affinity for protein kinase C which becomes maximally activated in their presence. On the other hand, aggregation and exocytosis can be induced also in the absence of protein kinase C activation, if the increase of cytosolic Ca^{2+} is high enough (Rink and Hallam, 1984; Rink et al., 1983). The sequence of events described for platelets, i.e. agonist-activated polyphosphoinositide breakdown and cytosolic Ca^{2+} increase as mediators in the process of stimulus-secretion coupling is now recognized as a general phenomenon, not solely involved in platelet physiology.

It has been reported (Vargaftig et al., 1985; White et al., 1977) that vitamin E, alone and maximally in association with the one electron acceptor nitroblue tetrazolium, inhibits platelet aggregation and exocytosis. These observations were generally discussed in terms of inhibition by these antioxidants of the cyclooxygenase, which is known to have antioxidant-sensitive free radical intermediates, leading to impaired synthesis of the powerful platelet activator thromboxane A_2. More recently it was discovered that the aggregation of platelets induced by soluble and particulate stimuli is enhanced by the addition of minute amounts of H_2O_2 and conversely that externally added catalase inhibits the aggregation induced by particulate stimuli and by phorbol esters. It was also shown that H_2O_2 is formed inside the platelets coincident with activation (Del Principe et al., 1985). These observations led us to investigate more in detail the action of antioxidant agents both on platelets (Alexandre et al., 1986) and on excitable systems such as the presynaptic nerve terminals (synaptosomes) where a depolarization of the plasma membrane rather than an hormone-receptor interaction promotes the influx of Ca^{2+} into the cytosol across the plasma membrane and the release of neurotransmitter-containing secretory granules.

Materials and Methods

Platelet rich-plasma obtained from fresh human blood as described by Alexandre et al. (1986) was incubated for 40 min at 37°C with 20 μM quin 2 acetoxymethyl ester. The platelets were pelleted by centrifugation at 500 x g at room temperature for 20 min. The cells were gently resuspended in prewarmed medium containing 145 mM NaCl, 5 mM KCl, 1 mM $MgSO_4$, 10 mM HEPES, 10 mM glucose, pH 7.4 and incubated for 20 min at 37°C with 100 μM aspirin. The platelet count was adjusted to about 1 x 10^8 cells/ml and the suspension left at room temperature. 5 min before the measurements, aliquots of the suspension were equilibrated at 37°C and the external calcium was adjusted by addition of $CaCl_2$ or EGTA.

Changes in the cytosolic free Ca^{2+} concentration were measured following the fluorescence of the indicator quin 2 as described by Tsien et al. (1982), with a Perkin-Elmer LS3 spectrofluorimeter in a cuvette termostatted at 37°C and magnetically stirred. Calibrations were performed according to Hallam et al. (1984 a). Simultaneous measurement of ATP secretion was carried out at 37°C with a LKB Luminometer by adding 10 μl of luciferin/luciferase reagent to 240 μl of quin 2 loaded aspirinated platelet suspension. Each trace was calibrated by addition of a standard ATP solution. Aggregation was evaluated in parallel at 37°C with an Elvi (Logos) aggregometer.

Synaptosomes from guinea pig cerebral cortex were prepared as previously described (Scott et al., 1980). The $^{45}Ca^{2+}$ content of synaptosomes incubated as described by Scott et al. (1980) was determined with $[^{14}C]$-polyethylene glycol as extrasynaptosomal marker followed by removal of superficial $^{45}Ca^{2+}$ by adding 2.5 mM EGTA plus 5 μM ruthenium red 10 sec before the centrifugation through silicon oil as described by Akerman and Nicholls (1981). The measurement of L-glutamate secretion from the synaptosomes was carried out in a cuvette termostated at 30°C and magnetically stirred using a Perkin-Elmer LS3 spectrofluorimeter (excitation at 340 nm and emission at 460 nm) as described by Nicholls and Sihra (1986). All types of experiments were performed with at least five independent preparations.

Results

Action of antioxidants on platelet function

In studies of the action of antioxidnts on platelet activation it is important that the effect of these substances on enzymes known to have free radical intermediates (such as the cyclooxygenase and lipoxygenases) may be ruled out. The treatment of platelets with aspirin inhibits the cyclooxygenase and thus prevents the synthesis of the powerful activator thromboxane A_2 from arachidonic acid (free arachidonic acid is invariably produced during platelet activation, secondary to the activation of a phospholipase A_2, promoted both by the increase of cytosolic Ca^{2+} and by the activation of protein kinase C). In the presence of aspirin arachidonic acid becomes inefficient as a platelet activator, while other stimuli, such as thrombin, vasopressin and platelet activating factor are still effective. These observations indicate that platelet activation does not necessarily involve metabolites of the cyclooxigenase, and that compounds formed via the lipoxygenase reaction are irrelevant for platelet activation, since aspirin, while preventing the arachinodic acid promoted activation, does not affect the lipoxygenase. For these reasons, all the experiments described below were performed with aspirinated platelets. Fig. 1 reports some results obtained with quin 2 loaded aspirinated platelets incubated in the presence of 1 mM external Ca^{2+} and activated with thrombin in the presence of various antioxidants (BHT, BHA, NDGA). Similar results are obtained with the one-elctron donor I,I'-dimethylferrocene. All the antioxidants tested strongly inhibit the thrombin-induced increase of cytosolic Ca^{2+}, as well as the shape change, aggregation and exocytosis (monitored as the release into the extracellular space of ATP contained in the secretory granules). 50% inhibition of the thrombin-promoted cytosolic Ca^{2+} increase is obtained at 20-30 μM BHT; ATP secretion and aggregation are affected at slightly higher concentrations.

BHT inhibits also the thrombin-induced increase of cytosolic Ca^{2+} originating from intracellular stores, as observed in experiments performed in the presence of the extracellular Ca^{2+} chelator EGTA (Fig. 2). Note that in these conditions the thrombin-induced increase of cytosolic Ca^{2+} is much lower than in the experiments of Fig. 1. This is largely due to the Ca^{2+}-buffering effect of quin 2.

The inhibition by antioxidants of platelet functions is observed not only with thrombin but also with different activating agents, such as vasopressin, platelet activating factor and ADP. Fig. 3 reports some experiments on the effects on cytosolic Ca^{2+}. These results indicate that the action of antioxidants is not thrombin-specific.

As already mentioned, phorbol esters as TPA are powerful activators of protein kinase C. They induce platelet aggregation and ATP secretion without increasing the cytosolic Ca^{2+} (Rink et al., 1983). These properties are taken as evidence that, if the protein kinase C is maximally activated, aggregation and exocytosis occur at resting or even below-resting cytosolic Ca^{2+} levels. It was important to study the effect of antioxidants on the phorbol ester promoted platelet activation, since in this process all the events normally preceding the activation of the protein kinase C (i.e. the agonist-receptor interaction leading to the activation of the phosphodiesterase) are bypassed. Besides, added catalase has been reported to interfere with the phorbol ester induced aggregation (Del Principe et al., 1985).

Fig. 4 shows that both the aggregation and the secretion of ATP evoked by TPA are markedly affected by the antioxidant BHA. Similar results were obtained with BHT, NDGA and 1,1'dimethylferrocene (plus ascorbate). These results indicate that the antioxidants have a direct effect on the process of exocytosis.

As already mentioned, the cyclooxygenase and lipoxygenase pathways of the arachidonic acid cascade are not directly involved in the activation of aspirinated platelets, whether promoted by physiological agonists or by phorbol esters. The finding (not shown) that the thrombin activation of aspirinated platelets is not affected by BW755C, a non specific inhibitor of the lipoxygenase, lends further support to this view. It can be concluded that the inhibitory action of antioxidants on platelet functions described here cannot be ascribed to the scavenging of free radicals involved in this type of reactions.

Platelet functions are sensitive to vitamin E (Vargaftig et al., 1975; White et al., 1977); H_2O_2 and possibly superoxide radicals potentiate the efficacy of platelet agonists; H_2O_2 and possibly superoxide radicals are produced upon platelet activation (Del Principe et al., 1985). Taken together with the results reported here, those observations suggest that some still undefined free radical-mediated reactions are involved in the process of platelet activation, both at the level of the events preceding the activation of protein kinase C and leading to the increase of cytosolic Ca^{++}, and at the level of the events, largely dependent on the activation of the protein kinase C, leading to aggregation and exocytosis.

These observations probably indicate that a cellular prooxidant state may be involved not only in the mediation of pathological events but also in the generation of physiological responses. Indeed it has been known for several years that the interaction of insulin with adipocytes promotes the synthesis of intracellular H_2O_2 (Ramasarma, 1982; Mukherjee and Lynn, 1977; May and de Haens, 1979), probably via the activation of a NADPH oxidase of the plasma membrane. This insulin-generated prooxidant state may be an important mediator of insulin's metabolic responses. In accordance, added H_2O_2 mimicks many of the responses evoked by insulin (Czech et al., 1974). Furthermore, it is now clear that the primary target of the tumor promoters phorbol esters is protein kinase C and that most of the effects of these agents are to be ascribed to a sustained uncontrolled activation of this protein kinase. Interestingly, many of the effects of the treatment with phorbol esters, such as the induction of some enzymatic activities (e.g. ornithine decarboxylase, poli (ADP ribose) synthetase) and the tumor promotion itself are strongly counteracted by antioxidative agents ranging from vitamins C and E, to the enzymes SOD and catalase, to BHT (Cerutti, 1985). The antioxidant inhibition of hormone induced cellular activation may be a much broader phenomenon that it appears now. Accordingly, experiments in progress in this laboratoty appear to indicate that the activation of polymorfonuclear leucocytes (induction of the NADPH oxidase activity leading to the superoxide production known as oxygen burst, exocytosis) may be controlled by antioxidative agents, similarly to what has just been described in platelets.

Action of BHT on the depolarization-induced activation of synaptosomes.

Neurotransmitter release from the synaptic vesicles of synaptosomes (isolated nerve terminals) is a type of exocytosis which is triggered by depolarization of the plasma membrane, rather than by the interaction of an hormone with a receptor on the cell surface. The depolarization-induced neurotransmitter release requires extracellular Ca^{++}. Calcium influx into cytosol from the extracellular space is in turn induced by the depolarization of the plasma membrane, which opens specific Ca^{++} channels.

The possibility that also these processes may be affected by some antioxidants was investigated in the experiments of Fig. 5 and Fig. 6. As reported in Fig. 5, a fast influx of Ca^{++} is observed when ^{45}Ca is added to the synaptosomes, if their plasma membrane is depolarized by incubation in high K^+ media. On the contrary, ^{45}Ca influx is slow and reaches a lower state when the plasma membrane is polarized, i.e. when the incubation medium is low in K^+. The high ^{45}Ca influx observed in high K^+ media is in turn strongly inhibited by inclusion of BHT, which appears to act like a Ca antagonist.

The effect of BHT on the depolarization-induced neurotransmitter release is shown in Fig. 6. In the experiments reported, a sudden

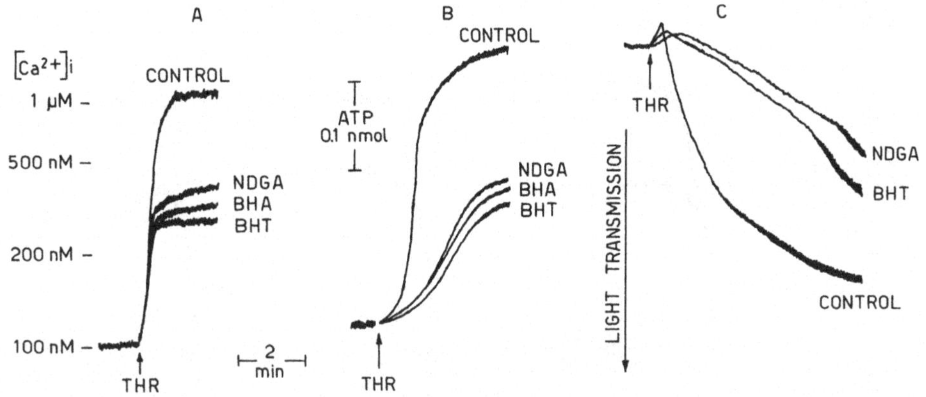

Fig. 1: Antioxidant inhibition of platelet functions. Quin 2-loaded aspirinated platelets were incubated with 1 mM $CaCl_2$ and stimulated with 0.15 U/ml thrombin (THR). When indicated 50 μM 2,3-ditert-butyl-4-methoxyphenol (BHT), 65 μM nordihydroguaiaretic acid (NDGA) and 65 μM 2,6-di-tert-butyl-4-methylphenol (BHA) were added 3 min before THR. A) Quin 2 fluorescence. B) ATP secretion. The traces are corrected for some quencing affect of the antioxidants. C) Platelet aggregation.

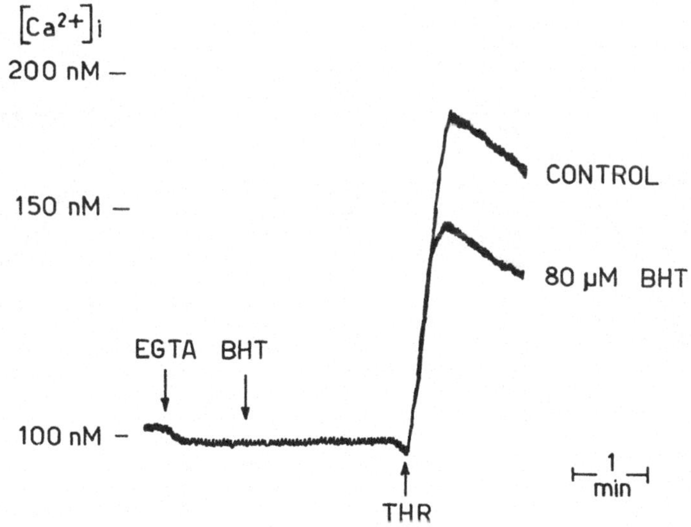

Fig. 2: The inhibitory effect of BHT on the increase of cytosolic Ca^{2+} induced by thrombin in quin 2-loaded platelets in the absence of external calcium. Experimental conditions as in Fig. 1 except that Ca^{2+} was replaced by EGTA (1 mM).

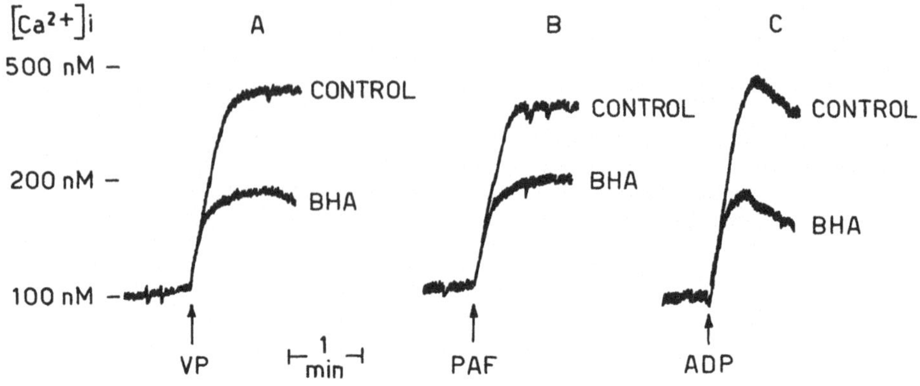

Fig. 3: BHA inhibition of agonist promoted cytosolic Ca^{2+} increase. Experimental conditions as in Fig. 1. When indicated 1 μM vasopressin (VP), 75 nM platelet activating factor (PAF) and 10 μM ADP were added BHA (70 μM) was added 3 min before the agonist.

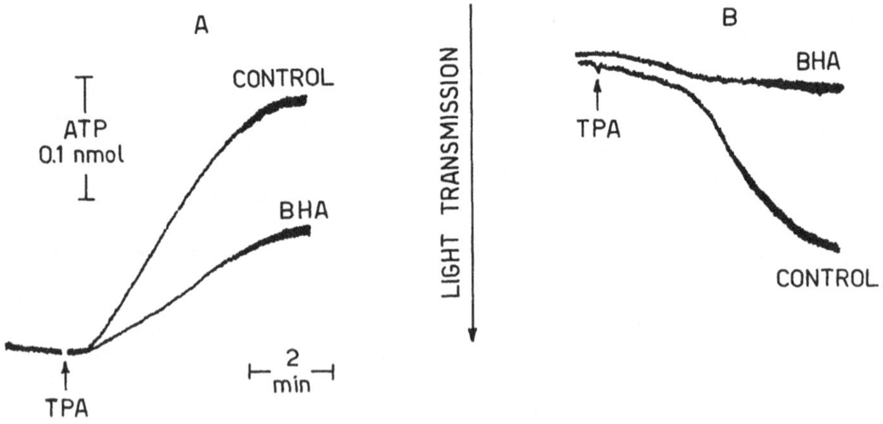

Fig. 4: BHA inhibition of phorbol ester-promoted ATP secretion (A) and aggregation (B). 12 nM 12-0-tetradecanoyl phorbol acetate (TPA) was added as indicated by the arrow; when present 100 μM BHA was added 3 min before TPA.

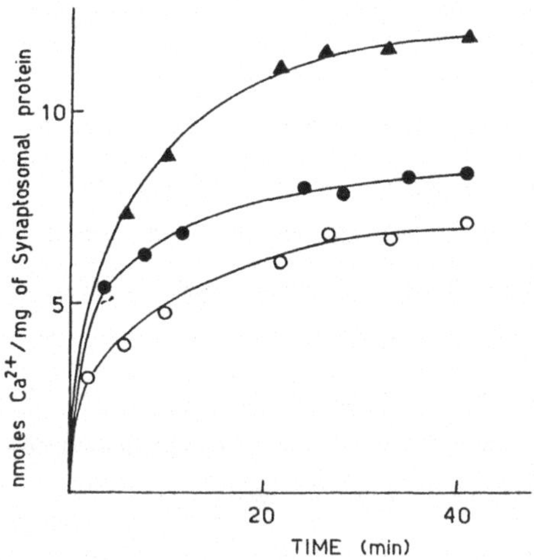

Fig. 5: Effect of BHT on depolarization-induced Ca^{++} uptake by synaptosomes. Synaptosomes (4.5 mg/ml) were preincubated 15 min in a medium containing 122 mM NaCl and 3.1 mM KCl as indicated in Materials and Methods. At zero time the synaptosomes were diluted to a final concentration of 1.5 mg/ml, 122 mM NaCl and 3.1 mM KCl (open symbols) or 42.7 mM NaCl and 82.4 mM KCl (closed symbols) together with $^{45}CaCl_2$ 1.3 mM (0.25 μC/ml). (●) 100 μM BHT added 5 min before zero time.

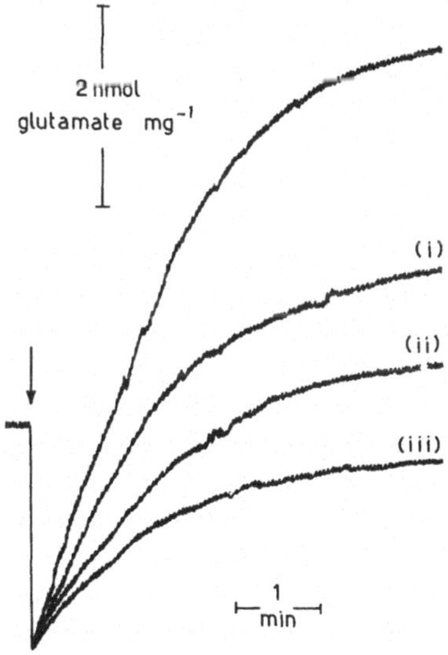

Fig. 6: The inhibitory effect of BHT on L-glutamate secretion induced by depolarization of synaptosomal plasma membrane. Synaptosomes (1.2 mg/ml) were incubated as indicated in Materials and Methods. 30 mM KCl was added at the arrow. BHT, added 2 min before KCl, was: (i) 30 μM; (ii) 90 μM; (iii) 120 μM.

increase of K^+ in the suspending medium determines a membrane depolarization which in turn triggers the rapid release of glutamate, which is a major excitatory neurotrasmitter in the central nervous system. The Ca-dependent exocytotic glutamate represents 15-20% of the total synaptosomal glutamate. It is monitored as the reduction of added NAD^+ in the presence of glutamate dehydrogenase (Nicholls and Sihra, 1986). Inclusion of BHT strongly depresses the rate and extent of glutamate relase. This experiment shows that also the depolarization-induced exocytosis of excitable cells is sensitive to antioxidants. Similar results were obtained with BHA and NDGA.

Conclusions.

The observations reported, that antioxidants interfere with Ca^{2+} movements and exocytosis, both in agonist-receptor activated and in depolarization activated systems, rise the possibility that free radical intermediates are involved in important cellular events. Accordingly a cellular prooxidant state may be required for the operation of physiological processes.

REFERENCES

Adunyah, S.E. and Dean, W.L., 1985. Inositol triphosphate-induced Ca^{++} release from human platelet membranes. Biochem. Biophys. Res. Comm., 128: 1274-1280.

Åkerman, K.E.O. and Nicholls, D.G., 1981. Calcium transport by intact synaptosomes. Eur. J. Biochem., 115: 67-73.

Alexandre, A., Doni, M.G., Padoin, E. and Deana, R., 1986. Inhibition by antioxidants of agonist evoked cytosolic Ca^{++} increase, ATP secretion and aggregation of aspirinated human platelets. Biochem. Biophys. Res. Commun., 139: 509-514.

Berridge, M.J. and Irvine, R.F., 1984. Inositol trisphosphate, a novel second messenger in cellular signal transduction. Nature, 312: 315-321.

Brass, L.F. and Joseph, S.K., 1985. A role for inositol triphosphate in intracellular Ca^{++} mobilization and granule secretion in platelets. J. Biol. Chem., 260: 15172-15179.

Cerutti, P.A., 1985. Prooxidant states and tumor promotion. Science,

227: 375-381.

Czech, M.P., Lawrence, J.C. Jr. and Lynn, W.S., 1974. Hexose transport in isolated brown fat cells. J. Biol. Chem., 249: 5421-5427.

Del Principe, D., Menichelli, A., De Matteis, W., Di Corpo, M.L., Di Giulio, S. and Finazzi-Agrò, A., 1985. Hydrogen peroxide has a role in the aggregation of human platelets. FEBS Lett., 185: 142-146.

Hallam, T.J., Sanchez, A. and Rink, T.J., 1984a. Stimulus-response coupling in human platelets. Changes evoked by platelet-activating factor in cytoplasmic free calcium monitored with the fluorescent calcium indicator quin 2. Biochem. J., 218: 819-827.

Hallam, T.J., Thompson, N.T., Scrutton, M.C. and Rink, T.J., 1984b. The role of cytoplasmic free calcium in the responses of quin 2 loaded human platelets to vasopressin. Biochem. J., 221: 897-901.

Israels, S.J., Robinson, P., Docherty, J.C. and Gerrard, J.M., 1985.Activation of permeabilized platelets by inositol-1,4,5-triphosphate. Thrombosis Res., 40: 499-509.

May, J.M. and de Haens, C., 1979. Insulin-stimulated intracellular hydrogen peroxide production in rat epididymal fat cells. J. Biol. Chem., 254: 2214-2220.

Mukherjee, S.P. and Lynn, W.S., 1977. Reduced nicotinamide adenine dinucleotide phosphate oxidase in adipocyte plasma membrane and its activation by insulin. Arch. Biochem. Biophys., 184: 69-76.

Nicholls, D.G. and Sihra, T.S., 1986. Synaptosomes posses an exocytotic pool of glutamate. Nature, 321: 772-773.

Nishizuka, Y., 1984. The role of protein kinase C in cell surface signal transduction and tumour promotion. Nature, 308: 693-698.

Ramasarma, T., 1982. Generation of H_2O_2 in biomembranes. Biochim. Biophys. Acta., 694: 69-93.

Rink, T.J. and Hallam, T.J., 1984. What turns platelets on? Trends Biochem. Sci., 9: 215-219.

Rink, T.J., Sanchez, A. and Hallam; T.J., 1983. Diacylglycerol and phorbol ester stimulate secretion without raising cytoplasmic free calcium in human platelets. Nature, 305: 317-319.

Scott, I.D., Åkerman, K.E.O. and Nicholls, D.G., 1980. Calcium-ion transport by intact synaptosomes. Biochem. J., 192: 873-880.

Tsien, R.Y., Pozzan, T. and Rink, T.J., 1982. Calcium homeostasis in intact lymphocytes: cytoplasmic free calcium monitored with a new, intracellularly trapped fluorescent indicator. J. Cell. Biol., 94: 325- 334.

Vargaftig, B.B., Tranier, Y. and Chignard, M., 1975. Blockade by metal complexing agents and by catalase of the effects of arachidonic acid on platelets: relevance to the study of anti-inflammatory mechanisms. Europ. J. Pharmacol., 33: 19-29.

White, J.G., Rao, G.H.R. and Gerrard, J.M., 1977. Effects on nitroblue tetrazolium and Vitamin E on platelet ultrastructure, aggregation and secretion. American J. Pathol., 88: 387-398.

PULMONARY VASCULAR INJURY FROM REACTIVE OXYGEN SPECIES

Bruce A. Freeman,[1,2] Peter Panus[1], Joseph S. Beckman[1], Sadis Matalon[3]
Departments of Anesthesiology[1] and Biochemistry[2], The University of Alabama at Birmingham, Birmingham, AL 35294, Department of Physiology[3], State University of New York, Buffalo, NY, 14214

INTRODUCTION

Vascular injury due to excess production of reactive oxygen species occurs secondary to diverse phenomena including trauma, acute inflammation, sepsis, tissue ischemia-reperfusion, oxygen toxicity and exposure to xenobiotics capable of redox cycling (Freeman et al., 1982a). Vascular lining cells, specifically the endothelium, can be both critical targets and sources of reactive oxygen species which can then yield other substances which activate inflammatory cells to exacerbate initial oxidant insults. Thus, the endothelium is an extremely critical site of oxidant injury since damage can be induced by diverse etiologic factors, resulting in losses of both microvascular metabolic function and barrier properties.

ULTRASTRUCTURAL AND FUNCTIONAL OBSERVATIONS

Since the discovery of the endothelium as a differentiated cellular unit having specific functional and structural roles in the maintenance of lung fluid balance, much recent interest has focused on the response of pulmonary endothelium to injury. In recent years the endothelium has been shown to have a primary role in oxygen-mediated tissue injury, because endothelial cells themselves are capable of producing and releasing highly reactive, partially reduced products of oxygen metabolism.

Animals with healthy lungs exposed to 100% O_2 at one atmosphere develop arterial hypoxemia (Matalon et al., 1981; Matalon et al., 1985) or progressive uncompensated respiratory acidosis (Erdmann et al., 1983; Matalon et al., 1982). Death from normobaric O_2 toxicity in all animals is secondary to massive protein-rich pulmonary edema, resulting from damage to both the alveolar epithelium (Matalon et al., 1981) and the capillary endothelium. Electron microscopic examination of the blood-gas barrier of rats exposed to 95% O_2 for 72 hours revealed progressive pulmonary capillary destruction, diminishing capillary area by 50% (Kistler et al., 1967).

A decrease in the metabolic activity of the pulmonary endothelium has also been used as an index of oxygen-induced damage to the pulmonary circulation.

Exposure of rats to 100% oxygen for 18 hrs decreased the clearance of serotonin by the pulmonary circulation (Block et al., 1977). After 24 hrs in hyperoxia there was significant decrease in the conversion of angiotensin I to angiotension II by canine pulmonary endothelium (Harabin et al., 1984). Angiotensin converting enzyme activity decreased to 77% of its control value after 16 hrs of exposure of conscious rabbits to 100% O_2, and to 66% of control value after 40 hrs in 100% O_2. At the same time intervals, the authors found a significant depression in the clearance of ^{14}C-5-hydroxytryptamine by the pulmonary circulation. No capillary damage accountable for these lesions could be identified by light or electron microscopic examination of lung tissue after 20 hrs in hyperoxia. Hyperoxia also decreased the plasma membrane fluidity of pulmonary artery and aortic endothelial cells in culture; the time course of this decrease paralleled the decrease in amine transport by these cells (Block et al., 1986).

BIOCHEMICAL MEDIATORS

Biochemical studies have shown that cellular oxygen toxicity is initiated by intracellular overproduction of reactive species of oxygen, including O_2^-, H_2O_2 and $OH\cdot$. It is energetically unfavorable for molecular oxygen to combine with spin-paired electrons, thus accounting for the relatively low reactivity of oxygen as an oxidant in the absence of catalysis. The thermodynamic barrier to acceptance of electrons by oxygen can be bypassed by one electron reductions sequentially yielding O_2^-, H_2O_2, $OH\cdot$ plus H_2O and $2H_2O$. Mitochondrial cytochrome *c* oxidase binds oxygen and transfers electrons to oxygen with no detectable release of reactive partially reduced species of oxygen. About 95% of the oxygen consumed by most mammalian cells can be accounted for by the catalytic reduction of oxygen to H_2O by cytochrome *c* oxidase.

Hyperoxia increases the cyanide-resistant (non-cytochrome *c* oxidase) oxygen consumption of lung tissue slices, lung homogenates, lung mitochondria and isolated and cultured cells (Barak et al., 1980; Freeman et al., 1981; Freeman et al., 1982b; Turrens et al., 1982; Beckman et al., 1986). This implies generally increased rates of partial reduction of oxygen to toxic intermediates in tissues. The cyanide-resistant respiration of cells also includes the more benign oxidation of substrates including amino acids, nucleotides and lipids. These processes do not involve radical intermediates in many cases, and are quantitatively minor compared to the contribution of oxygen radical generation to the net tissue cyanide-resistant respiration rate (Freeman et al., 1981; Turrens et al., 1982). Endothelial cells are unique in their capacity to generate reactive oxygen species, as determined from polarographic measurements of cellular cyanide resistant respiration. The non-mitochondrial oxygen consumption of endothelial cells was 19% of total oxygen consumption, compared with other cell or organ preparations, which had 5-8% of total oxygen consumption as cyanide-resistant (Crapo et al., 1983). This suggests that endothelial cells very actively utilize oxygen in biosynthetic and oxidative processes many of which can involve production of significant quantities of O_2^-, H_2O_2 and OH·.

<u>Cytosol</u>

Soluble cytoplasmic molecules are quantitatively important sources of intracellular production of reactive oxygen species. These molecules include thiols, hydroquinones, catecholamines, and flavins. In each instance, O_2^- is the primary radical generated by these substances (Freeman et al., 1985a). Hydrogen peroxide is a secondary product of O_2^- formation, via spontaneous or enzymatically catalyzed dismutation of O_2^-. Cytoplasmic enzymes can also generate O_2^- and H_2O_2 as byproducts of catalytic cycling. Xanthine oxidase, aldehyde oxidase, tryptophan dioxygenase, flavoprotein dehydrogenases, peroxisomal oxidases and hemoglobin are significant sources of O_2^- and H_2O_2. Free radical production by these sources almost universally increases directly as a function of oxygen tension.

<u>Organelle</u>

Membrane-bound proteins are also significant sources of cellular oxygen radical production. These sources exist in the nucleus, endoplasmic reticulum, mitochondria and plasma membrane. Free radicals generated by these sources probably account for many of the early morphological changes observed in subcellular organelles of oxygen-exposed lungs (Crapo et al., 1980). For example, it would be reasonable to expect that relatively high local concentrations of reactive oxygen species would react near the site of production since their inherent reactivity ensures that diffusion distances in biological milieu will be very short. Thus, the mitochondrial swelling and dilatation of the inner mitochondrial membrane observed in early stages of oxygen toxicity may be due to overproduction of reactive oxygen species by electron transport components located on the inner mitochondrial membrane. We have seen that the production of O_2^- by submitochondrial particles derived from lung increases directly as a function of oxygen tension (Turrens et al., 1982).

The nuclear membrane and the endoplasmic reticulum contain a number of components capable of O_2^- and H_2O_2 generation. These include cytochrome P_{450}, which generates O_2^- by autoöxidation and yields H_2O_2 by dissociation of peroxycytochrome P_{450}. Cytochrome b_5 can also autooxidize, yielding O_2^- and H_2O_2 (Estabrook et al., 1976; Archakov et al., 1980). In the case of nuclear membrane-derived reactive oxygen species, mechanisms of gene expression which regulate cell differentiation and growth will be at risk. Nuclei isolated from lung and maintained under hyperoxic conditions generate O_2^- at twice the rate of nuclei incubated in air saturated buffers (Yusa et al., 1984). Microsomes derived from endoplasmic reticulum generate O_2^- at a rate which increases 3-5 fold during hyperoxia (Freeman et al., 1982a). Extrapolation of in vitro observations of mitochondrial and microsomal H_2O_2 generation to what they could maximally contribute in whole lung tissue showed the H_2O_2 production rate was 2.9 (mitochondria) and 19.7 (microsomes) $nmol \cdot min^{-1} \cdot g\ lung^{-1}$.

Membrane

Most, if not all mitochondrial H_2O_2 is derived from dismutation of O_2^- generated intramitochondrially. Lung mitochondrial O_2^- does not escape the superoxide dismutase of this organelle to reach cytosolic spaces. Hydrogen peroxide can diffuse extramitochondrially and this rate increases as a function of oxygen tension. Thus, partial reduction of oxygen by mitochondria can damage other cytoplasmic components. Reactive oxygen species produced by the nuclear membrane in endoplasmic reticulum can undergo both intraorganelle reactions or diffuse directly into the cytosol.

Endothelial cell plasma membrane-derived free radical production has not been well defined. Cyclooxygenase-mediated oxidation of arachidonate has been proposed to yield both a carbon and an oxygen-centered free radical intermediate. The oxygen-centered radical formed during the breakdown of the hydroperoxide of PGG_2, initially proposed to be $OH^\cdot$ has recently been suggested to be a cyclooxygenase-hemoprotein radical, distinct from the oxygen-centered radical $OH^\cdot$ (Egan et al., 1976; Kalyanaraman et al., 1982). Free radical species are also involved in the conversion of prostaglandin endoperoxide (PGH_2) to thromboxanes, which is inhibited by the radical scavengers methional and nordihydroguiaretic acid (Moncada et al., 1977). It is interesting to note that the oxygen sensitive capillary endothelial cell is a major site of pulmonary eicosanoid synthesis. Because of the proximity of plasma membrane-located free radical sources to cell and organelle surfaces, membrane-derived reactive oxygen species can potentially affect intracellular membrane and extracellular compartments, depending on the solubility and diffusion distances of the reactive molecules. The high and indiscriminate reactivity of $OH^\cdot$ in biological milieu suggests that it will react within a few molecular radii of its site of generation. Superoxide is less reactive than $OH^\cdot$ but still exerts significant toxicity, in part because it may be able to diffuse to critical targets distal to its site of generation. Hydrogen peroxide is uncharged and less reactive than OH·. If H_2O_2 escapes cellular defense mechanisms, it is more likely to diffuse across organelle or plasma membranes to exert toxic effects distal to sites of generation than O_2^- or OH·. Thus, reactivity and toxicity are not necessarily directly linked.

Endothelial production of reduced oxygen species essentially obeys the Law of Mass Action. Many cellular components are available to reduce oxygen, and when the oxygen concentration increases, so does its rate of partial reduction. Experimental observations in general support the first order nature of lung O_2^- and H_2O_2 production, with respect to oxygen concentration (Freeman et al., 1982b; Freeman et al., 1981; Turrens et al., 1982; Yusa et al., 1984; Beckman et al., 1986). Other factors which would modify rates of lung cell oxygen radical production include enzyme inhibition or induction, cofactor availability, the concentration of substrate available for radical-producing enzymes and the presence of drugs or xenobiotics which are metabolized via free radical intermediates.

Intact Cells

Examination of monolayers of cultured pulmonary artery endothelium shows that both O_2- and H_2O_2 are released extracellularly. Extracellular O_2^- release can be quantified by measurement of vanadate-mediated cooxidation of NADH by O_2-. Hydrogen peroxide release was monitored by fluorescence detection of horseradish peroxidase-mediated oxidation of p-hydroxyphenylacetic acid. Endothelial cells and their medium equilibrated with 95% oxygen showed a significant increase in rates of O_2- and H_2O_2 release. The O_2- release by endothelial cells was inhibited by stilbene sulfonate derivatives which block the membrane anion channel. Additionally, 12-fold enhancement of intracellular catalase specific activity following treatment of endothelial cells with liposome-entrapped catalase resulted in complete inhibition of extracellular H_2O_2 release. Presumably, hyperoxia enhanced intracellular rates of O_2- and H_2O_2 production, which then gained access to extracellular spaces by diffusion across endothelial plasma membranes since no cell lysis was detected in the 30 min oxygen metabolite assay periods. The egress of O_2- and H_2O_2 from vascular lining cells exposes serum components to reactive oxygen species. This phenomenon can explain secondary effects of endothelial oxidant production, including modification of low density lipoprotein to a cytotoxic species (Steinbrecher et al., 1984) and formation of an albumin-bound lipid neutrophil chemoattractant (McCord et al., 1982). The dilemma of pulmonary oxygen toxicity, which results in primary free radical injury to lung cells and secondary injury due to infiltration of neutrophils, is an expected consequence of oxygen therapy. The observation that enhanced intracellular antioxidant enzyme activity prevents both hyperoxic injury to cells and animals (Freeman et al., 1983; Freeman et al., 1985b) and attenuation of the extracellular release of reactive oxygen species which could mediate inflammatory responses shows that pharmacologic modification of oxygen toxicity is possible.

Pretreatment of animals with superoxide dismutase and/or catalase results in significant, although incomplete, protection against subsequent ischemia-reperfusion injury, radionecrosis and carrageenan-induced granulomas (Michelson, 1982; Granger et al., 1986). Pretreatment with free superoxide dismutase or catalase does not protect rats against hyperoxia-induced toxicity when administered by intravenous or intraperitoneal injection (Crapo et al., 1977; Turrens et al., 1984), or by prior aerosolization of the free enzyme into the lungs (Padmanabham et al., 1985).

MODIFICATION OF ENDOTHELIAL DEFENSE MECHANISMS

Intracellular production and toxicity of O_2- and H_2O_2 during hyperoxia may in part explain the incomplete and/or lack of protection by free SOD and catalase. Superoxide dismutase and catalase are large molecules unable to cross cell membranes and are rapidly cleared by the kidneys. A mechanism which allows intracellular delivery of these enzymes to specific target cells will enhance their protective effects during situations of intracellular oxygen-mediated damage. Liposome-mediated delivery is one possible mechanism.

The general structure function, stability, and in vivo elimination of liposomes are discussed elsewhere (Yatvin et al., 1982; Gregoriadis, 1983). Intracellular delivery of liposome-entrapped superoxide dismutase is dependent upon the charge characteristics of the superoxide dismutase, the liposome lipid composition, and the target cell membrane. Michelson et al. (1980) demonstrated that acidic superoxide dismutase entrapped within cationic liposomes associates with erythrocytes more efficiently than similar liposomes containing basic superoxide dismutase. Fatty acid modification of the lecithin component in liposomes may also alter liposome binding to cellular membranes. Saturated fatty acid liposomes containing superoxide dismutase affix to erythrocytes more efficiently than similar liposome preparations consisting of unsaturated fatty acids. The optimum acyl chain length is 16, with acyl ether linkage as effective as ester linkage (Michelson et al., 1980). In vivo, the kidney and liver concentrate most of the superoxide dismutase per gram tissue, whether liposome-encapsulated or free (Tanswell and Freeman, in press; Michelson et al., 1981a; Michelson et al., 1981b). The liver demonstrates a preference for anionic liposome-entrapped superoxide dismutase (Michelson et al., 1981a; Michelson et al., 1981b). A preference by the kidney for free superoxide dismutase or superoxide dismutase in neutral liposomes is indicated. The lung concentrates cationic liposome-entrapped superoxide dismutase over other liposome lipid types.

Loss of pulmonary microvascular endothelial cell function may disrupt normal blood flow, resulting in lung edema and death. Porcine endothelial cells subjected to hyperoxia (95% oxygen) demonstrate a significant increase in cell death when compared to similar cells incubated under a normoxic (21% oxygen) state (Freeman et al., 1983). Pretreatment of cultured endothelium with exogenous superoxide dismutase was ineffective at preventing hyperoxia induced toxicity. Liposome-entrapped superoxide dismutase pretreatment of endothelial cells attenuated hyperoxia-induced cell death as well as cell death in normoxic and hypoxic states. Sonicated superoxide dismutase liposomes protected endothelial cells against the toxic effects of oxygen by increasing intracellular superoxide dismutase concentrations 6 to 9 fold over controls, an effect which extended several days after liposome treatment of the cells. Liposomes alone, with encapsulated inactive superoxide dismutase, or in the presence of unentrapped free superoxide dismutase marginally attenuate hyperoxia-induced cell injury. Attenuation of injury by these liposomes was due to the incorporation of liposome pholspholipid saturated fatty acids in to cell membranes, rendering them more resistant to the toxic effects of hyperoxia. Increasing target cell membrane saturated fatty acid content decreases hyperoxia-induced lipid peroxidation and lactate dehydrogenase release. Conversely, increasing unsaturated fatty acid content results in increased peroxidation and lactate dehydrogenase release (Freeman et al., 1983).

Injection of rats with reverse phase evaporation liposomes containing superoxide dismutase and catalase results in an increase in pulmonary superoxide dismutase and catalase concentrations which are maintained 15 times longer than the respective free superoxide dismutase or catalase with or without control liposomes (Turrens et al., 1984). Pretreatment with free superoxide dismutase or catalase by intravenous, intraperitoneal, or intratracheal routes does not afford rats protection against hyperoxia-induced mortality (Crapo et al., 1977; Turrens et al., 1984; Padmanabham et al., 1985). Intravenous injection of liposomes containing either superoxide dismutase or catalase alone did not significantly protect the animals from subsequent hyperoxia-induced mortality, however, liposomes containing both superoxide dismutase and catalase did protect rats from the toxic effects of hyperoxia

(Turrens et al., 1984). This suggested that increased survivorship in hyperoxia required both O_2^- and H_2O_2 to be reduced to H_2O. Furthermore, intratracheal instillation of either superoxide dismutase or catalase containing liposomes protected rats against hyperoxia induced mortality (Padmanabham et al., 1985). Again, enzyme-free liposomes alone were marginally effective in the above mentioned studies. Lungs from liposome-protected rats compared to those of control animals had less pleural effusion but a heavier wet lung weight, possibly due to longer survival times in hyperoxia resulting in more extensive pulmonary edema in particular regions of the lung.

Premature low birth weight infants are a high risk population for pulmonary effects of oxygen toxicity. Management of a variety of pulmonary disorders of newborns necessitate administration of higher than normal oxygen fractions in the inspired air. Thus, pharmacologic modification of the toxic effects of O_2 is of primary interest in newborn care. Intraperitoneal treatment of neonatal rats with reverse phase evaporation liposomes containing both catalase and superoxide dismutase prevented hyperoxia induced mortality when compared to oxygen-exposed animals receiving liposomal buffer or empty liposomes (Tanswell and Freeman, in press). Control liposomes again afforded some protection in these neonates due to either nutritional benefits of liposome lipids, or the protective effect of incorporation of saturated fatty acids into cell membranes or pulmonary surfactant. Superoxide dismutase-containing liposomes were no more effective than control liposomes. This implies that complete reduction of O_2^- and H_2O_2 to H_20 is required for adequate protection from oxygen toxicity.

Intracellular superoxide dismutase and catalase present within intact liposomes may protect the cell from toxicity due to reactive oxygen species via several potential mechanisms. Liposome-entrapped enzymes may protect the intracellular milieu by inactivating O_2^- and H_2O_2 which enter liposomes. H_2O_2 readily crosses lipid membranes, while the ability of O_2^- to cross lipid membranes is debated. Rumyantseva, et al., (1979) suggested that O_2^- is able to enter liposomes, dependent upon the structural state of the lipid bilayer membrane. However, other investigators (Takahashi et al., 1983; Turrens et al., 1984) were unable to demonstrate O_2^- passage across liposome membranes. Oxidation of unsaturated fatty acid-containing liposomes increases their passive permeability to small molecular weight solutes (Freeman et al., 1979). Knowing that O_2^- and H_2O_2 can peroxidize liposome membranes containing unsaturated fatty acids (Kellogg et al., 1977), one might suppose that enhanced oxidation of intact intracellular liposomes might result in enhanced scavenging activity of entrapped superoxide dismutase and catalase, or release of liposome contents after peroxidation-induced lysis. Thus, liposomes may release superoxide dismutase and catalase intracellularly, or alternatively, intact intracellular liposomes may sequester superoxide dismutase and catalase in an inactive depot form to be released intracellularly later, possibly when the cell undergoes stress from oxidant toxicity.

In vivo, liposome-entrapped superoxide dismutase and catalase may also modify oxidant mediated toxicity by inhibiting detrimental neutrophil recruitment and activation (McDonald et al., 1985), because free radicals derived from neutrophils often secondarily exacerbate primary oxidant tissue injury. These results have been disputed by other investigators who were unable to find inhibition of neutrophil function in vitro or in vivo by superoxide dismutase containing liposomes (Somiya et al., 1985).

MECHANISTIC INTERPRETATIONS

Antioxidant enzyme-inhibitable toxicity implies a role for a particular O_2 species in biological damage, whereas the source and mechanisms of toxicity of the O_2 species remain unresolved. Conversely the lack of a protective effect does not rule out the involvement of reduced O_2 species. It could simply be due to failure to deliver appropriate antioxidant enzymes in sufficient amounts to necessary locations. Some of the limitations inherent when using catalase and SOD to understand processes of oxidant injury to tissues are presented next.

Catalase

In several animal models of ischemia-reperfusion injury, no protective effect was found when catalase was added to the test systems, either with or without SOD (McCord 1985). This does not downplay the potential involvement of H_2O_2 in tissue injury. Hydrogen peroxide is sufficiently stable to diffuse considerable distances on a cellular scale and is soluble in lipids, thus enabling it to diffuse either into catalase-containing peroxisomes or out of cells into the circulation, where it may be consumed by serum reaction, red blood cell catalases and glutathione peroxidase. This suggests that cells can collaborate in antioxidant defense.

Catalase has a high Michaelis constant, making it a relatively poor scavenger of low levels of H_2O_2 (Chance et al., 1979a). In some situations it may be possible to enhance the H_2O_2 scavenging ability of catalase by adding ethanol (0.1-1 mM) to the system. Catalase normally reacts with two molecules of H_2O_2 in its catalytic cycle; the first molecule is rapidly reduced by catalase, but the second reacts slowly. Ethanol can react with the catalase intermediate to bypass the rate-limiting step of the catalytic cycle, thereby accelerating the decomposition of H_2O_2 (Chance et al., 1979b). Thus, adding ethanol to stimulate endogenous catalase may be more effective than adding catalase to a test system where low levels of H_2O_2 exert toxicity.

As an alternative to adding ethanol plus catalase to test systems, glutathione peroxidase plus glutathione can be used for H_2O_2 scavenging because glutathione peroxidase has a higher affinity for H_2O_2 than does catalase (Cohen et al., 1963). However, glutathione peroxidase also scavenges fatty acid peroxides and glutathione can be depleted in the absence of rereduction or can react directly with oxidants. This can cloud issues of whether protection is H_2O_2 dependent, when interpreting observations of protective effects in test systems.

Superoxide Dismutase

The protective effects observed in vivo with native SOD injected directly into the circulation [e.g., the intestinal model ischemia-reperfusion injury (McCord et al., 1982)] poses a dilemma. In this model, the putative source of O_2^- is tissue xanthine oxidase. One would expect native SOD to be protective only if O_2^- production occurs on the exofacial surface of the cell membrane. Available evidence, however, suggests that xanthine oxidase is a soluble cytoplasmic enzyme (Sackler, 1966) . There are also several proposed ways for the negatively charged and lipid-impermeable O_2^- to cross cell membranes, if tissue injury occurs after egress of intracellularly produced O_2^-. The existence of a region of low pH near the anionic polar groups of plasma membrane lipids, called the Gouy-Chapman-Stern boundary layer, may favor the protonation of O_2^- to the perhydroxyl radical ($HO_2^{\cdot}$).

$$O_2^- + H^+ \rightarrow HO_2^{\cdot}$$

The perhydroxyl radical is a stronger oxidant and is far more lipid soluble; thus it is more likely favored to cross cell membranes than is O_2^- (Fridovich 1983). However, dismutation of O_2^- is much faster at low pH and would compete with diffusion of O_2^- across the membranes. The O_2^- has been shown to diffuse through anion channels in red blood cells (Kellogg et al., 1977), but its diffusion through membranes of other cell types has not yet been demonstrated.

An equally plausible concept explaining extracellular phenomena occurring subsequent to intracellular O_2^- generation is that diffusible redox-active factors ($R^{\cdot}$) could leak from cells, which then undergo autoxidation externally to form O_2^-. For example, the SOD-inhibitable reduction of extracellular cytochrome *c* in *Escherichia coli* exposed to paraquat is due to extracellular diffusion of intracellularly reduced paraquat. Subsequently, molecular O_2 is reduce to O_2^- by paraquat in the extracellular milieu (Hassan et al., 1979). We have observed that menadione similarly participates in extracellular O_2^- generation by cultured vascular endothelial cells (Rosen et al., 1984). Menadione is reduced by intracellular reductases to its hydroquinone, which can diffuse extracellularly, dismute with menadione, and reduce molecular O_2 to O_2^-. Endogenous diffusible factors that could mediate the transport of O_2^- across endothelial cell membranes have not yet been described.

THERAPEUTIC USES OF ANTIOXIDANT ENZYMES

Therapeutic applications of antioxidant enzymes are receiving significant attention because of the demonstration of roles for reactive O_2 species in the pathobiology of disease processes, including adult respiratory distress syndrome, neonatal respiratory distress, loss of organ viability during transplantation, acute inflammation, myocardial infarction, and stroke. Damage to the endothelium plays an important role in many of these pathophysiologic states. Attractive aspects of antioxidant enzymes as pharmacological agents include their specificity for O_2^- and H_2O_2 metabolism, low toxicity, and availability of cloned human SOD. Drawbacks to clinical application of antioxidant enzymes are not insignificant. The bactericidal activity of phagocytic cells relies on O_2 radical-dependent microbial killing. Modification of antioxidant enzymes by liposome entrapment or conjugation with high-molecular-weight ligands may also have negative effects on host immune responses (McDonald et al., 1985; Richter et al., 1983). Short-term use of antioxidant enzymes for acute therapeutic needs, rather than chronic administration, may circumvent some of these problems.

Exogenous augmentation of antioxidant enzymes, despite many limitations, offers one of the most specific indicators of O_2 radical involvement available for biological systems. Although understanding the mechanisms of the protective action of antioxidant enzymes may not be of immediate concern in treating disease, a better understanding of the biochemical processes involved will foster more rational views of the pharmacological modification and pathobiology of oxidant injury.

ACKNOWLEDGEMENTS

We appreciate the assistance of Yvonne Lambott in preparation of the manuscript.

This work was supported by grants from the National Institutes of Health (NS-21782) and the Health Effects Institute.

REFERENCES

1. Archakov, A.I., Bachmanova, B.I., Isotaov, M.V. and Kuznetsova,C.P.,1980. Reduction of microsomal haemoproteins by superoxide radical generated by the NADPH-specific flavoprotein. In: Microsomes, Drug Oxidations and Chemical Carcinogenesis, (edited by RW Estabrook). New York, Academic Press, p289.

2. Barak, L.S., Yocum R.R., Nothnagel, E.A., and Webb, W.W., 1980. Fluorescence staining of the active cytoskelton in living cells with 7-nitrobenzo-2-oxa-1,3-diazole-phallacidin. Proc. Natl. Acad. Sci., 77:980-984.

3. Beckman, J.S., and Freeman, B.A., 1986. Antioxidant enzymes as mechanistic probes of oxygen-dependent toxicity. In Physiology of Oxygen Radicals, American Physiological Society, A. Taylor and S. Matalon, editors. pp39-53.

4. Block, E.R. and Fisher,A.B., 1977. Depression of serotonin clearance by rat lungs during oxygen exposure. J. Appl. Physiol., 42:33-38.

5. Block, E.R., Patel, J.M., Angelides, K.J., Sheridan, N.P., Garg, L.C., 1986. Hyperoxia reduces plasma membrane fluidity: A mechanism for endothelial cell dysfunction. J. Appl, Physiol., 60:826-835.

6. Chance, B., Sies, H., and Boveris, A., 1979a. Hyperoxia and hydroperoxide metabolism. In: Extrapulmonary Manifestations of Respiratory Disease, edited by E.D. Robins. New York: Dekker, pp185-605.

7. Chance B., Sies, H. and Boveris, A. 1979b. Hydroperoxide metabolism in mammalian systems. Physiol. Rev., 59:527-605.

8. Cohen, G., and Hochstein, P., 1963. Glutathione peroxidase: the primary agent for the elimination of H_2O_2 in erythrocytes. Biochemistry, 2:1420-1428.

9. Crapo, J.D., Delong, D.M., Sjostrom K., Hasler, G.R., and Drew, R.T., 1977. The failure of aerosolized superoxide dismutase to modify pulmonary oxygen toxicity. Am. Rev. Respir. Dis., 115:1027-33.

10. Crapo, J.D., Barry, B.E., Foscue, H.A., and Shelburne, J., 1980. Structural and biochemical changes in rat lungs occurring during exposures to lethal and adaptive doses of oxygen. Amer. Rev. Respir. Dis., 122:123.

11. Crapo, J.D., Freeman, B.A., Barry, B.E., Turrens, J.F., and Young, S.L., 1983. Mechanisms of hyperoxic injury to the pulmonary microcirculation. The Physiologist, 26:170-176.

12. Egan, R.W., Paxton,J., and Kuehl, F.A.,1976. Mechanism for irreversible self-deactivation of prostaglandin synthetase. J. Biol. Chem., 251:7329.

13. Erdmann J., III, Huttemeier, P.C., Landolt, C., and Zapol, W.M., 1983. Pure oxygen breathing increases sheep lung microvascular permeability. Anesthesiology, 58:153-158.

14. Estabrook, R.W., and Werringloer, J., 1976. Cytochrome P_{450}: its role in oxygen activation for drug metabolism. In: Drug Metabolism Concepts (edited by M.J. Donald, R.G. Robert, and D.C. Washington). American Chemical Society p 1.

15. Freeman, B.A., Sharman, M.C., and Mudd, J.B., 1979. Reaction of ozone with phospholipid vesicles and human erythrocyte ghosts. Arch. Biochem. Biophys., 197:264-72.

16. Freeman, B.A., and Crapo, J. D., 1981. Hyperoxia increases oxygen radical production in rat lungs and lung mitochondria. J. Biol. Chem., 256:10986-10992.

17. Freeman, B.A., and Crapo, J.D., 1982a. Biology of disease: Free radicals and tissue injury. Lab. Invest., 47:1-15.

17. Freeman, B.A., Topolosky, M.K., and Crapo, J.D., 1982b. Hyperoxia increases oxygen radical production in rat lung homogenates. Arch. Biochem. Biophys., 216:477-484.

18. Freeman, B.A., Young, S.L., and Crapo, J.D., 1983. Liposome-mediated augmentation of superoxide dismutase in endothelial cells prevents oxygen injury. J. Biol. Chem., 258:12534-12542.

19. Freeman, B.A., and Tanswell, A.K., 1985a. Biochemical and cellular aspects of pulmonary oxygen toxicity. Adv. Free Rad. Biol. Med., 1:133-164.

20. Freeman, B.A., Turrens, J.F., Mirza, Z., Crapo, J.D., and Young, S.L., 1985b. Modulation of oxidant lung injury by using liposome-entrapped superoxide dismutase and catalase. Fed. Proc., 44:2591-2595.

21. Fridovich, I., 1983. Superoxide radical: an endogenous toxicant. Ann. Rev. Pharmacol. Toxicol., 23:239-271.

22. Granger, D.N., Parks, D.A., and Hollwarth, M., 1986. Role of oxygen radicals in ischemic bowel disorders. Pediatr. Surg. Int., 1: 15-20.

23. Gregoriadis G., 1983. Liposomes as drug carriers. Pharm. Int., 4: 33-37.

24. Harabin, A.L., Homer, L.D., and Bradley, M.E., 1984. Pulmonary oxygen toxicity in awake dogs: metabolic and physiologic effects. J. Appl. Physiol., 57:1480-1488.

25. Hassan, H.M., and Fridovich, I., 1979. Paraquat and *Escherichia coli.* Mechanism of production of extracellular superoxide. J. Biol. Chem., 254:10846-10852.

26. Kalyanaraman, B., Mason, R.P., Tainer, B., and Eling, T.E, 1982. The free radical formed during the hydroperoxide-mediated deactivation of ram seminal vesicles is hemoprotein-derived. J. Biol. Chem., 257:4764.

27. Kellogg, E.W., and Fridovich, I., 1977. Liposome oxidation and erythrocyte lysis by enzymically generated superoxide and hydrogen peroxide.J. Biol. Chem., 252: 6721-8.

28. Kistler, G.S., Caldwell, P.R.B., and Weibel, E.R., 1967. Development of fine structural damage to alveolar and capillary lining cells in oxygen-poisoned rat lungs. J. Cell. Bio., 32:605-628.

29. Matalon, S., and Egan, E.A., 1981. Effects of 100% O_2 breathing on permeability of alveolar epithelium to solute. J. Appl. Physiol.: Respirat. Environ, and Exercise. Physiol., 859-863.

30. Matalon, S., and Cesar, M.A., 1985. Effects of 100% oxygen breathing on the capillary filtration coefficient in rabbit lungs. Microvasc. Res., 29:70-80.

31. Matalon, S., Nesarajah, M.S. and Farhi, L.E., 1982. Pulmonary and circulatory changes in conscious sheep exposed to 100% O_2 at 1 ATA. J.Appl.Physiol.:Respir. Environ. and Exercise Physiol., 53:110-116.

32. McCord, J.M., Wong, K, Stokes, S., Petrone, W., and English, D.,1980. Superoxide and inflammation: a mechanism for the anti-inflammatory activity of superoxide dismutase. Acta. Physiol. Scand. Suppl., 492:25-30.

43. McCord, J.M., and Roy, R.S, 1982. The pathophysiology of superoxide: roles in inflammation and ischemia. Can. J. Physiol. Pharmacol., 60:1346-1352.

44. McCord, J.B., 1985. Oxygen-derived free radicals in postischemic tissue injury. N. Engl. J. Med., 312:159-163.

45. McDonald, R.J., Berger, E.M., White, C.W., White, J.G., Freeman, B.A., and Repine, J.E., 1985. Effect of superoxide dismutase encapsulated in liposomes or conjugated with polyethylene glycol on neutrophil bactericidal activity in vitro and bacterial clearance in vivo. Am. Rev. Respir. Dis., 131: 633-7.

46. Michelson, A.M., Puget, K., Durosay, P., and Rouselet, A., 1980. Penetration of erythrocytes by superoxide dismutase, in The Significance of Superoxide and Superoxide Dismutase Vol.II. (Eds. E.H. Bannister and J.V. Bannister), pp. 348-366, Elsevier, New York.

47. Michelson, A.M., Puget, K., Perdereau, B., and Barbaroux, C., 1981a. Scintigraph studies on the localization of liposomal superoxide dismutase injected into rabbits. Mol. Physiol., 1:71-84.

48. Michelson, A.M., Puget, K., Perdereau, B., and Barbaroux, C., 1981b. Studies on of liposomal dismutase in rats. Mol. Physiol., 1:85-96.

49. Michelson, A.M., 1982. Oxygen radicals. Agents Actions (Suppl), 11: 179-201.

50. Moncada, S., Bunting, S., Mullane, K., Thorogood, P., Vane, J.R., Raz, A., Needleman, P., 1977. Imidazole: a selective inhibitor of thromboxane synthetase. Prostaglandins 13:611.

51. Padmanabham, R.V., Gudapaty, R., Liener, I.E., Schwartz, B.A., and Hoidal, J.R., 1985. Protection against pulmonary oxygen toxicity in rats by the intratracheal administration of liposome-encapsulated superoxide dismutase or catalase. Am. Rev. Respir. Dis., 132:164-7.

52. Richter, A.W., and Akerblom, E., 1983. Antibodies against polyethylene glycol produced in animals by immunization with monomethyxy polyethylene glycol modified proteins. Int. Arch. Allergy Appl. Immunol., 70:124-131.

53. Rosen, G.M., and Freeman, B.A. 1984. Detection of superoxide generated by endothelial cells. Proc. Natl. Acad. Sci. USA, 81:7269-7273.

54. Rumyantseva, G.V., Weiner, L.M., Molin, Y.N., and Budker, V.G., 1979. Permeation of liposome membrane by superoxide radical. FEBS Letters, 108:477-80.

55. Sackler, M.L., 1966. Xanthine oxidase from liver and duodenum of the rat: histochemical localization and electrophoretic heterogeneity. J. Histochem. Cytochem., 14:326-333.

56. Somiya, K., Niwa, Y., and Michelson, A.M., 1985. Effect of liposomal superoxide dismutase on human neutrophil activity. Free Rad. Res. Comm., 1:17-25.

57. Steinbrecher, U.P., Parthasarathy, S., Leake, D.S., and Steinberg, D., 1984. Modification of LDL by endothelial cells involves lipid peroxidation and degradation of LDL phospholipids. Proc. Nat. Acad. Sci., USA, 81:3883-3887.

58. Takahashi, M.A., and Asada, K., 1983. Superoxide anion permeability of phospholipid membranes and chloroplast thylakoids. Arch. Biochem. Biophys., 226:558-66.

59. Tanswell, A.K., and Freeman, B.A., (J. Appl. Physiol; in press). Liposome-entrapped antioxidant enzymes prevent lethal O_2 toxicity in the newborn rat.

60. Turrens, J.F., Freeman, B.A., Levitt, J.G., and Crapo, J.D., 1982. The effect of hyperoxia on superoxide production by lung submitochondrial particles. Arch. Biochem. Biophys., 217:401-410.

61. Turrens, J.F., Crapo, J.D., and Freeman, B.A., 1984. Protection against oxygen toxicity by intravenous injection of liposome-entrapped catalase and superoxide dismutase. J. Clin. Invest., 73:87-95.

62. Yatvin, M.B., and Lelkes, P.I., 1982. Clinical prospects for liposomes. Am. Assoc. Phys. Med., 9:149-75.

63. Yusa, T., Crapo, J.D., and Freeman, B.A., 1984. Hyperoxia enhances lung and liver nuclear superoxide generation. Biochim. Biophys. Acta., 798:167.

CHANGES OF ACTIVITY OF INTRACELLULAR ANTIOXIDANT ENZYMES OF HEART IN RESPONSE TO ISCHEMIA-REPERFUSION.

G.Rotilio, C.Guarnieri and I.Mavelli.

Department of Biology, University of Rome "Tor Vergata" and CNR Center for Molecular Biology, Rome (Italy), Institute of Biochemistry, University of Bologna, Bologna (Italy), and Institute of Biochemistry, University of Cagliari, Cagliari (Italy).

1) INTRODUCTION

The present review is aimed at a critical evaluation of possible role of the antioxidative enzyme systems in determining the observed effect of ischemia and reperfusion in experimental models of heart damage. In this context these enzyme systems include Cu, Zn- and Mn-superoxide dismutases (Cu, Zn-SOD, Mn-SOD), catalase (CAT), Se-dependent and non Se-dependent glutathione peroxidases (GSH-PX). These enzymes provide the cellular defense against the intermediates of dioxygen reduction (O_2^-, H_2O_2, $OH^{\cdot}$). They act in the following way:

$$2\ O_2^- + 2H^+ \xrightarrow{\text{SOD}} O_2 + H_2O$$

$$2\ H_2O_2 \xrightarrow{\text{CAT}} 2\ H_2O + O_2$$

$$2\ GSH + ROOH \xrightarrow[\text{non Se-GSH-PX}]{\text{Se-GSH-PX}} GSSG + ROH + H_2O \quad \text{(ROOH=Organic peroxide)}$$

$$2\ GSH + H_2O_2 \xrightarrow{\text{Se-GSH-PX}} GSSG + 2\ H_2O$$

These enzyme activities are cooperative in two respects. The first, and the most obvious one, is that SODs convert O_2^- into O_2 and H_2O_2, which has in turn to be removed by CAT and GSH-PX. Therefore the balance of the SOD activities versus that of H_2O_2-removing enzymes is crucial to keep low the steady state concentration of the oxygen radicals. The second kind of functional cooperation involves the protection of SOD by GSH-PX and CAT against inactivation by H_2O_2 (Rotilio et al. 1973, Bray et al 1974); reciprocally SOD may protect CAT and GSH-PX from inhibition by O_2^- (Kono and Fridovich 1983, Blum and Fridovich 1985). Moreover the extent of the selective inactivation of GSH-PX induced by treating cells with free radical-generating drugs (Mavelli et al. 1985) is related to the catalytic efficiency of CAT (Rotilio et al. 1986). The mutually supportive interaction among the antioxidative enzymes makes more critical the balance of their activities, specifically in pathological conditions or upon treatments with free radical-generating drugs. A further complication to be taken in consideration is the compartimentation of these enzyme activities in most cells. CAT is usually present in peroxisomes, where SOD and GSH-PX are missing, although evidence was reported for the presence of CAT activity in the mitochondrial matrix of rat heart (Nohl and Hegner 1978a). Mn-SOD seems to be a mitochondrial enzyme, while Cu,Zn-SOD is predominantly detected in the cytosolic fraction of cells (Fridovich 1983, Spanier et al. 1985). Se-dependent and non Se-dependent GSH-PX activities were found in the cytosol and in mitochondria as well (Mavelli and Rotilio 1984).

The interest in considering if and how the distribution and relative concentration of these enzymes play a role in the ischemic pathology of heart mostly lies in the established efficacy of SOD and/or CAT in protecting the heart tissue from damage, when added to the reperfusion medium (Shlafer 1982a, 1982b; Jolly et al. 1984; Myers et al. 1985; Burton 1985). This effect is related to the beneficial effects of other antioxidants of non-enzymic nature. Recently a great deal of attention has been payed to allopurinol, either as scavenger of oxy-radicals (Moorhouse et al. 1987) or as inhibitor of xanthine oxidase (Manning et al. 1984), which is considered a major source of oxy-radicals in ischemic tissues (Roy and McCord 1983). The available experimental data that represent a rationale for the therapeutic use of antioxidative enzymes in the ischemia-reperfusion syndrome may conveniently divided in two cathegories, which reflect the two major mechanisms by which oxidative damage occurs in tissues: an increased activity of the oxy-radical sources and/or a decreased efficacy of the tissue defense systems.

i) An obvious explanation for the efficacy of SOD and/or CAT in the heart ischemia-reperfusion syndrome is that in the reperfusion phase excess oxy-radicals are produced to an extent that overwhelms the defense capabilities of heart.

Under normal conditions, mitochondria form H_2O_2 as a dismutation product of the O_2^- formed during respiration (Nohl and Hegner 1978b, Turrens and Boveris 1980). In addition, H_2O_2 and O_2^- can be produced by the autoxidation of hemoglobin (Rotilio et al. 1977) and myoglobin (Satoh and Shikama 1981). The extremely reactive hydroxyl radical($OH^\cdot$) can be generated from H_2O_2 by an iron- catalyzed Fenton-like reaction, once iron has been reduced to the Fe(II) form by an increased flux of O_2^- for istance in the tissue storage protein ferritin (O'Connell et al. 1986).

Under ischemia-reperfusion conditions several events may lead to overproduction of oxygen free radicals. However it is extremely important to distinguish between sources that discharge oxy-radicals in the vascular lumen, where they are accessible to extracellularly added enzymes, and the intracellular sources. In fact, for extracellular proteins to be effective in the latter case, one should assume either outside diffusion of some radical species or some inside "penetration" of the enzyme effect (which may even be an intracellular response mediated by interactive events within membranes, with no physical permeation by the enzyme). Presently, both possibilities are purely hypothetical. The major extracellular source of the free radicals is from granulocytes (PMN's) which invade the ischemic tissue (Jolly et al. 1984, Romson et al. 1983). Moreover increased amounts of catecholamines are released from nerve terminals, and they accumulate in abnormally high concentration in ischemic myocardium (Munts et al. 1984). This may result in an increase of free radical production by catecholamine autoxidation. Intracellularly, mitochondria from ischemic cardiac muscle showed an increased NADH- dependent formation of O_2^-, concomitantly with their decreased ability to oxidize NAD- linked substrates. This could favor the maintenance at the reduced state of flavoproteins, which may be involved in O_2^- formation by spontaneous autoxidation (Guarnieri et al. 1985). There are no data available to decide if the activation of xanthine oxidase, which is likely to be a calcium-dependent proteolytic modification of xanthine dehydrogenase induced by ischemic conditions (Roy and Mc Cord 1983), is operating in human heart, while it was found to occur in coronary-occluded dog heart (Chambers et al. 1985) and rat isolated perfused heart (Schoutsen et al 1983). However, neither dehydrogenase to oxidase conversion nor allopurinol protection was detected in other comparable models including either coronary-occlusion of dog heart (Reimer and Jennings 1985) or isolated perfused rat heart (Kehrer et al. 1987).

ii)It is largely given for granted that ischemia-reperfusion induces a decrease of the antioxidant enzyme activities, which would be counteracted by the addition of the appropriate enzymes to the perfusate. The following discussion relates to this second point.

2) ANTIOXIDANT ENZYME DEFENSE SYSTEMS IN HEART

In order to evaluate the importance of the possibility that hypoxic and ischemic conditions induce a decrease of intracellular antioxidative enzymes, it is relevant to consider if heart is per se relatively poorly equipped as far as the antioxidative enzymes are concerned.

CAT is present at very low levels of activity in heart (Doroshow et al. 1980, Marklund et al. 1982), as compared to other organs. However a recent report presented evidence that it may have an important role in the detoxification of H_2O_2 in the myocardium (Thayer 1986). Cardiac metabolism of H_2O_2 was studied by determining the concentration dependence for H_2O_2-stimulated release of GSSG, an indicator for flux throughout GSH-PX pathway. Treatment of rats with aminotriazole inhibited heart CAT by 83% and shifted the dose-response curve for GSSG release toward lower H_2O_2concentration. In agreement with the hypothesis that CAT may function as a major route for H_2O_2 detoxification in the myocardium, especially under stress, conditions, Lazzarino et al. , 1987 found an apparently adaptive increase of CAT activity selectively in heart, in mice treated with a subchronic doses of daunomycin leading to augmented heart lipid peroxidation. Se-dependent GSH-PX activity is not much lower in heart than liver (Doroshow et al. 1980, Marklund et al. 1982), in contrast the non

Se-dependent enzyme was not detected in rat (Lawrence and Burk, 1978) and mouse (Doroshow *et al.* 1980) heart, while it has been recently found in human heart in much lower amount than liver (Di Ilio *et al.* 1986). Furthermore it has been found that the level of GSH in rat heart is about 5- fold lower than liver and also the capacity of the transport system for GSSG is substantially lower than in liver (Ishikawa and Sies 1984, Lazzarino *et al.* 1987). The Cu,Zn SOD activity is nearly four times lower than in liver, either in mouse (Doroshow *et al.* 1980) or in human heart, where it is comparable to that of brain, while the Mn-SOD activity is similar to that of liver (Marklund *et al.* 1982).

It can be concluded that heart has a limited capacity to destroy H_2O_2 which may be aggravated, in critical situations, by the relative efficiency of the SOD systems, especially Mn-SOD, leading to accelerated H_2O_2 production.

3) ANTIOXIDANT ENZYME SYSTEMS UNDER HYPOXIC CONDITIONS

A model for the ischemic damage of heart in natural pathology is the hypoxic heart preparation investigated by Guarnieri *et al.* 1979, 1980. This model involves nitrogen perfusion, with a Langendorff perfusion apparatus, and maintains a very low pO_2 (5-6 mm Hg). The results obtained with antioxidative enzymes and coenzymes are shown in Table I. There is a significant alteration of glutathione metabolism, consisting of reduction of the GSH content, due to its release in the perfusate (data not shown), and a marked decrease of GSH-PX activity. Moreover the SOD activity is significantly decreased as well. A comparable decrease of SOD and GSH-PX activities was recently reported also by Julicher *et al.* 1984, using the same model.

The decrease of GSH-PX activity may be related to the cellular GSH depletion, but it is not a direct result of membrane damage. In fact no GSH-PX activity was found in the hypoxic coronary effluent, but the GSH depletion could be crucial to make the enzyme more susceptible to proteolytic and/or oxidative inactivation. A protective effect of GSH on erythrocyte GSH-PX was shown in the case of oxidative damage induced by hydroquinone-quinone drugs (Ciriolo et al. 1986). Nevertheless no direct evidence is available for enhanced oxidative stress in this model, because increased GSSG was not detected (Guarnieri et al. 1979) and lipid peroxidation was found to be unaffected (Julicher et al. 1986).

TABLE I: Effect of Hypoxia on Myocardial Antioxidant Enzyme Systems (rat heart, paced 180 beats/min). Data from Guarnieri et al. 1979, 1980.

		Aerobic perfusion	95% N_2 - 5% CO_2 perfusion
SOD (Total)	10 min	3.9 ± 0.04	3.7 ± 0.03
(U/mg prot)	60 min	3.6 ± 0.06	2.2 ± 0.04
GSH-PX	10 min	0.21 ± 0.03	0.20 ± 0.03
(umol NADPH/min/ mg prot)	60 min	0.19 ± 0.04	0.14 ± 0.02
GSH	10 min	16.8 ± 1.5	14.1 ± 1.1
(nmol/mg prot)	60 min	16.2 ± 0.9	8.2 ± 2.1
GSSG	10 min	1.3 ± 0.2	1.5 ± 0.3
(nmol/mg prot)	60 min	1.1 ± 0.3	0.7 ± 0.2

4) ANTIOXIDANT ENZYME SYSTEMS UNDER ISCHEMIA/REPERFUSION CONDITIONS

In the most popular model of ischemia/reperfusion, ischemia is induced in isolated, perfused, electrically stimulated rabbit hearts, by reducing the coronary flow from 25 ml/min to 1 ml/min for 90 min. The effects of post-ischemic reperfusion are then followed for 30 min. Curello et al. , 1985, and Ferrari et al. , 1985, showed (table II) that ischemia caused 50% decrease of the Mn-dependent SOD activity, and reduction of GSH and protein SH groups. Reperfusion induced a further decrease of GSH, concomitant with an increase of GSSG. In the same experimental conditions a massive release of GSH and GSSG in the effluent and no recovery of heart mechanical function was reported (Ferrari et al. 1985). GSH-PX, CAT and Cu,Zn SOD activities were not affected by either ischemia or reperfusion (table II). In this model the GSH drop is accompanied by a parallel GSSG increase. In fact, a severe reduction of the GSH/GSSG ratio, due to enhanced GSSG production, was found, in spite of the marked release of GSSG induced by reperfusion. These data indicate that in the reperfusion model a myocardial oxidative stress mediated by H_2O_2 actually occurs. The additional data reported in table III are in line with this hypothesis: the levels of malondialdehyde and other fluorescent substances, which are used to determine the lipid peroxidation extent in biological systems (Chiu et al. 1982), are markedly increased upon post-ischemic reperfusion.

Mn-SOD is the only enzyme activity significantly decreased. Assuming its predominant mitochondrial localization, the decrease might be related to the mitochondrial damage found in this model by Guarnieri et al. 1985, which is associated to stimulation of O_2^- production by ischemic mitochondria. However this damage does not affect GSH-PX, which is also present in heart mitochondria

TABLE II: Effect of Ischemia and Reperfusion on Myocardial Antioxidant Defense Systems (rabbit heart, paced 180 beats/min).
CAT was assayed as in Mavelli et al. 1985. The other data are from Ferrari et al. 1985.

	Aerobic perfusion (120 min)	Ischemic perfusion (90 min)	Ischemic 90min + Aerobic perfusion 30min
Cu,Zn SOD (units/mg prot)	61.3 ± 3.1	54.4 ± 4.5	62.2 ± 8.2
Mn SOD (units/mg prot)	41.1 ± 4.0	24.6 ± 1.9	21.8 ± 3.8
CAT (umol H_2O_2/ min/mg prot)	41.8 ± 11.7	39.3 ± 11.8	40.5 ± 12.5
GSH-PX (umol NADPH/ min/mg prot)	0.21 ± 0.01	0.23 ± 0.02	0.23 ± 0.02
GSH (nmol/mg prot)	11.8 ± 0.7	6.6 ± 0.6	4.5 ± 0.6
GSSG (nmol/mg prot)	0.26 ± 0.08	0.17 ± 0.07	0.55 ± 0.02
PROTEIN SH (nmol/mg prot)	308 ± 11	105 ± 12	213 ± 12

On the basis of these results it is plausible that in the ischemia/reperfusion model the major event is actually overproduction of O_2^- /H_2O_2 may be predominantly in mitochondria, and that decrease of defense capabilities is not as important as in the hypoxic model.

TABLE III: Effect of Ischemia and Reperfusion on Lipid Peroxidation in Isolated Rabbit Heart

	nmol MDA/mg prot[1]	%Fluorescence/mg prot[2]
Whole tissue		
Aerobic perfusion (90min)	0.663 ± 0.01	1.5 ± 0.01
Ischemic perfusion (90min)	0.746 ± 0.10	1.2 ± 0.01
Reperfusion (20min)	0.951 ± 0.09	1.9 ± 0.01
Mitochondria		
Aerobic perfusion (90min)	0.385 ± 0.15	0.88 ± 0.30
Ischemic perfusion (90min)	0.410 ± 0.22	0.92 ± 0.42
Reperfusion (20min)	0.688 ± 0.17	1.88 ± 0.28

1) MDA was determined according to Ohkawa *et al.* 1979

2) Fluorescent substances were determined as in Tsushida *et al.* 1985

5) CONCLUSIONS

The hypoxic condition results in impairment of natural antioxidative enzymatic defense, which may play a role in the recovery of the heart upon the post-hypoxic reoxygenation. However, while in hypoxic conditions there is no evidence for augmented oxidative stress, this is the case in ischemia/reperfusion, and this increased oxy-radical flux may overwhelm the critically balanced enzyme pattern which is typical of heart (see section 2). The reduction of Mn-SOD activity under ischemic conditions is of difficult interpretation and doubtful relation to the observed effects. The strict dependence of the biochemical changes observed on the experimental model used is furtherly shown by the results obtained with a more "natural" model, although a less rigorously controlled one. In the early regional myocardial ischemia, induced by coronary occlusion (Rao et al. 1983), free-radicals of unspecified nature were shown to form in higher amounts than in the control normal tissue by EPR. Decrease of the GSH-PX activity and increase of malondialdehyde were also observed, providing evidence for augmented oxidative stress actually occurring in this model, which generates apparently intermediate results as compared to two models of perfused heart.

As a general conclusion from the results of all models, it may be concluded that, for oxidative damage to occur (increased GSSG, increased lipid peroxidation), augmented oxy-radical flux is more effective than decrease of both SOD and GSH-PX. It is however clear that the observed effects do not fit in a single trend, and none of them may be related to natural events. In any case these results do not offer a plane rationale to the use of antioxidative enzymes as therapeutic agents added to the perfusate. Their effects might even be related to extracellular phenomena not linked to changes of intracellular enzymes.

ACKNOWLEDGEMENTS

The authors wish to thank Mrs Daniela Buganza for her assistance in preparing the manuscript.

REFERENCES

Blum, J. and Fridovich I, 1985. Inactivation of glutathione peroxidase by superoxide radical. Arch. Biochem. Biophys., 240: 500-508.

Bray,R.C., Cockle, S.H., Fielden, E.M. Roberts, P.B. Rotilio G.,and Calabrese, L., 1974. Reduction and inactivation of superoxide dismutase by hydrogen peroxide, Biochem. J.,139: 43-48.

Burton,K.P., 1985. Superoxide dismutase enhances recovery following myocardial ischemia. Am. J. Physiol., 248 (Heart Circ. Physiol, 17) : H637-H643.

Chambers,D.E., Parks, D.A., Patterson, G., Mc Cord, J.M., Yoshida, S., Parmley, L.F., and Downey, J.M., 1985. Xanthine oxidase as a source of free radical damage in myocardial ischemia. J. Mol. Cell. Cardiol., 17: 145-152.

Chiu, D., Lubin, B., and Shohet, S.B., 1982. Peroxidative reactions in red cell biology. In: W.A. Pryor (Editor), Free Radicals in Biology, Vol.V. Academic Press, New York, pp. 115-159.

Ciriolo, M.R., Mavelli, I., and Rotilio, G., 1986. Effect of the redox state of the red blood cell components on the inactivation of glutathione peroxidase by divicine. Free. Rad. Res. Commun., 1: 297-304.

Curello, S., Ceconi, C., Bigoli, C., Ferrari, R., Albertini, A., and Guarnieri, C., 1985. Changes of the cardiac glutathione status after ischemia and reperfusion. Experientia, 41: 42-43.

Di Ilio, C., Sacchetta, P., Lo Bello, M., Caccuri, A.M., and Federici, G., 1986. Selenium independent glutathione peroxidase activity associated with cationic forms of glutathione transferase in human heart. J.Mol. Cell. Cardiol., 18: 983-991.

Doroshow,J.H., Locker, G.Y., and Myers, C.E., 1980. Enzymatic defenses of the mouse heart against reactive oxygen metabolites. Alterations produced by doxorubicin. J.Clin. Invest., 65: 128-135.

Ferrari, R., Ceconi, C., Curello, S., Guarnieri, C. Caldarera, C.M., Albertini, A., and Visioli, O., 1985. Oxygen-mediated myocardial damage during ischaemia and reperfusion: role of the cellular defences against oxygen toxicity. J. Mol. Cell. Cardiol., 17: 937-945.

Fridovich, I., 1983. Superoxide radical: an endogenous toxicant. Ann. Rev. Pharmacol. Toxicol., 23: 239-257.

Guarnieri, C., Flamigni, F., and Rossoni-Caldarera, C., 1979. Glutathione peroxidase activity and release of glutathione from oxygen-deficient perfused rat heart. Biochem. Biophys. Res. Commun., 89: 678-683.

Guarnieri, C., Flamigni, F., and Caldarera C.M., 1980. Role of oxygen in the cellular damage inducede by reoxygenation of hypoxic heart. J. Mol. Cell. Cardiol., 12: 797-801.

Guarnieri,C., Muscari, C., Ventura, C., and Mavelli, I., 1985. Effect of ischemia on heart submitochondrial superoxide production.Free Rad. Res. Commun., 1: 123-128.

Julicher, R.H.M., Sterremberg, L., Walenbergh, L.H.P., Bast,A., and Noordhoek, J., 1986. The effect of vitamin E -deficiency in isolated rat heart on the cellular defence system against free radicals during normal reperfusion after hypoxic, ischemic and Ca-free perfusion. Free Rad. Res. Commun., 1: 225-233.

Jolly, S.R., Kane, W.J., Bailie, M.B., Abrams, G.D.,and Lucchesi,B.R., 1984. Canine myocardial reperfusion injury. Its reduction by the combined administration of superoxide dismutase and catalase.Circ.

Res., 54: 277-285.
Kehrer, J.P., Piper, H.M., and Sies, H., 1987. Xanthine oxidase is not responsible for reoxygenation injury in isolated-perfused rat heart. Free Rad. Res. Commun., 3: 69-78.
Kono, Y. and Fridovich, I., 1982. Superoxide radical inhibits catalase J.Biol. Chem., 257: 5751-5754.
Lawrence, R.A., and Burk, R.F., 1978. Species, tissue and subcellular distribution of non Se-dependent glutathione peroxidase activity. J.Nutr., 108: 211-215.
Lazzarino, G., Viola, A.R., Mulieri, L., Rotilio, G., and Mavelli, I., 1987. Prevention by fructose-1.6-bisphosphate of cardiac oxidative damage induced in mice by subchromic doxorubicin treatment. Cancer Res., in press.
Manning, A.S., Coltart, D.J., and Hearse, D.J. 1984. Ischemia and reperfusion-induced arhythmias in the rat. Effects of xanthine oxidase inhibition with allopurinol. Circ. Res., 55: 545-548.
Marklund, S.L., Westman N.G., Lundgren, E., Roos, G., 1982. Copper-Zinc-containing superoxide dismutase, Manganese-containing superoxide dismutase, catalase, and glutathione peroxidase in normal and neoplastic human cell lines and normal human tissues. Cancer Res., 42: 1955-1961.
Mavelli, I., and Rotilio G., 1984. Enzymatic protection against intracellular oxidative process. In: A.Breccia, C.L.Greenstock and M. Tamba (Editors), Advances on Oxygen Radicals and Radioprotectors. Edizioni Scientifiche "Lo Scarabeo", pp. 65-80
Mavelli,I., Ciriolo, M.R., and Rotilio, G., 1985. Inactivation of red cell glutathione peroxidase by divicine and its relation to the hemolysis of favism. Biochem. Biphys. Acta, 847: 280-284.
Moorhouse, P.C., Grootveld, M., Halliwell, B., Quinlan, J.G., and Gutteridge J.M.C.,1987. Allopurinol and oxypurinol are hydroxyl radical scavangers. FEBS Lett., 213: 23-28.
Myers, M.L. Bolli, R., Lekich, R.F., Hartley, C.J., and Roberts, R., 1985. Enhancement of recovery of myocardial function by oxygen free-radical scavangers after reversible regional ischemia. Circulation, 72: 915-921.
Muntz, K.H., Hagler, H.K., Boulas, H.J., Willerson, J.T., and Buja, L.M., 1984. Redistribution of catecholamines in the ischemic zone of the dog heart. Am. J. Pathol. 114: 64-78.
Nohl, H., Hegner, D., 1978a. Evidence for the existance of catalase in the matrix space of rat-heart mitochondria. FEBS Lett., 89: 126-130.
Nohl, H. and Hegner, D., 1978b. Do mitochondria produce oxygen radicals in vivo?. Eur. J. Biochem., 82: 563-567.
O'Connell, M., Halliwell, B., Moorhouse, C.P., Aruoma, O.I. Baum, H., and Peters, T.J., 1986. Formation of hydroxyl radicals in the presence of ferritin and haemosiderin. Is haemosiderin formation a biological protective mechanism?. Biochem. J., 234: 727-731.
Ohkawa, H., Ohishi, N., and Yagi, K.,1979. Assay for lipid peroxides in animal tissues by thiobarbituric acid reaction. Anal. Biochem., 95: 351-358.
Rao, P.S., Cohen, M.V., and Mueller H.S., 1983. Sequential transcardiac changes in free radicals, catecholamines and lipid peroxides in early myocardial ischemia. In:R.A.Greenwald and G.Cohen (Editors), Oxy Radicals and Their Scavanger Systems. Vol.II: Cellular and Medical Aspects.Elsevier Sc. Publ. Co., Inc., New York, pp.357-360.

Reimer, K.A., and Jennings, R.B., 1985. Failure of the Xanthine oxidase inhibitor allopurinol to limit infarct size after ischemia and reperfusion in dogs. Circulation, 71: 1069-1075.

Romson, J.L. Hook, B.G., Kunkel, S.L., Abrams, G.D., Schork, M.A., and Lucchesi B.R., 1983. Reduction of the extent of ischemic myocardial injury by neutrophil depletion in the dog. Circulation, 67: 1016-1023.

Rotilio, G., Morpurgo, L., Calabrese L., and Mondovi' B., 1973. On the mechanism of superoxide dismutase reaction of the bovine enzyme with hydrogen peroxide and ferrocyanide. Biochim. Biophys. Acta, 302: 229-235.

Rotilio, G., Fioretti, E., Falcioni, G., and Brunori, M., 1977. Generation of superoxide radical by heme protein and its biological relevance. In: A.M. Michelson, J. M. Mc.Cord and I.Fridovich (Editors), Superoxide and Superoxide Dismutase. Academic Press, New York pp. 239-244.

Rotilio, G., Ciriolo, M.R., and Mavelli, I.,1986. Inactivation of erythrocyte glutathione peroxidase as a mechanism of red cell damage by hydroquinone and quinone drugs. In: A.J.G. Swaak and J.F. Koster (Editors), Free Radicals and Arthritic diseases. EURAGE, Rijswijk, pp. 185-189.

Roy, R.S. and Mc Cord, J.M., 1983. Superoxide and ischemia: conversion of xanthine dehydrogenase to xanthine oxidase. In: R.A. Greenwald and G. Cohen (Editors), Oxy Radicals and Their Scavenger Systems. Vol.II: Cellular and Medical Aspects. Elsevier Sc. Publ. Co.,Inc., New York, pp. 145-153.

Satoh, Y., and Shikama, K., 1981. Autoxidation of oxymyoglobin. A nucleophilic displacement mechanism. J. Biol. Chem., 256: 10272-10275.

Schoutsen, B., De Jong, J.W., Harmsem, E., De Tombe, P.P., and Achterberg,P.W., 1983. Myocardial xanthine oxidase/dehydrogenase. Biochim. Biophys. Acta, 762: 519-524.

Shlafer, M., Kane, P.F. and Kirsh, M.M., 1982a. Superoxide dismutase plus catalase enhance the efficacy of hypothermic cardioplegia to protect the globally ischemic, reperfused heart. J.Thorac. Cardiovasc. Surg., 83: 830-839.

Shlafer, M., Kane, P.F., Wiggins, V.Y. and Kirsh, M.M., 1982b. Possible role for cytotoxic oxygen metabolites in the pathogenesis of cardiac ischemic injury. Circulation, 66: 85-92.

Spanier, A.M., Weglicki, W.B., Stiers, D.L. and Misra, H.P., 1985. Superoxide dismutase: tissue, cellular, and subcellular distribution in adult canine heart. Am. J. Physiol., 259 (Cell. Physiol.,18): c379- c384.

Thayer, W.S., 1986. Role of catalase in metabolism of hydrogen peroxide in the perfused rat heart. FEBS lett., 202: 137-140.

Tsushida, M., Miura, T., Mizitani, K., Aibara, K., 1985. Fluorescent substances in mouse and human sera as a parameter of in vivo lipid peroxidation. Biochim.Biophys.Acta, 834: 196-202.

Turrens, J.F. and Boveris, A., 1980. Generation of superoxide anion by the NADH dehydrogenase of bovine heart mitochondria. Biochem. J., 191: 421-427.

ENZYMATIC DEFENSE SYSTEMS AGAINST HYDROPEROXIDES AND OXYGEN-CENTERED RADICALS IN MAMMALS: GLUTATHIONE PEROXIDASE AND SUPEROXIDE DISMUTASES

L. Flohé, W. Straßburger, W.A. Günzler
Grünenthal GmbH, Center of Research, Zieglerstr. 6, D-5100 Aachen, Fed. Rep. of Germany

INTRODUCTION

Hydrogen peroxide, other hydroperoxides, superoxide radicals and further radicals derived therefrom are normally formed in the organism, but, in case of unbalanced production, they play a deleterious role. The most topical pathological events putatively attributed to hydroperoxides and oxygen-centered radicals are mutagenesis, inflammation and reperfusion injury. If produced simultaneously, hydroperoxides and superoxide interact with each other to give an aggressive mixture of pro-oxidant compounds including the hydroxyl radical. Overexposure to such pro-oxidant compounds is also referred to as "oxidative stress" (Sies, 1985).

Nature was wise enough to develope various enzymatic devices to cope with these hazards imminent to aerobic life. The longest known example is catalase, a heme enzyme catalyzing the dismutation of H_2O_2 into molecular oxygen and water. In most tissues, however, catalase appears restricted to special organels, the peroxisomes, and is responsoble for the removal of H_2O_2 there formed by several enzymatic processes. In mitochondria and cytosol of mammals another H_2O_2 netabolizing enzyme prevails, glutathione peroxidase (Flohé, 1982), which requires continuous regeneration of reduced glutathione needed for H_2O_2 reduction. Apart from H_2O_2 it can also reduce a large variety of other hydroperoxides.

H_2O_2 is formed in the organism either directly or as a product resulting from dismutation of the superoxide radical. Superoxide, .OOH, in fact dismutates spontaneously very rapidly to form O_2 and H_2O_2, but as an acid it is present in biological environment largely as the superoxide radical anion, $.O_2^-$. This radical anion resists spontaneous dismutation due to electrostatic repulsion, but is catalytically removed by enzymes called superoxide dismutases (Steinman, 1982). This catalysis is brought about by transition metals coordinated to the protein such as copper, manganese or iron. In the cytosol of mammals a superoxide dismutase is found which contains both Cu and Zn, whereas the mitochondrial enzyme contains Mn.

Superoxide dismutases and peroxidases probably supported by vitamin E and retinoids build up a system of partially redundant, partially complementary scavengers of peroxides and free radicals. The present review is to summarize the structural and functional characteristics of two important constituents of this defense system, glutathione peroxidase and Cu/Zn superoxide dismutase.

CU-ZN SUPEROXIDE DISMUTASE

Reaction catalysed

Superoxide dismutase activity was discovered to be associated with already long known copper containing proteins, the cupreins, by McCord and Fridovich in 1969. The function consists in the facilitation of the dismutation of two superoxide radical anions:

$$2\ .O_2^- + 2H^+ \longrightarrow H_2O_2 + O_2$$

Till now, this activity has remained the only one unambiguously established for the cupreins.

Structure

Cu-Zn superoxide dismutases have been isolated from representatives of all classes of living organisms. They are phylogenetically old proteins which have conserved characteristic structural elements during evolution.

Cu-Zn superoxide dismutases are dimeric proteins consisting of identical subunits each containing one Cu and one Zn ion. The three-dimensional structure of the bovine enzyme has been elucidated Richardson _et al._, 1975) and, with regard to the pronounced sequence

Table 1: Amino acid sequences of eleven Cu-Zn superoxide dismutases isolated from different species. Boxed residues are conserved in all sequences. Asterisks mark metal ligands. Data are taken from Steffens et al., 1986.

```
                   1                                    20
Cabbage                A K G V A V L N S S I G V K G T I F F T H E G N G - A
Man             Ac-A T K A V C V L K G D G P V Q G I I N F E Q K E S N G P
Cattle          Ac-A T K A V C V L K G D G P V Q G T I H F E A K G D - - T
Pig             Ac-A T K A V C V L K G D G P V Q G T I Y F E L K G E K - T
Horse           Ac-A L K A V C V L K G D G P V H G V I H F E Q Q Q E G G P
Rat             Ac-A M K A V C V L K G D G P V Q G V I H F E Q K A S G G P
Swordfish          V L K A V C V L R G A G E T T G T V Y F E Q E G N A N A
Fruitfly           V V K A V C V I M G D A K G T V F F E Q I S S G T - - P
Yeast                V Q A V A V L K G D A G V S G V V K F E Q A S E S E P
Neurospora           V K A V A V V R G D S N V K G T V I F E Q E S E S A P
P.leiognathi         Q D L T V K M T D L Q T G K P V G T I E L S Q N K Y G

                                        40
                                                       *   *
Cabbage            T T V T G T V S G - L R P G L H G F H V H A L G D N T N
Man                V K V W G S I K G - L T E G L H G F H V H E F G D N T A
Cattle             V V V T G S I T G - L T E G D H G F H V H Q F G D N T Q
Pig                V L V T G T I K G - L A E G D H G F H V H Q F G D N T Q
Horse              V V L K G F I E G - L T K G D H G F H V H E F G D N T Q
Rat                V V V S G Q I T G - L T E G E H G F H V H Q Y G D N T Q
Swordfish          V G K G I I L K G - L T P G E H G F H V H G F G D N T N
Fruitfly           V K V S G E V C G - L A K G L H G F H V H E F G D N T N
Yeast              T T V S Y E I A G N S P N A E R G F H I H E F G D A T N
Neurospora         T T I T Y D I S G N D P N A D K G F H I H T F G D N T N
P.leiognathi       V V F T P E L A D - L T P G M H G F H I H Q N G - - - -

                        60                                      80
                                                         *
Cabbage            G C M S - - - - - - - - - - - - T G P H F N P - D G K T
Man                G C T S - - - - - - - - - - - - A G P H F N P - L S R K
Cattle             G C T S - - - - - - - - - - - - A G P H F N P - L S K K
Pig                G C T S - - - - - - - - - - - - A G P H F N P - E S K K
Horse              G C T T - - - - - - - - - - - - A G A H F N P - L S K K
Rat                G C T T - - - - - - - - - - - - A G P H F N P - H S K K
Swordfish          G C I S - - - - - - - - - - - - A G P H F N P - A S K K
Fruitfly           G C M S - - - - - - - - - - - - S G P H F N P - Y G K E
Yeast              G C V S - - - - - - - - - - - - A G P H F N P - F K K T
Neurospora         G C T S - - - - - - - - - - - - A G P H F N P - H G A T
P.leiognathi       S C A S S E K D G K V V L G G A A G G H Y D P E H T N K

                   *                 *     *    100
Cabbage            H G A P E D A N R H A G D L G N I I V G D D G T A T F T
Man                H G G P K D E E R H V G D L G N V T A D K D G V A D V S
Cattle             H G G P K D E E R H V G D L G N V T A D K N G V A I V D
Pig                H G G P K D Q E R H V G D L G N V T A G K D G V A T V Y
Horse              H G G P K D E E R H V G D L G N V T A D E N G K A D V D
Rat                H G G P A D E E R H V G D L G N V A A G K D G V A N V S
Swordfish          H A G P K D E D R H V G D L G N V T A D A N G V A K I D
Fruitfly           H G A P V D E N R H L G D L G N I E A T G D C P T K V N
Yeast              H G A P T D E V R H V G D M G N V K T D E N G V A K G S
Neurospora         H G D R T A E V R H V G D L G N I E T D A Q G N A K G T
P.leiognathi       H G F P W T D D N H K G D L P A L F V S A N G L A T N P

                                120                          *          140
Cabbage            I T D S Q I P L S G P N S I V G R A I V V H A D P D D L
Man                I E D S V I S L S G D H C I I G R T L V V H E K A D D L
Cattle             I V D P L I S L S G E Y S I I G R T M V V H E K P D D L
Pig                I E D S V I A L S G D H S I I G R T M V V H E K P D D L
Horse              M K D S V I S L S G K H S I I G R T M V V H E K Q D D L
Rat                I E D R V I S L S G E H S I I G R T M V V H E K Q D D L
Swordfish          I T D - K I S L T G P Y S I I G R T M V I H E K A D D L
Fruitfly           I T D S K I T L F G A D S I I G R T V V V H A D A D D L
Yeast              F K D S L I K L I G P T S V V G R S V V I H A G Q D D L
Neurospora         V T D N L V K L I G P E S V I G R T V V V H A G T D D L
P.leiognathi       V L A P R L T L K - - - E L K G H A I M I H A G G D N H

                                                        160
Cabbage            G K G G H E L S L S T G N A G G R V A C G I I G L Q G
Man                G K G G N E E S T K T G N A G S R L A C G V I G I A Q
Cattle             G R G G N E E S T K T G N A G S R L A C G V I G I A K
Pig                G R G G N E E S T K T G N A G S R L A C G V I G I T Q
Horse              G K G G N E E S T K T G N A G S R L A C G V I G I A T
Rat                G K G G N E E S T K T G N A G S R L A C G V I G I A Q
Swordfish          G R G G N E E S L K T G N A G S R L A C G V I G T E -
Fruitfly           G Q G G H E L S K S T G N A G A R I G C G V I G I A K
Yeast              G K G D T E E S L K T G N A G P R P A C G V I G L T N
Neurospora         G K G G N E E S L K T G N A G P R P A C G V I G I S Q
P.leiognathi       - - - - S D M P K A L G G G G A R V A C G V I Q - - -
```

homology between different species, may be considered representative for all Cu-Zn superoxide dismutases. Apart from a single loop, helical structures are absent (Fig. 1a). Most characteristic is the prevalence of β-structures forming a rigid barrel-like central core. The arrangement of the β-strands is fixed by a single disulfide bond and the coordinated metals. Calculations of the surface charge of the enzyme molecule revealed that a channel of steadily increasing positive charge centers onto the copper (Getzoff et al., 1983). The main contributor to this electrostatic channel is Arg141. Table 1 shows that a total of ca. 25 % of the amino acid residues are conserved in homologous position on the superoxide dismutases of 11 species including such diverse organisms as bacteria, plants, insects and vertebrates. The putative role of some conserved residues may be derived from Fig. 1b. In this computer graphic the conserved residues are marked in the three-dimensional peptide backbone of the seven histidines and an aspartate chelating the metals, the disulfide bridge and the positively changed arginine. It can be assumed that these residues are indispensible for structural and functional integrity of the enzyme (Steffens et al., 1986).

Fig. 1: Views of the threedimensional structure of the Cu-Zn superoxide subunit from cattle. The computer graphics were prepared by means of CHEMX software (Chemical Design, Ltd., Oxford, UK).

Fig. 1a: Peptide backbone of the subunit showing elements of secundary structure: purple = helix; green = β-strands; blue = β-turns and random structure; yellow = disulfide bond. Orange and green balls represent the copper and zinc ion, respectively.

Fig. 1b: Some view of the subunit showing conserved amino acid residues (red).

Fig. 1c: Active site of Cu-Zn superoxide dismutase with its substrate $\cdot O_2^-$ (purple) located between Arg141 (blue) and the copper ion (orange).

Fig. 1d: Close-up of Fig. 1c with van der Waals radii covered by a net (yellow).

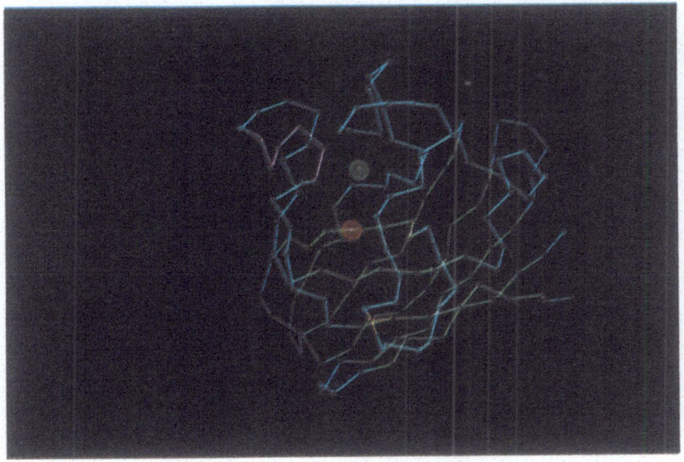

Fig. 1a

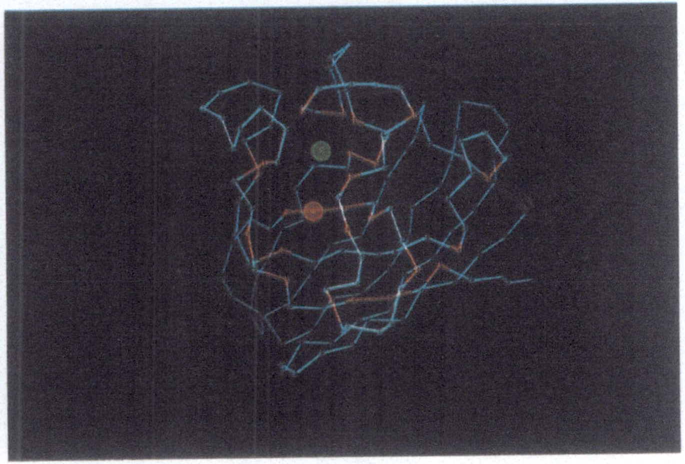

Fig.1b

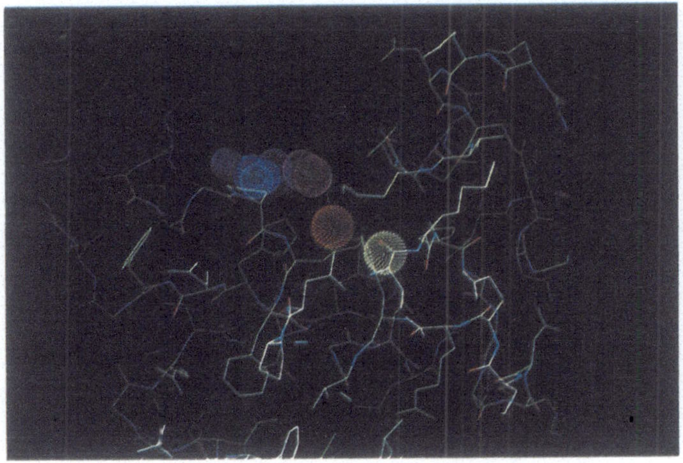

Fig. 1c

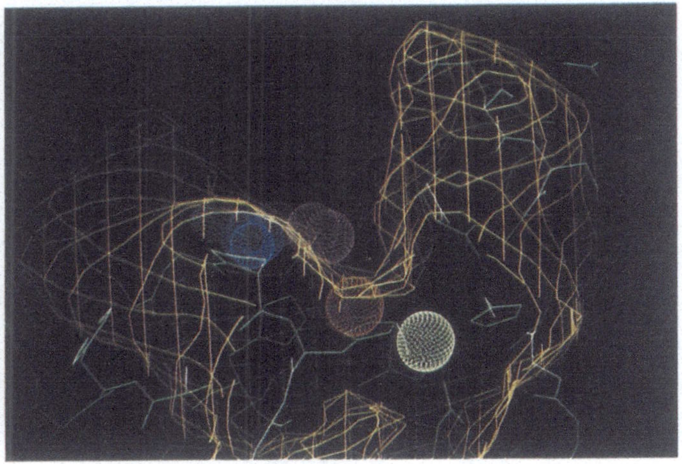

Fig.1d

Mechanism of action

Metal substitution experiments proved that the copper of Cu-Zn superoxide dismutase is the crucial catalytically active constituent. It is by now accepted that the catalysis consists of two consecutive redox reactions as follows:

$$\cdot O_2^- + EnzCu^{2+} \longrightarrow O_2 + EnzCu^+$$
$$\cdot O_2^- + EnzCu^+ + 2H^+ \longrightarrow H_2O_2 + EnzCu^{2+}$$

Thus mediated by the protein-bound copper the electrostatic repulsion of the superoxide anions is overcome. The above mentioned positive surface charge increasing towards the active center attracts the negatively charged substrate molecule thereby mimimizing futile collisions. The figures 1c and d are to demonstrate how exactly the $\cdot O_2^-$ molecule fits between the arginine residue and the copper ion. By means of this "clever" arrangement of surface changes the attraction of changed substrate and the release of unchanged products is optimized to an extent that the electron transition at the copper can procede with "inorganic velocity". In fact, the rate constants are in the range of $2 \times 10^9\ M^{-1}\ sec^{-1}$, i.e. limited by collision frequency (Klug et al., 1972).

GLUTATHIONE PEROXIDASE

Reaction catalysed

In 1957 Mills first described the enzymatic reduction of H_2O_2 by GSH in red blood cells:

$$H_2O_2 + 2GSH \longrightarrow 2H_2O + GSSG$$

Later it was discovered that glutathione peroxidase can actually also reduce a large variety of organic hydroperoxides (for review see Flohé, 1982):

$$ROOH + 2GSH \longrightarrow ROH + GSSG + H_2O_2$$

Table 2: Amino acid sequences of glutathione peroxidases. Asterisks mark residues potentially involved in substrate binding or catalysis. Data are taken from Chambers et al. 1986, Condell and Tappel 1982, and Günzler et al. 1984.

	1 … 10 … 20
Mouse	Met-Cys-Ala-Ala-Arg-Leu-Ser-Ala-Ala-Ala-Gln-Ser-Thr-Val-Tyr-Ala-Phe-Ser-Ala-Arg-Pro-Leu-
Cattle	Ala-Ala-Ala-Leu-Ala-Ala-Ala-Ala-Pro-Arg-Thr-Val-Tyr-Ala-Phe-Ser-Ala-Arg-Pro-Leu-
Rat	Gly-Ala-Val-Ala-Gln-Ser-Thr-Val-Tyr-Ala-Phe-Ser-Ala-Arg-Pro-Leu-

	30 … 40
Mouse	Thr-Gly-Gly-Glu-Pro-Val-Ser-Leu-Gly-Ser-Leu-Arg-Gly-Lys-Val-Leu-Leu-Ile-Glu-Asn-
Cattle	Ala-Gly-Gly-Glu-Pro-Phe-Asn-Leu-Ser-Ser-Leu-Arg-Gly-Lys-Val-Leu-Leu-Ile-Glu-Asn-
Rat	Ala-Gly-Gly-Glu-Pro-Val-Ser-Leu-Gly-Ser-Leu-Arg-Gly-Lys-Val-Leu-Leu-Ile-Glu-Asn-

	* … *50 … 60
Mouse	Val-Ala-Ser-Leu-Sec-Gly-Thr-Thr-Ile-Arg-Asp-Tyr-Thr-Glu-Met-Asn-Asp-Leu-Gln-Lys-
Cattle	Val-Ala-Ser-Leu-Sec-Gly-Thr-Thr-Val-Arg-Asp-Tyr-Thr-Gln-Met-Asn-Asp-Leu-Gln-Arg-
Rat	Val-Ala-Ser-Leu-Sec-Gly-Thr-Thr-Thr-Arg

	70 … 80
Mouse	Arg-Leu-Gly-Pro-Arg-Gly-Leu-Val-Val-Leu-Gly-Phe-Pro-Cys-Asn-Gln-Phe-Gly-His-Gln-
Cattle	Arg-Leu-Gly-Pro-Arg-Gly-Leu-Val-Val-Leu-Gly-Phe-Pro-Cys-Asn-Gln-Phe-Gly-His-Gln-

	90 … * … 100
Mouse	Glu-Asn-Gly-Lys-Asn-Glu-Glu-Ile-Leu-Asn-Ser-Leu-Lys-Tyr-Val-Arg-Pro-Gly-Gly-Gly-
Cattle	Glu-Asn-Ala-Lys-Asn-Glu-Glu-Ile-Leu-Asn-Cys-Leu-Lys-Tyr-Val-Arg-Pro-Gly-Gly-Gly-

	110 … 120
Mouse	Phe-Glu-Pro-Asn-Phe-Thr-Leu-Phe-Glu-Lys-Cys-Glu-Val-Asn-Gly-Glu-Lys-Ala-His-Pro-
Cattle	Phe-Glu-Pro-Asn-Phe-Met-Leu-Phe-Glu-Lys-Cys-Glu-Val-Asn-Gly-Glu-Lys-Ala-His-Pro-

	130 … 140
Mouse	Leu-Phe-Thr-Phe-Leu-Arg-Asn-Ala-Leu-Pro-Thr-Pro-Ser-Asp-Asp-Pro-Thr-Ala-Leu-Met-
Cattle	Leu-Phe-Ala-Phe-Leu-Arg-Glu-Val-Leu-Pro-Thr-Pro-Ser-Asp-Asp-Ala-Thr-Ala-Leu-Met-

	150 … 160
Mouse	Thr-Asp-Pro-Lys-Tyr-Ile-Ile-Trp-Ser-Pro-Val-Cys-Arg-Asn-Asp-Ile-Ala-Trp-Asn-Phe-
Cattle	Thr-Asp-Pro-Lys-Phe-Ile-Thr-Trp-Ser-Pro-Val-Cys-Arg-Asn-Asp-Val-Ser-Trp-Asn-Phe-

	170 … * * 180
Mouse	Glu-Lys-Phe-Leu-Val-Gly-Pro-Asp-Gly-Val-Pro-Val-Arg-Arg-Tyr-Ser-Arg-Arg-Phe-Arg-
Cattle	Glu-Lys-Phe-Leu-Val-Gly-Pro-Asp-Gly-Val-Pro-Val-Arg-Arg-Tyr-Ser-Arg-Arg-Phe Leu

	190 … 198
Mouse	Thr-Ile-Asp-Ile-Glu-Pro-Asp-Ile-Glu-Thr-Leu-Leu-Ser-Gln-Gln-Ser-Gly-Asn-Ser
Cattle	Thr-Ile-Asp-Ile-Glu-Pro-Asp-Ile-Glu-Thr-Leu-Leu-Ser-Gln-Gly-Ala-Ser-Ala

The substrates of glutathione peroxidase comprise hydroperoxides of unsaturated fatty acids, steroids, and nucleic acids. Peroxo groups of intact lipids, however, are commonly not accessible to glutathione peroxidase probably due to steric hindrance. But a low molecular weight glutathione peroxidase variant from porcine tissue has been reported to directly interact with peroxidized lipid bilayers (Ursini et al., 1982).

Structure

Glutathione peroxidase is a tetrameric enzyme of a molecular weight of 84000 consisting of four identical subunits. Each subunit contains one selenocysteine residue firmly integrated in the protein backbone. It represents the catalytic element of the enzyme (see below).

The complete amino acid sequence of bovine glutathione peroxidase was elucidated by Günzler et al. (1982), an N-terminal fragment of the rat enzyme has been sequenced (Condell and Tappel, 1983) and the total sequence of the mouse enzyme became recently available as an transcript of the corresponding structural gene (Table 2) (Chambers et al., 1986). From this investigation it can be derived that the nucleic acid sequence encoding selenocysteine is TGA, formerly considered a nonsense or termination codon.

X-ray analysis of the bovine glutathione peroxidase revealed the structure shown in Fig. 2a. The subunit is composed of each four helices and β-strands connected by β-turnes or random elements. The selenium atom is exposed at the surface of a flat impression which is surrounded by four arginine residues (Fig. 2b). The lack of pronounced structural differentiation near the active site is striking and may explain the poor specificity of glutathione peroxidase for hydroperoxides.

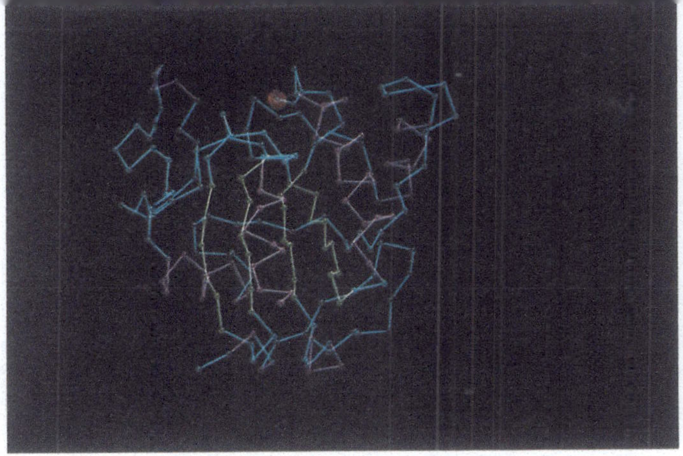

Fig. 2a

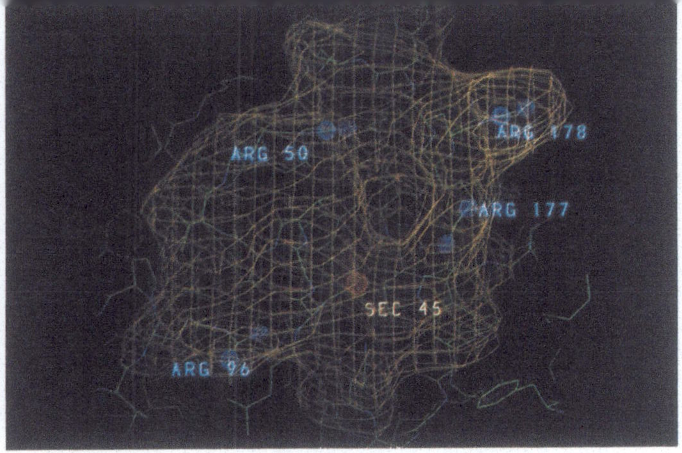

Fig. 2b

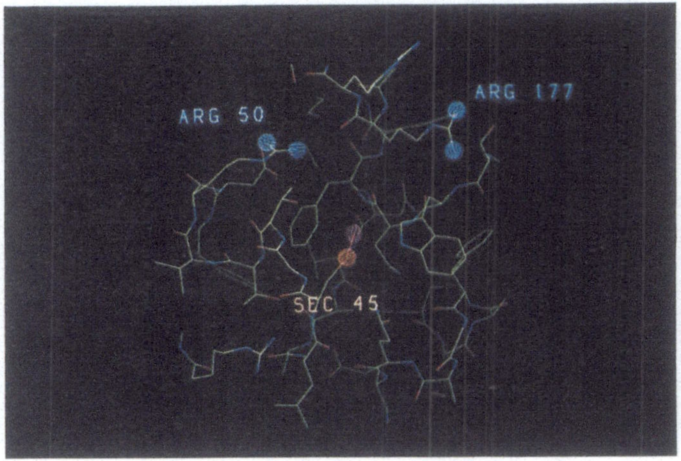

Fig. 2c

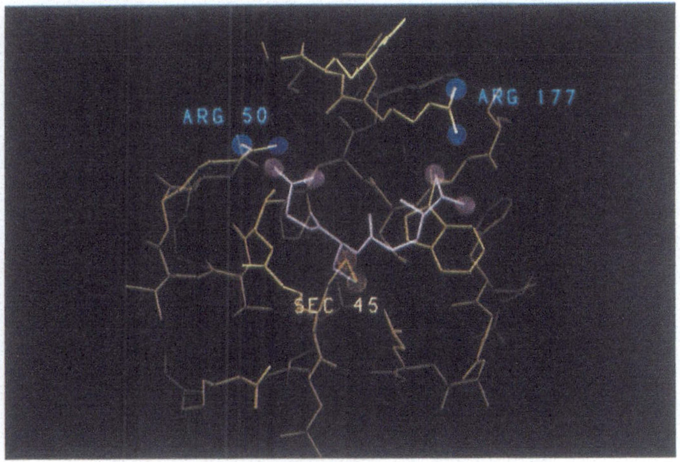

Fig. 2d

Fig. 2: Views of the three-dimensional structure of the glutathione peroxidase subunit of cattle according to Ladenstein et al. 1986. The computer graphs were prepared by means of CHEMX software (Chemical Design, Ltd., Oxford, UK).

Fig. 2a: shows the elements of secondary structure and the selenium atom (orange). Helices are shown in purple, β-strands in green, turns and random structure in blue.

Fig. 2b: Active site with van der Waals radii covered by a net (yellow). Note the lack of structural differentiation around the selenium atom (sec 45).

Fig. 2c: Amino acid residues constituting the active site (oxidized form). (Colour code: blue balls = guanidine nitrogens of Arg50 and Arg177; orange ball = selenium; purple ball = oxygen; green = carbon; red = oxygen; blue = nitrogen)

Fig. 2d: Active site with GSH molecule (purple) bound covalently to selenium. The caboxylic groups of GSH are electrostatically linked to the positively changed guanidine residues of Arg50 and Arg177.

Mechanism of action

Unfortunately the limited sequence information on glutathione peroxidases do not yet allow a definition of essential structural elements. But by means of kinetic studies complemented with the structural information a putative reaction mechanism can be deduced. The experimental evidence supporting this mechanism has been recently discussed in detail (Flohé, in press).

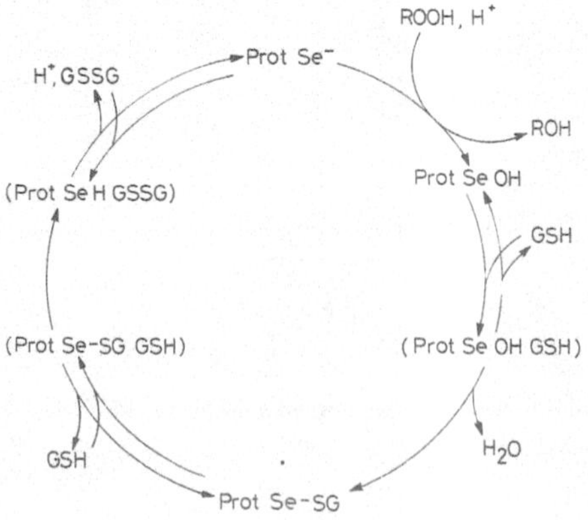

Fig. 3: Catalytic cycle of glutathione peroxidase

The catalytic cycle (Fig. 3) starts with the reaction of the selenocysteine residue by a hydroperoxide. This step is considered a simple bimolecular reaction not rendered specific by previous formation of a typical enzyme substrate complex. The rate constants depend on the nature of the hydroperoxide and decrease with sterical shielding of the hydroperoxo group, but are extraordinarily high for small hydroperoxides (10^7 - 10^8 M^{-1} sec^{-1}). The product of this first step is water or an alcohol and an oxidized enzyme, very likely a selenenic acid derivative. This intermediate of the catalytic cycle forms a weak complex with glutathione, whereby the negative carboxy groups of the substrate bind electrostatically to two arginine residues flanking the active site (Fig. 2c,d). By this orientation the sulfur of the reducing substrate gets into an ideal position to react with the selenenic acid group of the enzyme and then forms a new intermediate, wherein a selenadisulfide bridge links the substrate to the enzyme (Fig. 2d). The second glutathione molecule has to split this selenadisulfide bond to regenerate the reduced enzyme form, i.e. that with the selenocysteine group (Fig. 3).

MEDICAL ASPECTS

Superoxide dismutase has been widely used experimentally to investigate pathological phenomena supposed to be mediated by $.O_2^-$. In *in vivo* experiments, the free enzyme proved particularly helpful in elucidating effects of superoxide released into the extracellular space, as e.g. by stimulated phagocytes. If superoxide is believed to arise from intracellular compartments injection of the enzyme cannot be considered a revealing approach. In this case special technique such as liposome encapsulation may be applied (see B. Freeman, this volume).

The concept to remove extracellular superoxide by injection of superoxide dismutase has found therapeutic application in the treatment of various inflammatory disorders (Puhl and Sies, 1984). But the full scope of therapeutic options for superoxide dismutase has not yet been explored, primarily since so far only a heterologuous protein, bovine superoxide dismutase, has been made available. An authentic human superoxide dismutase from genetically transformed yeast is now being developed and will soon be available for clinical trials (Flohé et al., 1986).

Glutathione peroxidase is not an ideal experimental tool to investigate the role of hydroperoxides *in vivo*, since its cosubstrate, glutathione, is only present extracellularly at very low concentrations and there is not regenerated. Therefore the catalytic hydroperoxide removal, even in the presence of massive amounts of glutathione peroxidase, will stop after a few cycles.

More interesting is the modulation of glutathione peroxidase activity by restricting or optimizing selenium supply. A considerable proportion of the well known selenium deficiency symptoms in life stock or experimental animals are probably due to an impaired hydroperoxide removal (Flohé, 1982, Flohé, in press). At least, glutathione perxodase activity can be used as a reliable marker of the selenium status in animals and man.

Selenium fortification of animal food is now commonly accepted due to the economic impact of the deficiency diseases in life stock. In human medicine the benefit of extra selenium supply is still debated, since relevant deficiencies in populations on mixed food have not been demonstrated. In isolated selenium-deficient areas acute selenium deficiency is observed in humans and may lead to severe or even fatal diseases, as exemplified by the Keshan disease endemic in some parts of China. However, selenium supplementation in man will remain critical due to its narrow therapeutic window, but the possibility to monitor the treatment by glutathione peroxidase determinations may help to solve this problem.

ACKNOWLEDGEMENT

This work was supported by the *Bundesministerium für Forschung und Technologie* (Grant PTB 8663).

REFERENCES

Chambers, I., Frampton, J., Goldfarb, P., Affara, N., McBain, W. and Harrison, P.R., 1986. The structure of the mouse glutathione peroxidase gene: the selenocysteine in the active site is encoded by the "termination" codon, TGA. EMBO J., 5: 1221-1227.

Condell, R.A. and Tappel, A.L., 1982. Amino acid sequence around the active-site selenocysteine of rat liver glutathione peroxidase. Biochim. Biophys. Acta., 709: 304-309.

Flohé, L., 1982. Glutathione peroxidase brought into focus. In: W.A. Pryor (Editor), Free Radicals in Biology. Academic Press, New York and London, pp. 223-253.

Flohé, L. In: D. Dolphin, Poulson, R., Avramovic, O. (Eds.), Coenzymes and Cofactors, Vol. III "Glutathione", John Wiley & Sons, Inc. Publishers, New York (in press).

Flohé, L., Günzler, W.A. and Schock, H.H., 1973. Glutathione peroxidase: A selenoenzyme. FEBS Lett. 32: 132-134.

Flohé, L., Kim, S.-M.A., Ötting, F., Saunders, D., Schwertner, E., Steffens, G.J.; Blacher, R., Masiarz, F., Scandella, C. and Hallewell, R., 1986. In: G. Rotilio (Editor), Superoxide and Superoxide Dismutase in Chemistry, Biology and Medicine. Elsevier Science Publishers, Amsterdam, New York, Oxford, pp. 266-269.

Ge, K., Xue, A., Bai, J. and Wang, S., 1983. Keshan disease - an endemic cardiomyopathy in China. Virchows Arch. (Pathol. Anat.), 401: 1-15.

Getzoff, E.D., Tainer, J.A., Weiner, P.K., Kollman, P.A., Richardson, J.S. and Richardson, D.C., Nature, 306: 287- .

Günzler, W.A., Steffens, G.J., Grossmann, A., Kim, S.-M.A., Ötting, F., Wendel, A. and Flohé, L., 1984. The amino-acid sequence of bovine glutathione peroxidase. Hoppe-Seyler's Z. Physiol. Chem., 365: 195-212.

Klug, D.; Rabani, J. and Fridovich, I., 1972. A direct demonstration of the catalytic action of superoxide dismutase through the use of pulse radiolysis. J. biol. Chem., 247: 4839-4842.

Ladenstein, R., Epp, O., Günzler, W.A. and Flohé, L., 1986. Glutathione peroxidase on approval. Life Chem. Rep., 4: 37-55.

McCord, J.M. and Fridovich, I., 1969. Superoxide dismutase. An enzymic function for erythrocuprein (hemocuprein). J. Biol. Chem., 244: 6049-6055.

Mills, G.C.H., 1957. Hemoglobin catabolism. I. Glutathione peroxidase, an erythrocyte enzyme which protects hemoglobin from oxidative breakdown. J. Biol. Chem., 229: 189-197.

Puhl, W. and Sies, H. (Editors), 1984. Biochemie und Klinik der Superoxid-Dismutase. perimed Fachbuch-Verlagsgesellschaft mbH, Erlangen.

Richardson, J.S., Thomas, K.; Rubin, B.H. and Richardson, D.C., 1975. Crystal structure of bovine Cu,Zn superoxide dismutase at 3 Å resolution: Chain tracing and metal ligands. Proc. Natl. Acad. Sci., 72: 1349-1353.

Sies, H. (Editor), 1985. Oxidative Stress. Academic Press, London.

Steffens, G.J., Michelson, A.M., Ötting, F., Puget, K., Straßburger, W. and Flohé, L., 1986. Primary structure of Cu-Zn superoxide dismutase of *Brassica oleracea* proves homology with corresponding enzymes of animals, fungi and prokaryotes. Biol. Chem. Hoppe-Seyler, 367: 1007-1016.

Steinman, H.M., 1982. In: L.W. Oberley (Editor). Superoxide Dismutase. Vol. 1, CRC Press, Inc., Boca Raton, Florida, pp. 11-68.

Ursini, F., Maiorino, M., Valente, M., Ferri, L. and Gregolin, C., 1982. Purification from pig liver of a protein which protects liposomes and biomembranes from peroxidative degradation and exhibits glutathione peroxidase activity on phosphatidylcholine hydroperoxides. Biochim. Biophys. Acta, 710: 197-211.

ANTIOXIDANT MECHANISMS IN THE HEART: THE POTENTIAL INVOLVEMENT OF MYOGLOBIN

PAUL HOCHSTEIN
INSTITUTE FOR TOXICOLOGY
UNIVERSITY OF SOUTHERN CALIFORNIA
LOS ANGELES, CALIFORNIA 90033

All aerobic biological systems are exposed to a variety of oxidants and oxygen-derived free-radicals. These reactive chemical species may arise from exogenous sources, e.g., xenobiotics and radiation. Alternatively, they may come from endogenous metabolic events and constituents, e.g., electron transport processes and the peroxidation of the fatty acid components of lipids. Living cells are protected from such substances by one or more important scavenger and compensatory systems. However, when the rates of oxidant formation exceed the capacity of detoxification systems, then pathology in the form of altered cellular function and ultimate cell death results. Oxidants are presumed to be the basis for several pathological and toxicological states. In particular, they seem to characterize ischemic-reperfusion disease in several organs including the heart. In this organ oxidant damage is thought to be the basis for deaths associated with coronary artery disease and myocardial infarction.

It should be noted that most cellular macromolecules (lipids, proteins, and nucleic acids) are inherently, albeit differentially, sensitive to oxidants. This is also the case for many small molecules (fatty acids, amino acids, and carbohydrates). For these reasons and because many potential oxidants are short-lived chemical species, the extent of damage to cellular proceses and structures will depend on the specific sites of association or formation of each oxidant. Therefore, the operation of protective and repair mechanisms in localized areas of the cell may be the critical determinants of ultimate damage. On the other hand, for more long-lived oxidants, e.g., hydrogen peroxide and organic hydroperoxides, the total protective capacity of the cell, as often determined by nutritional and genetic status, may be of primary importance. While these distinctions are often difficult to draw experimentally, they are of considerable interest in the understanding of antioxidant mechanisms as well as in the development of therapeutic modalities.

As indicated above, the total protective capacity of a tissue such as the heart is likely to depend on a number of systems which operate at distinctive sites, either simultaneously or sequentially, to ameliorate the effects of oxidants. It is our view that it is not helpful to view these systems as "primary" or "secondary". Depending upon the oxidant, the molecular target and the organelle they all may be essential in the maintenance of appropriate metabolic functions. These systems are listed below:

DETOXIFYING ENZYMES:	GLUTATHIONE PEROXIDASES SUPEROXIDE DISMUTASES DT DIAPHORASE
SCAVENGER MOLECULES:	VITAMIN E CAROTENE URIC ACID GLUTATHIONE
REPAIR SYSTEMS FOR:	PROTEINS LIPIDS NUCLEIC ACIDS MEMBRANE SUFHYDRYLS
"OXIDANT SINKS":	PROTEINS (NON-METAL) HEMOGLOBIN MYOGLOBIN

The incompleteness of this list should first be apparent. There are other enzymes that undoubtedly participate in maintaining cellular homeostasis in the presence of oxidative challenges. Additionally, many small molecules (including water!) exhibit reactivities, concentrations, and turnovers sufficient to permit them to serve as non-essential, and hence protective, oxidant targets. It is also not our intention to review the literature on the occurrence, operation, and importance of the systems that are listed. However, we do call attention to the last category of substances. These are the "oxidant sinks". Their potential importance has received too little attention. For example, it is unfortunate that most studies on oxidants in ischemic-reperfusion injury are carried out in the absence of extracellular proteins such as albumin. This is particularly regrettable since the contemporary view of the events associated with injury is that oxidants are generated outside of the myocyte by endothelial or white cells. Plasma or interstitial proteins might serve as a critical sink for these oxidants in transit to targets. Their capacity to react with a variety of oxidants is well-known and their concentrations are high.

A similar capacity undoubtedly exists in the case of both intracellular and membrane proteins. Since the concentration of these proteins is low and they may have critical enzymatic or structural capacities, the recognition, removal, and repair of these molecules would necessarily be an essential aspect of their antioxidant functions as targets.

The situation with respect to intracellular proteins such as myoglobin, which contain easily oxidized and reduced transition metals as "oxidant sinks", has not been carefully evaluated. We take the view that the oxidation of iron to higher valance states in myoglobin might be an important protective device in muscle. This concept is enhanced by newly described experiments which illustrate the capacity of intracellular reduced glutathione (GSH) to rapidly reduce the iron of myoglobin (1).

Our view that myoglobin might participate in the detoxification of hydrogen peroxide and organic hydroperoxides through a "glutatione peroxidase-like" activity is based upon the scheme as shown below:

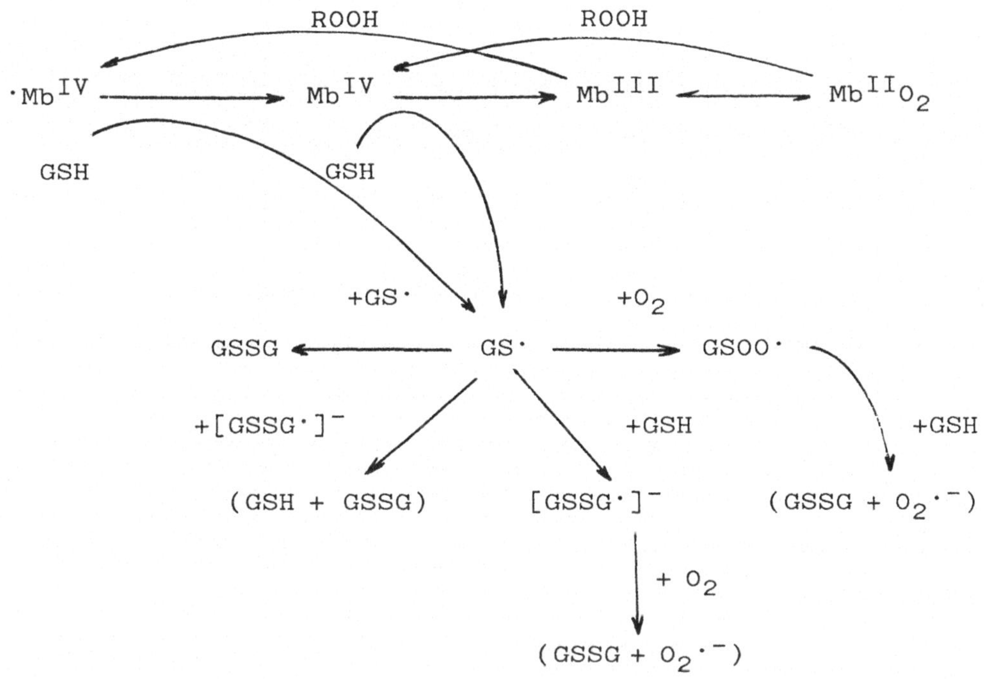

A rapid oxidation of GSH that takes place when MB^{III} is exposed to either H_2O_2 or linoleate hydroperoxide. This "GSH peroxidase" activity is dependent upon the conversion of Mb to ferryl states. It is of interest because ferryl species of Mb have been implicated in the causation of cellular damage under conditions in which $O_2^{\cdot -}$ and H_2O_2 might be formed. The potential for such damage has been demonstrated in model systems (2-4). However, in living cells the presence of reducing agents or enzyme systems (5,6) with the capacity to convert ferrylmyoglobin to lower valence states, might be crucial determinants of damage. In this context, GSH is of obvious interest because of its high concentration (ca. 2 mM) in myocytes and because of the low glutathione peroxidase activity of these cells (7). Although the above diagram focuses on the different redox transitions of GSH involving Mb, the participation of the protein should be regarded in a catalytic rather than stoichiometric fashion.

The reduction of either $\cdot Mb^{IV}$ or Mb^{IV} by GSH is a one-electron event and thiyl radicals (GS·) are produced. It should be noted that horseradish peroxidase and prostaglandin synthase (but not glutathione peroxidase) have been recently shown to oxidize GSH by one electron (8,9). In the presence of air, GS· may react with GSH and O_2 giving rise to GSSG and $O_2^{\cdot -}$ as end products, within a set of reactions involving different intermediates. Under such circumstances, the ultimate formation of H_2O_2 might result in a continuous reoxidation of Mb and eventual depletion of cellular GSH. Of course, this acceleration of GSH depletion might well sensitize cells to H_2O_2 and to the direct oxidizing effects of Mb^{IV} states. On the other hand, when the availability of O_2 is decreased, the reactions of GS· which produce GSSG without $O_2^{\cdot -}$ formation and in stoichiometric amounts to H_2O_2 added would be favored. By these means, damage to sensitive cellular constituents by Mb^{IV}, as well as by H_2O_2 and its decomposition products, might be prevented. It should be noted that the intracellular concentration of O_2 is indeed much lower than that of aerated solutions with a rather steep gradient from the capilaries through the plasma membrane to the mitochondria (10). Thus, relative anaerobiosis may favor GSSG formation without $O_2^{\cdot -}$ and H_2O_2 generation. The contribution of cellular reducing systems or agents, which might not generate $O_2^{\cdot -}$ or other free radicals must also be considered in the evaluation of whether Mb ultimately participates in the initiation of damaging reactions.

Under appropriate circumstances, Mb may be a component in the defense against oxidant-induced damage in muscle cells, rather than an initiator of such damage. On the basis of our experiments, this former possibility seems equally tenable and merits further investigation.

Acknowledgements - This work was supported, in part by a grant from the National Institutes of Health (ES03816).

REFERENCES

(1) Galaris, D., Cadenas, E., and Hochstein, P. (1987) Submitted for publication.

(2) Kanner, J. and Harel, S. (1985) Arch. Biochem. Biophys. 237, 314-321.

(3) Grisham, M.B. (1985) J. Free Radicals Biol. Med. 1, 227-232.

(4) Kanner, J. and Harel, S. (1985) Lipids 20, 625-628.

(5) Taylor, D. and Hochstein, P. (1982) J. Mol. Cell Cardiol. 14 133-140.

(6) Hagler, L., Coppes, R.I. and Herman, R.H. (1979) J. Biol. Chem. 254 6505-6514.

(7) Mills, G.C. (1960) Arch. Biochem. Biophys. 86, 1-5.

(8) Eling, E.T., Curtis, J.F., Harman, L.S. and Mason, R.P. (1986) J. Biol. Chem. 261, 5023-5028.

(9) Harman, L.S., Carrer, D.K., Schreiber, J. and Mason, R.P. (1986) J. Biol. Chem. 261, 1642-1648.

(10) Jones, D.P. and Kennedy, F.G. (1982) Biochem. Biophys. Res. Commun. 105, 419-424.

THE CARDIAC DEFENSE SYSTEM ASSOCIATED WITH GLUTATHIONE

Toshihisa Ishikawa

Institut für Physiologische Chemie I, Universität Düsseldorf,
Moorenstrasse 5, D-4000 Düsseldorf, F.R.G.

In the living cell glutathione peroxidase plays a significant role in reducing hydrogen peroxide (H_2O_2) as well as organic hydroperoxides. Glutathione peroxidase (selenium-dependent) activity in the heart is similar to that in liver, whereas the glutathione reductase activity is relatively low, corresponding to only 10 % of the hepatic one. The redox balance of glutathione (GSH)/glutathione disulfide (GSSG) in the heart is readily shifted towards oxidation even upon a slight increase in the glutathione peroxidase reaction. It has been estimated that extra H_2O_2 generation in the heart with a rate exceeding only 0.4 % of the oxygen consumption rate of the tissue leads to a substantial increase in the intracellular GSSG level and GSSG release from the heart. The GSSG release is considered as a sensitive indicator for the assessment of extra H_2O_2 generation in the heart.

The relationship between the GSSG release rate and the intracellular GSSG level exhibited a saturation kinetic with an apparent K_m value of 30 nmol x g heart^{-1} and a maximal release rate of 7.5 nmol x min^{-1} x g heart^{-1}. The maximal rate of the GSSG release was temperature-sensitive (Q_{10} = 1.8) and dependent on the cytosolic energy state, i.e. cytosolic free ATP/ADP ratio. The existence of an energy-linked membrane transport system for GSSG was suggested. The physiological meaning of the GSSG transport may be in maintaining a low level of intracellular GSSG because of the low activity of cardiac glutathione reductase.

Glutathione S-transferase activity, on the other hand, presents one of the body's most important defense mechanisms against endogenously generated electrophilic intermediates as well as numerous xenobiotics. There was a remarkable difference in the isozyme pattern between rat heart and liver glutathione S-transferases. One major isozyme (pI = 6.9) of cardiac glutathione S-transferases was found to have a significantly high activity towards *trans*-4-hydroxynon-2-enal (4-hydroxynonenal) which is a cytotoxic and mutagenic carbonyl compound originating from the peroxidative breakdown of polyunsaturated fatty acids. The rate of the enzyme-catalyzed conjugation reaction in the heart was estimated to be more than 30 times the rate of the spontaneous reaction, the half-life of 4-hydroxynonenal being less than 4 sec.

The resulting glutathione S-conjugate was subsequently released from the cardiac cells. A mutual competition between the glutathione S-conjugate and GSSG effluxes was found, and it has been suggested that the glutathione S-conjugate is released *via* the identical membrane transport system for GSSG. The transport of the glutathione S-conjugate is considered important not only in interorgan glutathione metabolism but also in diminishing the inhibitory effect of the glutathione S-conjugate on glutathione S-transferases and glutathione reductase.

INTRODUCTION

The heart is the organ continuously exposed to freshly oxygenated blood from the lung, and is first exposed to reactive compounds which may have escaped from hepatic and pulmonary detoxication systems. As cardiomyopathy resulting from oxidative damage inflicted by hyperoxia or by administration of anticancer drugs, such as adriamycin, has been well documented (Balentine, 1982; Doroshow and Hochstein, 1982), it is without doubt of importance and necessity to study cardiac defense mechanisms which prevent the tissue itself from possible damages brought about by endogenously generated or exogenously elicited reactive metabolic intermediates.

In recent years, our interest has been focused upon glutathione and glutathione-related enzymes in the heart, which are considered to play physiologically significant roles in the protection of cardiac cells against oxidative damage. In order to gain insight into the mechanism and capacity of the cardiac defense system associated with glutathione, the following items have been studied; (i) intracellular redox state of glutathione in the heart. (ii) the capacity of cardiac glutathione peroxidase system in hydroperoxide metabolism and its ancillary systems. (iii) GSSG release from the heart as a highly specific indicator for the assessment of H_2O_2 generation in the cardiac cell. (iv) cardiac glutathione S-transferases and their potency in detoxication of cytotoxic lipid peroxidation products. (v) characterization of the energy-linked membrane transport system for the release of glutathione disulfide and glutathione S-conjugates, and its physiological meaning.

Here, the nature of the glutathione-associated cardiac defense system is discussed with results concerning these points as well as recent progresses in this field.

MATERIAL AND METHODS

Isolated perfused rat heart: A physiological model system for the assessment of cardiac defense capacity

The isolated perfused heart has been widely used in the study on the energy metabolism and hormonal regulations in this organ, to offer a useful physiological model system which bridges a gap between *in vitro* and *in vivo* experiments. Fig. 1 shows the heart perfusion system used in the author's laboratory. The heart of male Wistar rats (180 - 250 g body weight) was perfused according to Langendorff's method under a constant hydrostatic pressure of 80 cm H_2O. The perfusion medium was Krebs-Henseleit bicarbonate buffer solution containing 10 mM glucose and 0.2 mM pyruvate, which was equilibrated with 95 % O_2 + 5 % CO_2 or 95 % N_2 + 5 % CO_2 at 37°C. The system was devised for the purpose to assess readily both biochemical and physiological parameters; for example (i) the system is a non-recycling system. (ii) the effluent perfusion medium is cooled immediately on an ice-cooled funnel, and collected into plastic tubes kept at 0°C. (iii) test compounds can be infused at constant concentrations in the perfusion medium, being independent of changes in the coronary flow rate. (iv) the left ventricular pressure, heart beat rate, coronary flow and oxygen consumption rate are continuously measured to monitor the performance of cardiac function. They are 70 - 80 mm Hg (systolic pressure), 240 - 260 beats x min^{-1}, 9 - 11 ml x min^{-1} x g $heart^{-1}$ and 4.5 - 5.2 µmol x min^{-1} x g $heart^{-1}$, respectively, and they were maintained constant for at least 2 hours under

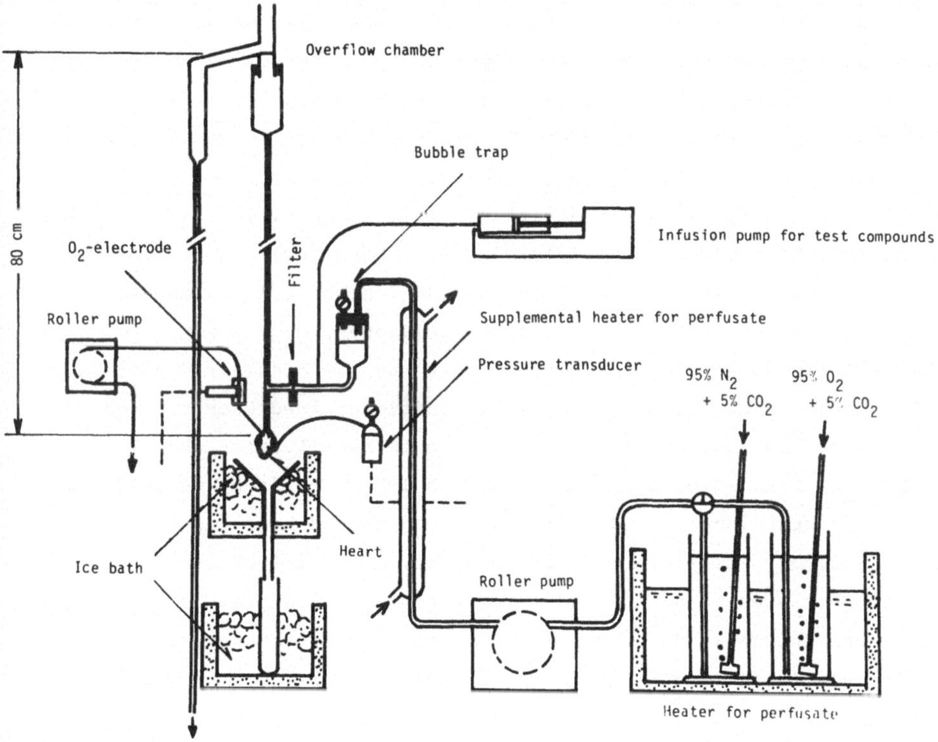

Fig. 1. Schematic illustration of rat heart perfusion system.

the standard perfusion condition.

^{31}P-NMR measurement of isolated perfused rat heart

This was performed with a Bruker WH 360 NMR spectrometer (Leibfritz et al., 1985; Ishikawa et al., 1986d).

Assay of metabolites in heart

GSH, GSSG, glutathione S-conjugates, ATP, ADP, AMP, creatine and creatine phosphate in the perfused heart were assayed as described in Ishikawa and Sies (1984a) and in Ishikawa et al. (1986c; 1986d). The subcellular distribution of total glutathione (GSH + GSSG) was analyzed by subfractionation of the tissue in non-aqueous solvents according to Soboll and Bünger (1981).

RESULTS AND DISCUSSION

Redox state of glutathione in heart

Glutathione (GSH) is a tripeptide (γ-Glu-Cys-Gly), which is the most abundant non-protein thiol in the living cell. In the cell GSH is synthesized by two cytosolic enzymes, γ-glutamylcysteine synthetase and glutathione synthetase, where 2 mols of ATP are expended for 1 mol of GSH synthesized (Snoke and Bloch, 1952). The rate of GSH synthesis and the intracellular GSH level is influenced by the availability of intracellular cysteine (Bannai and Tateishi, 1986, for recent review). The γ-glutamylcysteine synthetase step is inhibited by GSH (Jackson, 1969) and the inhibition is released by glutathione S-conjugates, e.g. 2,4-dinitrophenyl glutathione (Kondo et al., 1984). The first step is considered rate-limiting and there may be a physiologically significant feed back control of GSH synthesis (Meister and Tate, 1976). The intracellular stability of GSH is favored by the γ-glutamyl linkage, which is not split by α-peptidase.

Total glutathione (GSH + 2GSSG) in the perfused heart is 1.2 μmol x g heart^{-1}, almost one-fifth of that in liver. About 1 % of the total glutathione is present as GSSG (15 nmol x g heart^{-1}); the redox state of cardiac glutathione is in a predominantly reduced state under the standard perfusion condition (Ishikawa and Sies, 1984a). About 90 % of the total glutathione was found in the extra-mitochondrial space, the concentration being about 3 mM.

Glutathione peroxidase and its ancillary systems

H_2O_2 generation in the biological system was first reported in the isolated heart mitochondria (Kaplan-Bresler, 1965; cf. Loschen et al., 1971) and subsequently in the peroxisome of rat liver (Sies and Chance, 1970). The discovery afforded to the conceptional basis in our consideration of the mechanism of H_2O_2 generation in the living cells (Chance et al., 1979). The disposition of H_2O_2, on the other hand, has great general interest with respect to oxidative pathologies for the reason that H_2O_2 can become a direct precursor of hydroxyl radical (OH·) which is generally accepted to be a highly reactive oxygen species to initiate a series of processes leading the cell to the oxidative damage.

In the living cell, glutathione peroxidase is localized in the cytosol and the mitochondrial matrix (Flohé and Schlegel, 1971) to reduce H_2O_2 as well as organic hydroperoxides, while catalase is spatially and functionally restricted to the peroxisome (Leighton et al., 1968; Oshino and Chance, 1977). Glutathione peroxidase is a tetrametric protein consisting of four identical subunits arranged almost in a plane. Each contains a single selenium atom at the active site, and the selenocysteine residue is intimately involved in the catalytic process of the enzyme (Ladenstein et

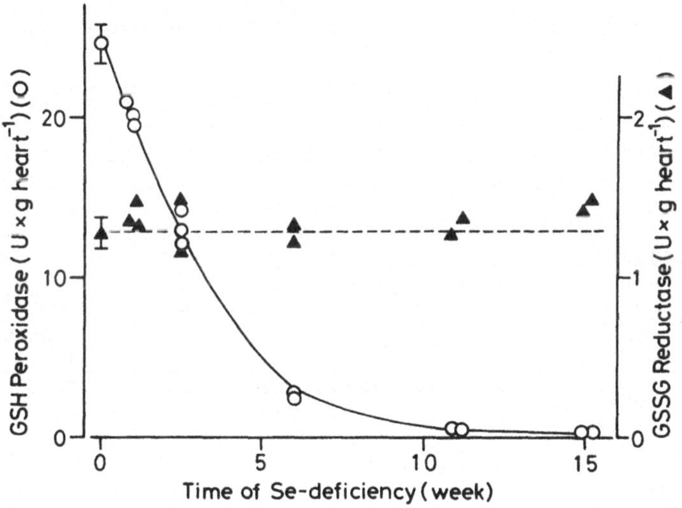

Fig. 2. Effect of Se-deficient diet on the activities of glutathione peroxidase and of glutathione reductase in rat heart.

Male Wistar rats (100 - 120 g body weight) were maintained on selenium-deficient diet during the period indicated. The enzyme activities were measured according to Ishikawa and Sies (1984a). One unit is 1 µmol of NADPH oxidized per min.

al., 1979). The activity of glutathione peroxidase in the tissue depends on the nutritional state of selenium uptake. As shown in Fig. 2, glutathione peroxidase activity in rat heart decreased substantially when the rat was maintained on selenium-deficient diet, whereas the glutathione reductase activity was little changed during the period studied.

Keshan disease is known as an endemic cardiomyopathy in China which is characterized by the multiple focal myocardial necrosis scattered throughout the heart muscle. It occurs most frequently in children under 15 years of age and women of child-bearing age. Recent works have shown that selenium deficiency is a pathological cause, and an implication to the low activity of glutathione peroxidase was suggested (Chen et al., 1980).

In the glutathione peroxidase reaction, GSH serves as the electron donor to reduce hydroperoxides. GSSG, thus formed, is subsequently reduced back to GSH by glutathione reductase at the expense of NADPH, or eliminated out of the cell. Glutathione peroxidase activity in the heart is 25 µmol x min^{-1} x g $heart^{-1}$, being similar to that in liver, whereas the glutathione reductase activity is 1.2 µmol x min^{-1} x g $heart^{-1}$, only 10 % of the hepatic one. About 70 % of their activities were found in the cytosol fraction (Table 1). Reducing equivalents for NADPH to regenerate GSH in the cytosol is considered to be mainly supplied by $NADP^+$-dependent isocitrate dehydrogenase (Pfeifer et al., 1986). In contrast to liver, the hexose monophosphate

Table 1. Subcellular distribution of GSH peroxidase and GSSG reductase in rat heart.

The activities of GSH peroxidase and GSSG reductase were measured as described in Ishikawa and Sies (1984a). The activities of lactate dehydrogenase (cytosolic marker enzyme) and of citrate synthase (mitochondrial marker enzyme) as well as protein were assayed according to Bergmeyer (1983) and Lowry et al., (1951).

	Precipitate			Supernatant
Enzyme	300 x g	10 000 x g	105 000 x g	105 000 x g
	(Activity: nmol x min^{-1} x mg $protein^{-1}$)			
GSH peroxidase	52	92	10	240
GSSG reductase	2.4	3.5	0.1	9.5
Lactate dehydrogenase	260	66	190	9 350
Citrate synthase	470	800	17	50
Protein (mg x g $heart^{-1}$)	63.4	40.8	4.9	70.8

shunt in the heart is not a significant pathway to provide the reducing equivalent; its main function seems to be the supply of ribose phosphate for nucleotide synthesis. In the heart, about 80 % of the total cellular nicotinamide adenine dinucleotide phosphate ($NADP^+$ + NADPH) is localized in the mitochondria (Klingenberg, 1961), where NADPH is considered to be regenerated in the nicotinamide nucleotide transhydrogenase reaction (Rydström et al., 1976).

GSH peroxidase rection and GSSG efflux from heart

Under the standard perfusion condition GSH and GSSG are released from the heart at rates of 0.37 and 0.11 nmol x min^{-1} x g $haert^{-1}$, respectively (Ishikawa and Sies, 1984a). When glutathione peroxidase reaction in the heart was enhanced by infusing hydroperoxide into the organ, a substantial increase in intracellular GSSG level and in GSSG efflux was observed. There was a threshold for the increase of GSSG efflux at a hydroperoxide infusion rate of 20 nmol x min^{-1} x g $heart^{-1}$ (Fig. 3). No significant difference was observed in the kinetics of the GSSG release between the infusions of H_2O_2 and *t*-butyl hydroperoxide. Although the existence of microperoxisome and catalase activity in cardiac cells was reported (Herzog and Fahimi, 1974), the activity is extremely low. GSH peroxidase is supposed to be the most responsible enzyme in the reduction of H_2O_2. It is deduced from the result that extra H_2O_2 generation, exceeding only 0.4 % of the oxygen consumption

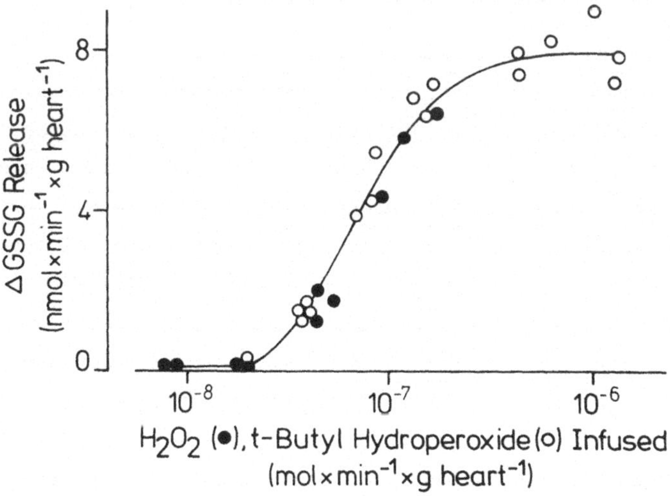

Fig. 3. Relationship between GSSG release and hydroperoxide infusion rate

of the perfused heart, leads to a substantial increase of GSSG efflux. Namely, the GSSG efflux is considered as a highly specific indicator for the assessment of intracellular H_2O_2 production (Ishikawa, 1986e).

Redox cycling and H_2O_2 generation in heart

Redox cycling associated with quinone compounds has been well documented for the production of $O_2^{\cdot-}$ and H_2O_2 in biological systems (Kappus, 1986, for recent review). Cardiotoxicity of antineoplastic drugs with a quinone structure, e.g. adriamycin, has also been discussed with this regard (Doroshow and Hochstein, 1982).

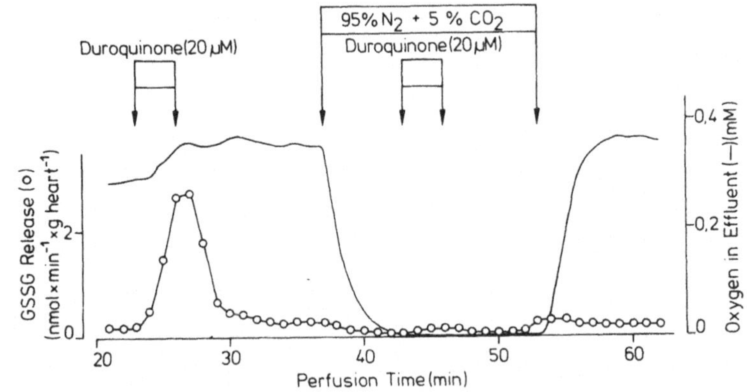

Fig. 4. GSSG release from heart upon perfusion with duroquinone (tetramethyl-*p*-benzoquinone) under aerobic and anaerobic conditions.

As shown in Fig. 4, GSSG release from the heart was enhanced on perfusion with quinone compounds, such as tetramethyl-*p*-benzoquinone (duroquinone), under the aerobic perfusion condition. The increase of GSSG release was accompanied by an enhancement of the oxygen consumption. On the other hand, no significant change in GSSG efflux was observed under the anaerobic condition. The result exemplifies a quinone-elicited H_2O_2 generation in the heart, which may have resulted from divalent reduction of molecular oxygen and/or from $O_2^{\cdot-}$-dismutation reaction catalyzed by superoxide dismutase. Similar results were obtained with menadione (2-methyl-1,4-naphthoquinone). It has been shown in intact hepatocytes that menadione-mediated oxygen uptake predominantly ($>$90 %) results from electron transfer in the mitochondrial respiration chain by menadione and that the complex I is the definitive site of mitochondrial menadione reduction (De Groot et al., 1985).

The importance of the mitochondrial complex I has been also implied in the formation of H_2O_2 and $O_2^{\bar{\cdot}}$ by anthracycline compounds (Davis and Doroshow, 1986; Doroshow and Davis, 1986). However, it should be noted that adriamycin, which was shown *in vitro* to be activated by a similar redox cycling mechanism, promoted no GSSG efflux and no increase of intracellular GSSG level in either perfused rat heart or liver. The hypothesis for the cardiotoxicity of adriamycin associated with redox cycling is still a matter of controversy.

Mechanism of cardiac GSSG release: Energy-linked membrane transport

The relationship between the rate of GSSG efflux and the intracellular GSSG level showed a saturation kinetics with an apparent K_m value of 30 nmol x g heart^{-1} and a maximal release rate of 7.5 nmol x min^{-1} x g heart^{-1} (Fig. 5). The maximal rate was temperature-sensitive (Q_{10} = 1.8) and the activation energy for the release has been estimated to be 12 kcal x mol^{-1}; this value is too high for the simple diffusion. The existence of a membrane transport system for GSSG release was suggested.

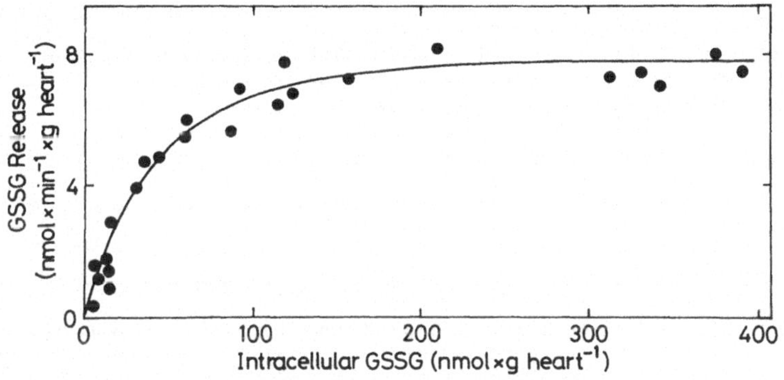

Fig. 5. Relationship between GSSG release rate and intracellular GSSG level. (Data from Ishikawa and Sies, 1984a)

The GSSG release was substantially restricted when the mitochondrial respiration of the perfused heart was inhibited by KCN, antimycin A or rotenone. Studies with ^{31}P-NMR have shown that the GSSG release rate is dependent on the cytosolic energy state, i.e. free ATP/ADP ratio. The transport is half maximal at ATP/ADP(free) $\approx$ 10 (Fig. 6; Ishikawa et al., 1986d). On the other hand, the GSSG transport was not affected by a potassium-induced cardiac arrest nor by the infusion of epinephrine, norepinephrine or dibutyryl cyclic AMP. Thus, the GSSG transport in the heart is considered to be closely linked to the cytosolic energy state, being independent of the membrane potential and of the hormonal regulation associated with adrenergic hormones.

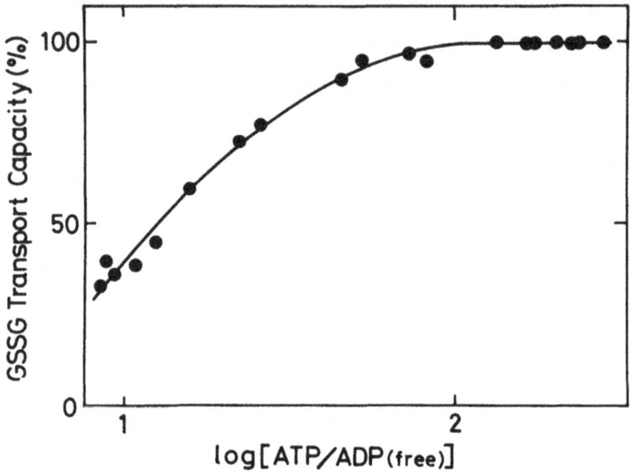

Fig. 6. GSSG transport capacity as a function of cytosolic free ATP/ADP. ATP/ADP(free) was 180 ± 11 (n = 4) for the heart perfused under the standard condition. 100 % transport capacity corresponds to 7.5 ± 0.2 nmol x min^{-1} x g $heart^{-1}$. (Data from Ishikawa et al., 1986d)

When a substrate for glutathione S-transferase, e.g. 1-chloro-2,4-dinitrobenzene, was infused into the heart, the release of the corresponding glutathione S-conjugate was observed. Interestingly, there was a mutual competition between the glutathione S-conjugate and GSSG releases (Ishikawa and Sies, 1984a). It has been suggested that the glutathione S-conjugate is released *via* the identical transport system for GSSG, and that the transport system may play a role in the elimination of glutathione S-conjugate generated from the glutathione S-transferase reaction.

Cardiac glutathione S-transferases

In the living cell, various electrophilic compounds, such as epoxides or α,β-unsaturated aldehydes, are generated from endogenous and exogenous sources *via* various oxidative reactions. Glutathione S-transferases are of importance in preventing cell damage resulting from the electrophilic attack of such reactive compounds (Ishikawa et al., 1986a).

The hitherto most extensively studied class of glutathione S-transferases is that of rat liver cytosol. More than ten glutathione S-transferase isozymes have been recognized as binary combinations of eight apparently distinguishable subunits with molecular weights of 24 000 to 28 000; i.e. Yα, Yk, Ya (subunit 1), Yn (subunit 6), Yb_1 (subunit 3), Yb_2 (subunit 4), subunit 5 and Yc (subunit 2), in order of increasing molecular weight (Mannervik, 1985, for recent review). In addition to them, a new isozyme was recently found in the liver with primary hepatoma, not being apparent in normal liver (Kitahara et al., 1984). Peptide mapping experiments (Hayes, 1983; Beale et al., 1982), N-terminal sequence analysis (Frey et al., 1983) and the application of recombinant DNA technique have revealed that the subunits are derived from separate genes, and that the expression of each subunit is independently regulated prior to the level of mRNA processing (Tu et al., 1984; Pickett et al., 1984). The isozyme patterns of glutathione transferases in extrahepatic organs differ significantly from that of the hepatic forms (Tu et al., 1983), and the physiological meaning in the different occurrence of the isozymes remains to be elucidated.

Rat heart lacks the major basic isozymes found in the liver, such as transferase 1-1 (YaYa), 1-2 (YaYc) and 2-2 (YcYc). Transferases 3-3 (Yb_1Yb_1) and 3-4 (Yb_1Yb_2) are present in negligible amounts. The most part of glutathione S-transferase activity in the heart is associated with near-neutral and anionic proteins (Ishikawa and Sies, 1984b). One major isozyme of the cardiac glutathione transferases with a isoelectric point of 6.9 was purified to homogeneity. Studies on the molecular and immunological properties of the isozymes have shown that it is identical with one hepatic isozyme consisting of two Yb_2 subunits (Ishikawa et al., 1986b), and a physiologically significant role of the isozyme in the both organs was suggested.

Interestingly, the neutral isozyme purified from rat heart and liver was found active for glutathione conjugation of 4-hydroxynonenal (Ishikawa et al., 1986b) which is a major aldehyde product of lipid peroxidation in rat liver microsomes (Esterbauer et al., 1982; Poli et al., 1985). Its specific activity was significantly higher than the other major basic isozymes recognized in rat liver. The kinetic parameters for the reaction (1) were: K_m = 50 μM for 4-hydroxynonenal, k_{cat} = 460 mol x min^{-1} x mol $enzyme^{-1}$. However, the isozyme can be competitively inhibited by the resulting glutathione S-conjugate (K_i = 85 μM).

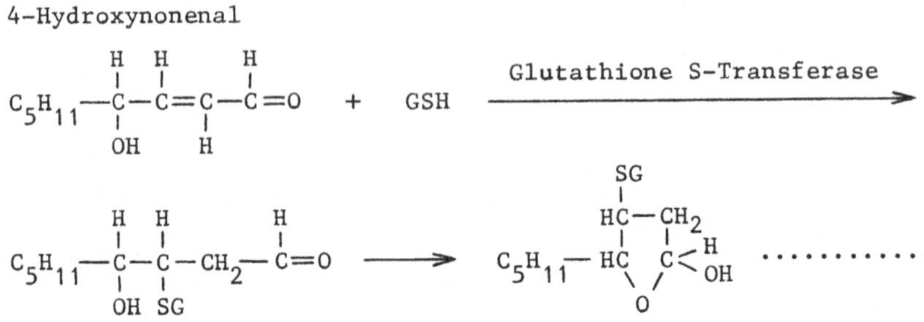

(1)

The role of cardiac glutathione S-transferases and glutathione S-conjugate export system

Hydroxyalkenals including 4-hydroxynonenal are generated from peroxidative breakdown of polyunsaturated fatty acids (Esterbauer et al., 1982), and they are considered of importance in the cause of cytotoxicity and mutagenicity (Benedetti et al., 1980; Marnett et al., 1985). In addition, the chemotactic activity of the alkenals for polymorphonuclear neutrophils has been recently shown (Curzio et al., 1986). The hydroxyalkenals with an α,β-unsaturated carbonyl structure are fairly electrophilic and readily react with thiol groups of cysteine, coenzyme A and proteins.

The capacity of the glutathione S-transferase for glutathione conjugation of 4-hydroxynonenal was investigated with the isolated perfused rat heart, and the rate of the conjugation reaction in the heart was estimated to be more than 30 times the rate of the spontaneous uncatalyzed reaction, the half-life of 4-hydroxynonenal being less than 4 sec (Ishikawa et al., 1986c).

The glutathione S-conjugate of 4-hydroxynonenal, thus formed, was released from the cardiac cells, and the existence of a common export system for the glutathione S-conjugate and GSSG has been proven (Ishikawa et al., 1986c). The transport of the glutathione S-conjugate is important in interorgan glutathione metabolism, e.g. mercapturic acid formation in the kidney. Moreover, it diminishes the inhibitory effect of the glutathione S-conjugate on glutathione reductase and glutathione S-transferases; these enzymes are inhibited competitively by glutathione S-conjugates (Bilzer et al., 1984; Ishikawa et al., 1986c), and more deleterious effect can be brought about from the inhibition (Fig. 7). These results show the physiological significance of cardiac glutathione S-transferases and of the glutathione S-conjugate export system in the detoxication of electrophilic compounds which may be endogenously generated from oxidative reactions.

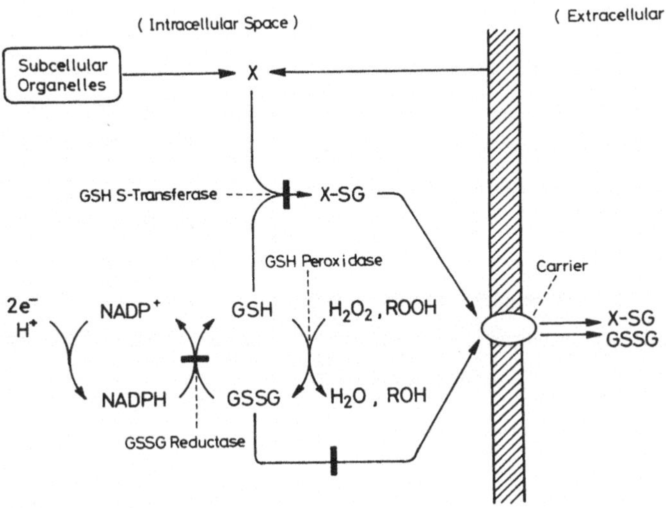

Fig. 7. Schematic illustration of cardiac defense system associated with glutathione. (Scheme is based on Ishikawa et al., 1986c)

X, endogenously generated electrophiles (e.g. 4-hydroxyalkenals), X-SG, glutathione S-conjugates of the electrophiles; ROOH, organic hydroperoxides. Steps inhibited by X-SG are indicated by solid bars.

CONCLUSIONS

This paper summarizes some recent studies on glutathione-associated defense mechanisms in the heart, especially on the glutathione peroxidase, glutathione S-transferases and on the transport system for GSSG and glutathione S-conjugates. It is becoming apparent that oxidation is a common mechanism underlying many pathological and mutagenic conditions at the cellular level, and contributes in the aging process. Endogenously reactive oxygen species (O_2^-, H_2O_2, OH· or $^1O_2$) are generated even during normal metabolism by the electron transfer chain, by oxidases and in the neutrophil inflammatory response (Sies, 1985, for review). Oxidation products of lipids are also important agents in the propagation of oxidative damage. In this respect, the abovementioned glutathione-related enzyme systems must be a physiologically significant defense in the heart. Of course, they are not all that counteracts oxidative challenges. GSH itself is an intracellular water soluble reductant to protect the thiol group of a variety of proteins from the possible oxidation and S-alkylation. This function of GSH may be of importance in maintaining the homeostasis of the cellular metabolism, intracellular ion balances and also probably in the regulation of force generation of the cardiac cell. Oxidation of thiol groups in sarcoplasmic reticulum resulted in an impairment of Ca^{2+}-ATPase function (Scherer and Deamer, 1986). Disulfide bonds can be formed by oxidation of thiol groups between the chains within a portion of myosin rod molecules, which may lead to a local unfolding of the coiled-coil myosin rod (Nyitray et al., 1985). In fact, depletion of GSH in the perfused heart led to a remarkable disorder in the cardiac functions (Ishikawa, unpublished work). It is likely that GSH protects the essential thiol group of the functional and structural proteins in the organ, and this point would be an interesting object to study in future.

ACKNOWLEDGEMENTS

The author is grateful to Prof. H. Sies for his generous support throughout this study.

REFERENCES

Balentine, J.D., 1982. Pathology of Oxygen Toxicity, Academic Press, New York.

Bannai, S. and Tateichi, N., 1986. Role of membrane transport in metabolism and function of glutathione in mammals. J. Membrane Biol., 89: 1-8.

Beale, D., Meyer, D.J., Taylor, J.D. and Ketterer, B., 1982. Evidence that the Ya and Yc subunits of glutathione transferase B (ligandin) are the products of separate genes. Eur. J. Biochem., 126: 459-463.

Bergmeyer, H.U. (Editor), 1983. Methods of Enzymatic Analysis, Verlag Chemie, Weinheim.

Benedetti, A., Comporti, M. and Esterbauer, H., 1980. Identification of 4-hydroxynonenal as a cytotoxic product originating from the peroxidation of liver microsomal lipids. Biochim. Biophys. Acta, 620: 281-296.

Bilzer, M., Krauth-Siegel, R.L., Schirmer, R.H., Akerboom, T.P.M., Sies, H. and Schulz, G.E., 1984. Interaction of a glutathione S-conjugate with glutathione reductase kinetic and X-ray crystallographic studies. Eur. J. Biochem., 138: 373-378.

Chance, B., Sies, H. and Boveris, A., 1979. Hydroperoxide metabolism in mammalian organs. Physiol. Rev., 59: 527-605.

Chen, X., Yang, G., Chen, J., Chen, X., Wen, Z. and Ge, K., 1980. Studies on the relations of selenium and Keshan disease. Biol. Trace Element Res., 2: 91-107.

Curzio, M., Esterbauer, H., Mauro, C.D., Cecchiniti, G. and Dianzani, M.U., 1986. Chemotactic activity of the lipid peroxidation product 4-hydroxynonenal and homologous hydroxyalkenals. Biol. Chem. Hoppe-Seyler, 367: 321-329.

Davis, K.J.A. and Doroshow, J., 1986. Redox cycling of anthracyclines by cardiac mitochondria: I. Anthracycline radical formation by NADH dehydrogenase. J. Biol. Chem., 261: 3060-3067.

De Groot, H., Noll, T. and Sies, H., 1985. Oxygen dependence and subcellular partitioning of hepatic menadione-mediated oxygen uptake; Studies with isolated hepatocytes, mitochondria and microsomes from rat liver in an oxystat system. Arch. Biochem. Biophys., 243: 556-562.
Doroshow, J. and Hochstein, P., 1982. Redox cycling and the mechanism of action of antibiotics in neoplastic diseases. In: Autor, A.P. (Editor), Pathology of Oxygen, Academic Press, New York, pp. 245-275.
Doroshow, J.H. and Davis, K.J.A., 1986. Redox cycling of anthracyclines by cardiac mitochondria: II. Formation of superoxide anion, hydrogen peroxid and hydroxyl radical. J. Biol. Chem., 261: 3068-3074.
Esterbauer, H., Cheeseman, K.H., Dianzani, M.V., Poli, G. and Slater, T.F., 1982. Separation and characterization of the aldehydic products of lipid peroxidation stimulated by ADP-Fe^{2+} in rat liver microsomes. Biochem. J., 208: 129-140.
Flohé, L. and Schlegel, W., 1971. Glutathion-Peroxidase IV, Intrazelluläre Verteilung des Glutathion-Peroxidase-Systems in der Rattenleber. Hoppe-Seyler's Z. Physiol. Chem., 352: 1401-1410.
Frey, A.B., Friedberg, T., Oesch, F. and Kreibich, G., 1983. Studies on the subunit composition of rat liver glutathione S-transferases. J. Biol. Chem., 258: 11321-11325.
Hayes, J.D., 1983. Rat liver glutathione S-transferases; A study of the structure of the basic YbYb-containing enzymes. Biochem. J., 213: 625-633.
Herzog, V. and Fahimi, H.D., 1974. Microbodies (peroxisomes) containig catalase in myocardium; Morphological and biochemical evidence. Science, 185: 271-273.
Ishikawa, T. and Sies, H., 1984a. Cardiac transport of glutathione disulfide and S-conjugate: Studies with isolated perfused rat heart during hydroperoxide metabolism. J. Biol. Chem., 259: 3838-3843.
Ishikawa, T. and Sies, H., 1984b. The isozyme pattern of glutathione S-transferases in rat heart. FEBS Lett., 169: 156-160.
Ishikawa, T., Akerboom, T.P.M. and Sies, H., 1986a. Role of key defense systems in target organ toxicity. In: Cohen, G.M. (Editor), Target Organ Toxicity, CRC Press, Baca Raton, pp. 129-143.
Ishikawa, T., Milbert, U., Oesch, F. and Sies, H., 1986b. The major isozyme of rat cardiac glutathione transferases; Its correspondence to hepatic transferase X. Eur. J. Biochem., 154: 299-305.
Ishikawa, T., Esterbauer, H. and Sies, H., 1986c. Role of cardiac glutathione transferase and of glutathione S-conjugate export system in biotransformation of 4-hydroxynonenal in the heart. J. Biol. Chem., 261: 1576-1581.
Ishikawa, T., Zimmer, M. and Sies, H., 1986d. Energy-linked cardiac transport system for glutathione disulfide. FEBS Lett., 200: 128-132.
Ishikawa, T., 1986e. Die Freisetzung von Glutathiondisulfid im Herzen: Ein hochspezifischer Indikator für die Beurteilung einer H_2O_2-Bildung in Herzzellen und der zugrundeliegende Mechanismus. In: Elstner, E.F. (Editor), Reaktive Sauerstoffspezies in der Medizin, Springer Verlag, Berlin, in press.
Jackson, R.C., 1969. Studies in the enzymology of glutathione metabolism in human erythrocytes. Biochem. J., 111: 309-315.
Kaplan-Bresler, A.E., 1965. Metmyoglobin oxidation during electron transport reaction in mitochondrion. J. Gen. Physiol., 48: 685-698.
Kappus, H., 1986. Overview of enzyme systems involved in bioreduction of drugs and in redox cycling. Biochem. Pharmacol., 35: 1-6.
Kitahara, A., Satoh, K., Nishimura, K., Ishikawa, T., Ruike, K., Sato, K., Tsuda, H. and Ito, N., 1984. Changes in molecular forms of rat hepatic

glutathione S-transferase during chemical hepatocarcinogenesis. Cancer Res., 44: 2698-2703.
Klingenberg, M., 1961. Zur Bedeutung der freien Nukleotide. In: 11. Mosbacher Kolloquium, Springer Verlag, Berlin, pp. 82-106.
Kondo, T., Taniguchi, N. and Kawakami, Y., 1984. Significance of glutathione S-conjugate for glutathione metabolism in human erythrocytes. Eur. J. Biochem., 145: 131-136.
Ladenstein, R., Epp, O., Bartels, K., Jones, A., Huber, R. and Wendel, A., 1979. Structure analysis and molecular model of the selenoenzyme glutathione peroxidase at 2.8 Å resolution. J. Mol. Biol., 134: 199-218.
Leibfritz, D., Offermann, W., Kuhn, W., Ishikawa, T., Wolf, K.U. and Becker, J., 1985. P-31-NMR studies on perfused rat organs (heart, diaghram, gaster) and on human erythrocytes. In: Govil, Khetrapal and Saran (Editors), Magnetic Resonance in Biology and Medicine, McGraw-Hill, New Delhi, pp. 417-427.
Leighton, F., Poole, B., Beaufay, H., Baudhuin, P., Caffey, J.W., Fowler, S. and de Duve, C., 1968. The large scale separation of peroxisomes, mitochondrion and lysosomes from the livers of rats injected with Triton WR-1339. J. Cell. Biol., 37: 482-513.
Loschen, G., Flohé, L. and Chance, B., 1971. Repiratory chain linked H_2O_2 production in pigeon heart mitochondria. FEBS Lett., 18: 261-264.
Lowry, O.H., Rosebrough, N.J., Farr, A.L. and Randall, R.J., 1951. Protein measurement with the Folin phenol reagent. J. Biol. Chem., 193: 265-275.
Mannervik, B., 1985. The isoenzymes of glutathione transferases. Adv. Enzymol. Relat. Areas Mol. Biol., 57: 357-417.
Marnett, L.J., Hurd, H.K., Hollstein, M.C., Levin, D.E., Esterbauer, H. and Ames, B.N., 1985. Naturally occurring carbonyl compounds are mutagens in Salmonella tester strain TA 104. Mutation Res., 148: 25-34.
Meister, A. and Tate, S.S., 1976. Glutathione and related γ-glutamyl compounds; Biosynthesis and utilization. Annu. Rev. Biochem., 45: 559-604.
Nyitray, L., Mocź, G. and Bálint, M., 1985. Localization of a new proteolytic site accessible in oxidized myosin rod. FEBS Lett., 181: 353-356.
Oshino, N. and Chance, B., 1977. Properties of glutathione release observed during reduction of organic hydroperoxide, demethylation of aminopyrine and oxidation of some substances in perfused rat liver and their implications for the physiological function of catalase. Biochem. J., 162: 509-525.
Pfeifer, R., Karl, G. and Scholz, R., 1986. Does the pentose cycle play a major role for NADPH supply in the heart? Biol. Chem. Hoppe-Seyler, 367: 1061-1068.
Pickett, C.B., Telakowski-Hopkins, C.A., Ding, G.J.-F., Argenbright, L. and Lu, A.Y.H., 1984. Rat liver transferases; Complete nucleotide sequenz of a glutathione S-transferase mRNA and the regulation of the Ya, Yb, and Yc mRNAs by 3-methylcholanthrene and phenobarbital. J. Biol. Chem., 259: 5182-5188.
Poli, G., Dianzani, M.V., Cheeseman, K.H., Slater, T.F., Lang, J. and Esterbauer, H., 1985. Separation and characterization of the aldehydic products of lipid peroxidation stimulated by carbontetrachloride or ADP-iron in isolated rat hepatocytes and rat liver microsomal suspensions. Biochem. J., 227:629-638.
Rydström, J., Hoek, J.B. and Ernster, L., 1976. Nicotinamide nucleotide transhydrogenase. In: Boyer, P.D. (Editor), The Enzymes, Academic Press, New York, vol. 13, pp. 51-88.

Scherer, N.M. and Deamer, D.W., 1986. Oxidative stress impairs the function of sarcoplasmic reticulum by oxidation of sulfhydryl group in the Ca^{2+}-ATPase. Arch. Biochem. Biophys., 246: 589-601.
Sies, H. and Chance, B., 1970. The steady state level of catalase compound I in isolated hemoglobin-free perfused rat liver. FEBS Lett., 11: 172-176.
Sies, H. (Editor), 1985. Oxidative Stress, Academic Press, Orlando.
Snoke, J.E. and Bloch, K., 1952. Formation and utilization of γ-glutamylcysteine in glutathione synthesis. J. Biol. Chem., 199: 407-414.
Soboll, S. and Bünger, R., 1981. Compartmentation of adenin nucleotide in the isolated working guinea pig heart stimulated by noradrenaline. Hoppe-Seyler's Physiol. Chem., 362: 125-132.
Tu, C.-P., Weiss, M.J., Li, N. and Reddy, C.C., 1983. Tissue-specific expression of the rat glutathione S-transferases. J. Biol. Chem., 258: 4659-4662.
Tu, C.-P., Lai, H.-C., Li, N., Weiss, M. and Reddy, C.C., 1984. The Yc and Ya subunits of rat liver glutathione S-transferases are the products of separate genes. J. Biol. Chem., 259: 9434-9439.

LIPID PEROXIDES AS A CAUSE OF ATHEROSCLEROSIS

Kunio Yagi
Institute of Applied Biochemistry, Yagi Memorial Park,
Mitake, Gifu 505-01, Japan

ABSTRACT

Lipid peroxides increased in the blood initiate atherogenesis by injuring arterial endothelial cells. This injury induces platelet aggregation, and the adherence of the aggregates is facilitated by the inhibition of prostacyclin biosynthesis in the endothelium by lipid peroxides. Smooth muscle cells, which migrate from their normal medial site in the arterial wall to the intima and proliferate there in response to migration and proliferation factors released from the aggregated platelets, are affected by the lipid peroxides in that they show increased uptake of low density lipoprotein as well as increased degradation of its apoprotein. This leads to the formation of lipid-laden cells from the smooth muscle cells. Macrophages efficiently take up low density lipoprotein, if it is affected by lipid peroxides, thus becoming lipid-laden cells as well. These lipid-laden cells contribute to the formation of the atheromatous plaque. From these facts, it is clear that lipid peroxides increased in the blood by any cause act as an initiator and a promoter of atherogenesis.

INTRODUCTION

For prolongation of our lives, atherosclerosis is one of the most important diseases to be prevented or cured. Thus, this disease has obviously become one of the main targets for researchers in medicine, especially in medical biochemistry.

Fortunately, a great deal of morphological data has been accumulated on human and experimental atherosclerosis. These data clearly indicate the events occurring during atherogenesis. It is well accepted that the initial event is injury to the endothelial cells of the intima of the artery and that the final one is the maturation of the atheromatous plaque. From the initial to the final step, there occur many successive and interrelated events.

Now, biochemists are asked to answer such questions as "What is the cause of the injury?" and "What are the biochemical bases for the successive events following the injury?" In answering these questions, the author has reached the conclusion that lipid peroxides increased in the blood are the cause of the initial injury to the endothelial cells. This conclusion was derived from experimental data that are summarized in the present communication.

The above conclusion was supported by clinical investigation. By use of a simple method devised by the author (Yagi, 1976) for the assay of serum lipid peroxide levels, many clinical data have been obtained regarding lipid peroxide levels in patients with vascular disorders. Miki and his co-workers (personal communication) found an increase in serum lipid peroxide levels in patients suffering from atherosclerosis. Kibata et al. (1977) reported that the serum lipid peroxide levels of patients having had a recent stroke were higher than those of normal subjects, whereas patients whose levels were measured some time after their stroke showed values not different from those of normal subjects. Kagami et al. (1978) and Kawamoto et al. (1986) measured the serum lipid peroxide levels of patients with apoplexy and found that the levels were high in both cases of cerebral bleeding and cerebral infarction at hospitalization. The levels remained high in those patients who died, whereas the levels decreased to the normal ones within one month in patients who survived. Yoshikawa et al. (1982) reported similar results. Sato et al. (1979) carried out a study on patients with diabetes and reported that plasma lipid peroxide levels were significantly higher in the patients than in healthy subjects and that the levels in diabetic patients with angiopathy were markedly higher than in those without it.

The author's conclusion was even further supported by the results obtained by Tomita et al. (1979) on stroke-prone spontaneous hypertensive rats (SHRSP): the serum lipid peroxide levels were remarkably elevated just before an apoplectic stroke.

The present communication also describes other contributions made by lipid peroxides to the events that occur during atherogenesis.

INJURY TO AORTIC INTIMA BY LIPID PEROXIDES

To examine the author's hypothesis that lipid peroxides increased in the blood injure the intima of the artery, we conducted a model experiment to increase directly the lipid peroxides in the bloodstream. For this purpose, we prepared linoleic acid containing its hydroperoxide and injected it intravenously into a rabbit through the ear vein (Yagi et al., 1981).

The changes in the serum lipid peroxide level after the injection are shown in Fig. 1. As seen in the figure, the level was elevated immediately after the injection and remained high for a few hours thereafter. No significant increase was found when linoleic acid was injected. The lipid peroxide levels in several organs were also measured 24 hours after the injection, and a significant increase was found in the aorta, as summarized in Table 1. Morphological changes observed by scanning electron microscopy are shown in Fig. 2. The profile of the endothelial surface of the thoracic aorta of a rabbit without injection was normal and smooth; rhomboidal endothelial cells were arranged along the longitudinal axis oriented in the direction of blood flow. Upon injection of linoleic acid, minute, but recognizable, injury to the endothelial cells was detected, as shown in Fig. 2 left. However, after linoleic acid containing its hydroperoxide was injected, marked damage to the endothelial cells was observed (Fig. 2 right). Many holes were seen in the cells and some cells were even enucleated. In some areas, subendothelial fibrous tissue was exposed. The aggregated platelets exhibiting pseudopodia appeared to be adhering to the injured site. The minute change caused by the injection of linoleic acid

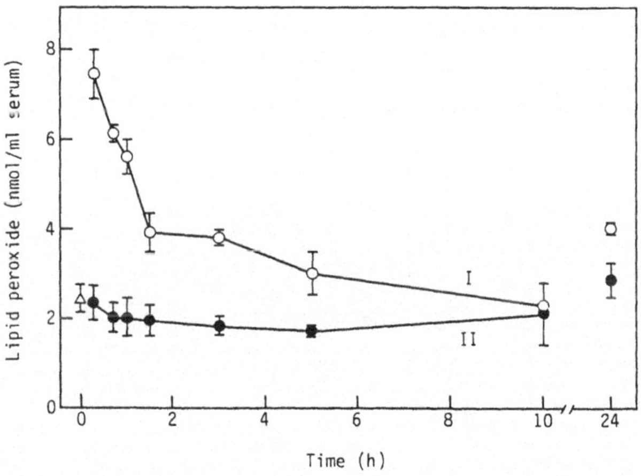

Fig. 1. Changes in lipid peroxide level of rabbit serum after injection of linoleic acid hydroperoxide. Linoleic acid containing its hydroperoxide (peroxide value, 2000 meq/kg) was administered to rabbits by a single intravenous injection through the ear vein at a dose of 25 mg/kg body weight. The level of thiobarbituric acid reactive substances in the serum (Yagi et al., 1981) was expressed in terms of malondialdehyde (nmol/ml serum). Mean ± SE (n=4). I, After injection of linoleic acid containing its hydroperoxide; II, after injection of linoleic acid. Triangle shows the level before injection.

Table 1. Lipid peroxide levels in various tissues 24 h after injection of linoleic acid hydroperoxide[a]

	Lipid peroxide level[b]	
	Linoleic acid hydroperoxide	Linoleic acid
Aorta	3.54 ± 0.27[c,*]	1.62 ± 0.30
Vein	7.99 ± 0.87	7.20 ± 0.59
Retina	14.0 ± 1.76	14.3 ± 1.64
Liver	6.78 ± 1.60	8.49 ± 1.22
Lung	7.65 ± 0.23	8.70 ± 1.08
Spleen	15.8 ± 1.83	16.3 ± 2.29

[a]The administration of the hydroperoxide was performed as described in the legend to Fig. 1.
[b]Measured according to Ohkawa _et al_. (1979) and expressed in terms of malondialdehyde (nmol/100 mg wet weight).
[c]Mean ± SE (n=4). $^{*}p < 0.01$.

may be ascribed to a small amount of its hydroperoxide either contained in the linoleic acid sample tested or formed _in vivo_.

Cutler and Schneider (1974) had administered linoleate hydroperoxide to rabbits by repeated subcutaneous injections and produced aortic lesions. The peroxide content of the aorta was raised. By contrast, linoleate or the secondary degradation products of linoleate hydroperoxide had little or no effect. They supposed that the hydroperoxide had been transported,

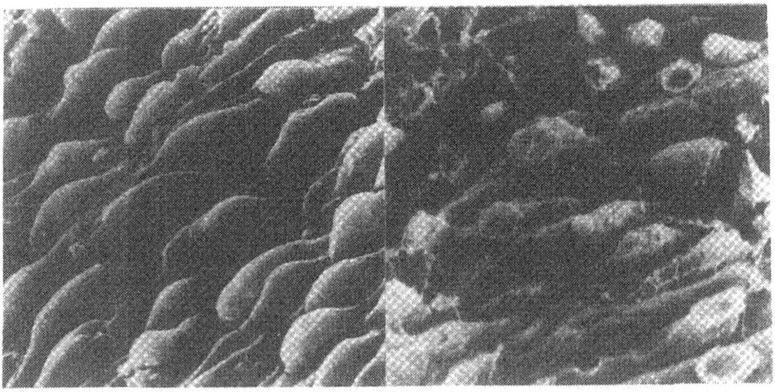

Fig. 2. Scanning electron micrographs of aortic endothelium. The administration was performed as described in the legend to Fig. 1. Left, 24 h after injection of linoleic acid; right, 24 h after injection of linoleic acid containing its hydroperoxide.

presumably by the blood, to produce its effect on the aorta.

Sedar *et al.* (1978) examined the effects of fatty acids on the endothelial cells of rabbit ear veins and observed the provocation of similar damage by linoleic acid or other fatty acids. These results could be due to hydroperoxides contained in their samples or formed from their samples *in vivo*.

EFFECT OF LIPID PEROXIDES ON CULTURED ENDOTHELIAL CELLS AND SMOOTH MUSCLE CELLS

The injury to endothelial cells by linoleic acid hydroperoxide was further studied with cultured endothelial cells from human umbilical cord vein (Sasaguri *et al.*, 1984). A representative electron micrograph of the endothelial cell is shown in Fig. 3. Elongated mitochondria, which are one of the characteristic features of the cells, are clearly evident. When the cells were incubated in culture medium containing 0.05, 0.1, 0.5, 1.0, 5.0, or 7.5 nmol/ml (measured by thiobarbituric acid reaction [Yagi, 1976] and expressed in terms of malondialdehyde) of linoleic acid hydroperoxide at 37°C for 3 h, no morphological change was observed up to 0.1 nmol/ml of the hydroperoxide. However, when the cells were incubated with 0.5 nmol/ml of the hydroperoxide, a slight but definite increase in the number of cellular organelles and decreased electron density of the matrix of some mitochondria were observed. When the concentration of the hydroperoxide was

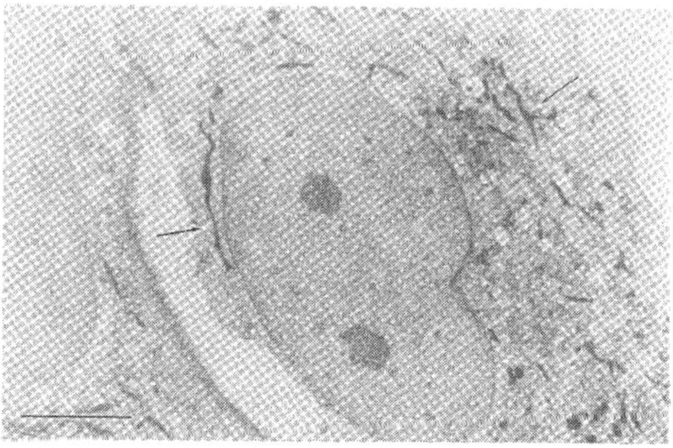

Fig. 3. Transmission electron micrograph of endothelial cells cultured from human umbilical cord vein. Arrows show elongated mitochondria. Bar, 5 μm.

increased to 1.0 nmol/ml, these changes became pronounced. As shown in Fig. 4A, the number of organelles increased, especially near the nucleus. And Fig. 4B demonstrates the remarkable decrease in electron density of the matrix of some mitochondria. This morphological change suggests disorder of mitochondrial functions such as a decrease in mitochondrial respiration. In addition, the rough-surfaced endoplasmic reticulum showed signs of dilatation and cysts containing electron-dense materials. This suggests a disorder in protein synthesis.

When the concentration of linoleic acid hydroperoxide was increased to 5.0 nmol/ml, the morphological features were enormously changed; the number

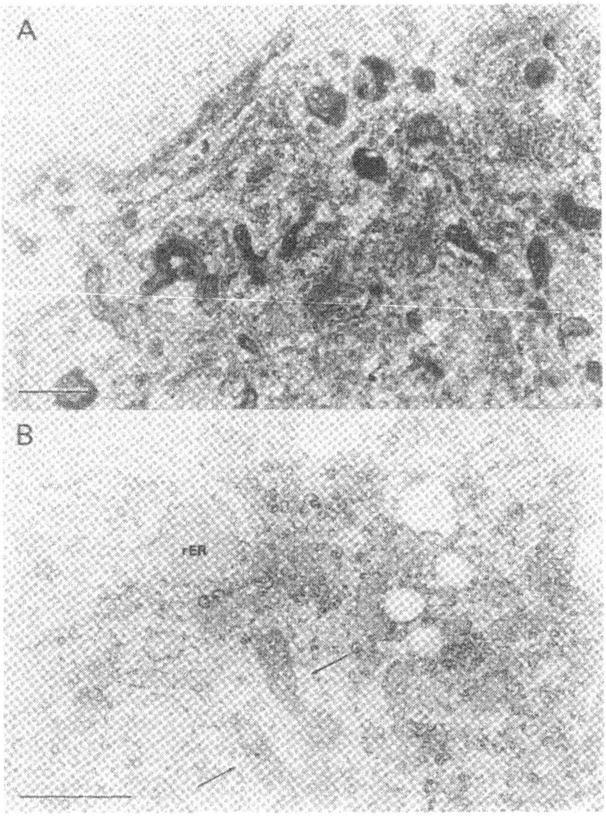

Fig. 4. Transmission electron micrographs of endothelial cells cultured from human umbilical cord vein and incubated with 1.0 nmol/ml of linoleic acid hydroperoxide. A shows the increased number of organelles around the nucleus. B shows changes in the peripheral region of the cell. rER indicates an enlarged rough-surfaced endoplasmic reticulum. Arrows show mitochondria. Bar, 1 μm.

Table 2. Effect of linoleic acid hydroperoxide on respiration of cultured endothelial and smooth muscle cells from fetal calf aorta

Linoleic acid hydroperoxide (nmol/ml)	Cell respiration (nmol O_2/min/10^6 cells)	
	Endothelial cells	Smooth muscle cells
None	161 (100)[a]	619 (100)
0.05	142 (88)	617 (100)
0.1	99 (62)	543 (88)
0.5	72 (45)	467 (75)
1.0	22 (14)	331 (54)

[a]The values in parentheses are percentages; the values obtained without addition of linoleic acid hydroperoxide were set equal to 100%.

of organelles was rather decreased, differing from the cases in which lower concentrations of linoleic acid hydroperoxide were used. On the other hand, the rough-surfaced endoplasmic reticulum was markedly dilated and contained translucent cisternae. Upon a further increase of the concentration of linoleic acid hydroperoxide to 7.5 nmol/ml, the cytoplasm of the endothelial cell was filled with numerous vacuoles that seemed to be derived from denatured rough-surfaced endoplasmic reticulum. Another remarkable finding was the change in the form of the mitochondria: the normally elongated shape of the mitochondria had changed to a round form.

Then, the effect of linoleic acid hydroperoxide on cultured smooth muscle cells from human umbilical cord artery was studied (Sasaguri et al., 1985a). The cells were characterized by their "hill and valley" growth, and electron microscopic observation revealed the occurrence in their cytoplasm of abundant microfilaments with dense bodies, which are characteristic fine structures of cultured smooth muscle cells. Electron microscopic examination of the hydroperoxide-treated cultured smooth muscle cells revealed that incubation of the cells with 5.0 nmol/ml (in terms of malondialdehyde) of the hydroperoxide for 3 h caused a decrease in electron density of the mitochondrial matrix and that dilatation of the rough-surfaced endoplasmic reticulum occurred when the cells were incubated with 10 nmol/ml of the hydroperoxide. These concentrations are higher by one order of magnitude than those required for the same effects on cultured endothelial cells from human umbilical cord vein. A similar difference in susceptibility to injury by linoleic acid hydroperoxide was found between cultured endothelial and smooth muscle cells from fetal calf aorta.

To verify further the difference in susceptibility to lipid peroxides between endothelial cells and smooth muscle cells, we carried out an experiment to measure cellular respiration. As summarized in Table 2, the inhibitory effect was dose-dependent for both endothelial and smooth muscle cells, and the effect clearly manifested itself in the endothelial cells at a lower concentration than in the smooth muscle cells.

These results indicate that the smooth muscle cells are more resistant to lipid peroxides than are the endothelial cells and that they can survive when the endothelial cells are killed by lipid peroxides.

INHIBITION OF PROSTACYCLIN BIOSYNTHESIS BY LIPID PEROXIDES

When the intima of the artery is injured, platelet aggregation is provoked and aggregates adhere to the injured site, as demonstrated by the animal experiment described in a previous section. Relating to this phenomenon, it should be mentioned that prostacyclin synthesized in the artery has a potent inhibitory effect on both platelet aggregation and adherence of aggregated platelets to the luminal surface of the artery. Again lipid peroxides have a deleterious effect in this respect, for it has been reported that lipid peroxides inhibit prostacyclin biosynthesis in isolated rabbit aorta (Moncada *et al.*, 1976a), rat aorta (Bunting *et al.*, 1976; Szczeklik and Gryglewski, 1980; Valentovic *et al.*, 1982), bovine coronary artery (Szczeklik and Gryglewski; 1980), pig aortic microsomes (Gryglewski

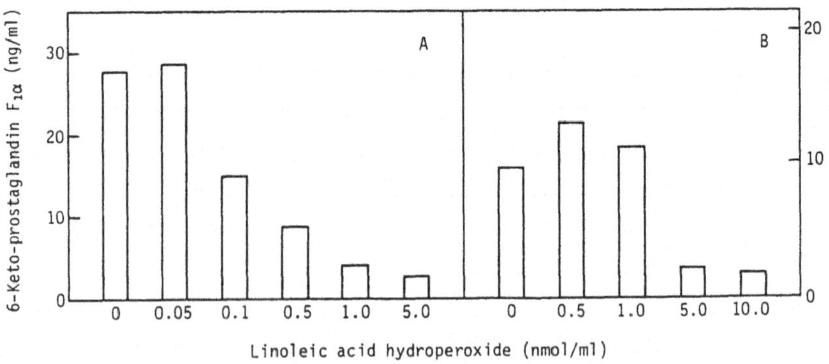

Fig. 5. Effect of linoleic acid hydroperoxide on prostacyclin biosynthesis in cultured endothelial cells from human umbilical cord vein (A) and in cultured smooth muscle cells from rabbit aorta (B). Prostacyclin synthesized per dish was shown by the amount of its stable product, 6-keto-prostaglandin $F_{1\alpha}$ (ng/ml). Mean of three experiments is given.

et al., 1976; Moncada *et al.*, 1976b), and cultured endothelial cells form human umbilical cord (Marcus *et al.*, 1978). We also examined the effect of linoleic acid hydroperoxide on prostacyclin biosynthesis in the endothelial cells in comparison with that in the smooth muscle cells (Sasaguri *et al.*, 1985b). The results are shown in Fig. 5. As can be seen in Fig. 5A, incubation of the endothelial cells with linoleic acid hydroperoxide up to 0.05 nmol/ml had no effect on the amount of prostacyclin synthesized, whereas that with above 0.1 nmol/ml of the hydroperoxide inhibited prostacyclin biosynthesis. The inhibition was dose-dependent. The effect in the case of the smooth muscle cells is shown in Fig. 5B. By increasing the concentration of linoleic acid hydroperoxide, we observed that the amount of prostacyclin synthesized was not changed by incubation of the cells with up to 1.0 nmol/ml of the hydroperoxide and that the amount finally decreased when the cells were incubated with over 5.0 nmol/ml of the hydroperoxide. Comparing the data obtained with cultured endothelial cells with those obtained with cultured smooth muscle cells, we noted that, in the absence of linoleic acid hydroperoxide, the amount of prostacyclin synthesized per dish was larger in the endothelial cells than in the smooth muscle cells, and that inhibition of prostacyclin biosynthesis in the endothelial cells occurred at lower concentrations of linoleic acid hydroperoxide than those required for similar inhibition in the smooth muscle cells. In other words, the endothelial cells are more susceptible to the inhibitory effect of the hydroperoxide on prostacyclin biosynthesis than are the smooth muscle cells. Although arterial smooth muscle cells *in vivo* would probably still be active in prostacyclin biosynthesis when the endothelial cells had become inactive due to lipid peroxide-induced injury, the decreased synthesis of prostacyclin in the latter cells would facilitate the aggregation of platelets and their adherence to the injured site. From these aggregates, a growth factor which causes smooth muscle cells to proliferate is released (Baumgartner and Studer, 1977, Moore *et al.*, 1977; Ross and Vogel, 1978). Chemoattractants, such as 12-L-hydroxy-5,8,10,14-eicosatetraenoic acid, released from platelets force smooth muscle cells to migrate from their normal medial site to the intima (Nakao *et al.*, 1983). Judging from the lower susceptibility to lipid peroxides of the smooth muscle cells, it is reasonable to consider that they are active when the endothelial cells are injured. Therefore, upon reaching the intima, they proliferate, take up cholesterol, and synthesize connective tissue proteins, resulting in the thickening of the intima and the ultimate formation of the atheromatous plaque.

EFFECT OF LIPID PEROXIDES ON UPTAKE OF LOW DENSITY LIPOPROTEIN BY SMOOTH MUSCLE CELLS

When endothelial cells are injured as mentioned above, lipid peroxides as well as lipoproteins such as low density lipoprotein (LDL) might reach the medial cell layer more easily, and a direct effect of the hydroperoxides on the smooth muscle cells there can be expected. This effect can also be expected when the smooth muscle cells migrate and proliferate as described in the previous section. To study this problem, we used cultured smooth muscle cells from rabbit aorta (Nishigaki et al., 1984).

Figure 6 shows the effect of linoleic acid hydroperoxide on the binding of LDL to cultured smooth muscle cells. The cells were incubated with ^{125}I-labelled LDL ([^{125}I]LDL) at 4°C for the periods indicated. As represented by curve I, the binding was not significant in the absence of the hydroperoxide. However, when the cells were incubated with [^{125}I]LDL in the presence of 3 nmol/ml of the hydroperoxide, a definite amount of the lipoprotein was bound to the cells, as indicated by curve II. In the presence of 6 nmol/ml, the binding was further increased, as shown by curve

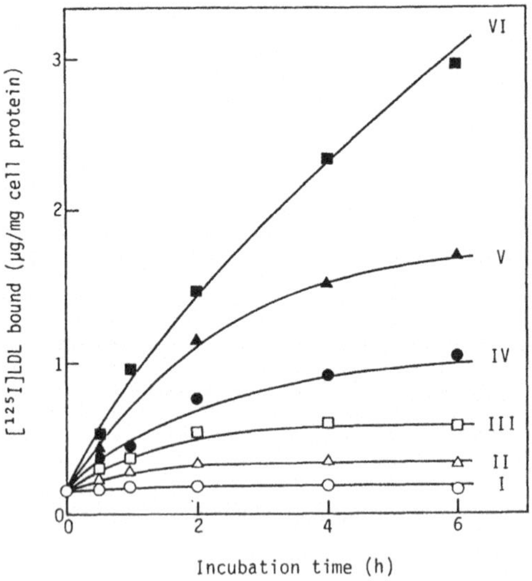

Fig. 6. Effect of linoleic acid hydroperoxide on binding of [^{125}I]LDL to cultured smooth muscle cells from rabbit aorta. Cells were incubated for the indicated times with 10 μg/ml of [^{125}I]LDL either at 4°C (open symbols) or 37°C (closed symbols) in the absence (I,IV) or presence of 3 nmol/ml (II,V) or 6 nmol/ml (III,VI) of linoleic acid hydroperoxide. After the incubation, cells were separated from the medium, washed, and their radioactivity measured.

III. When incubation was carried out at 37°C, a considerable binding of [^{125}I]LDL occurred in the absence of the hydroperoxide (curve IV). The binding was increased in the presence of 3 nmol/ml of the hydroperoxide (curve V) and further increased in the presence of 6 nmol/ml of it (curve VI).

Figure 7 shows the effect of linoleic acid hydroperoxide on the degradation of LDL taken up by cultured smooth muscle cells from rabbit aorta. After the cells were incubated with [^{125}I]LDL at 37°C for the periods indicated, the radioactivity of the degraded apoprotein of LDL appearing in the medium was measured. The degradation rate of the control is shown by curve I. On incubation in the presence of 3 nmol/ml of linoleic acid hydroperoxide, the rate of degradation was increased as indicated by curve II, and further increased in the presence of 6 nmol/ml of the hydroperoxide (curve III). This acceleration of the internalization and degradation seems to depend on that of the uptake of LDL by the cells.

To determine whether the hydroperoxide interacts predominantly with LDL or the cells to produce its effect on binding of LDL to the cells, treatment of [^{125}I]LDL or the cells with the hydroperoxide prior to the

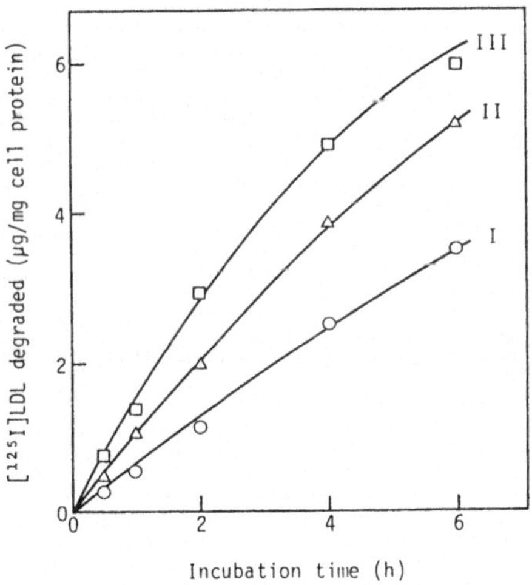

Fig. 7. Effect of linoleic acid hydroperoxide on degradation of [^{125}I]LDL in cultured smooth muscle cells from rabbit aorta. Cells were incubated for the indicated times with 10 µg/ml of [^{125}I]LDL at 37°C in the absence (I) or presence of 3 nmol/ml (II) or 6 nmol/ml (III) of linoleic acid hydroperoxide. After the incubation, the medium was separated from the cells, and the radioactivity in the trichloroacetic acid-soluble fraction of the medium was measured.

binding was carried out. The pretreatment of [^{125}I]LDL was performed by its incubation with definite concentrations of the hydroperoxide at 25°C for 3 h, followed by gel filtration on a Sephadex G-25 column; and the pretreatment of the cells, by their incubation with the hydroperoxide at 37°C for 3 h, followed by washing of the cells three times with Eagle's MEM. Figure 8 shows the binding of hydroperoxide-pretreated [^{125}I]LDL to the cells. As shown in the figure, treatment with low concentrations of the hydroperoxide slightly increased the binding. However, the binding was rather decreased at higher concentrations (3-6 nmol/ml) of the hydroperoxide. Figure 9 shows the binding of [^{125}I]LDL to the cells pretreated with the hydroperoxide, in which case the binding was remarkably increased. These results suggest that the effect of the hydroperoxide on LDL uptake by cultured smooth muscle cells occurs mainly *via* its action on the cells.

It is well known that LDL carries cholesterol into cells (Brown and Goldstein, 1976; Goldstein and Brown, 1977; Goldstein *et al.*, 1979). If we neglect any change in the metabolic processing of cholesterol in the smooth muscle cells, the increase in the binding of LDL to the cells, followed by

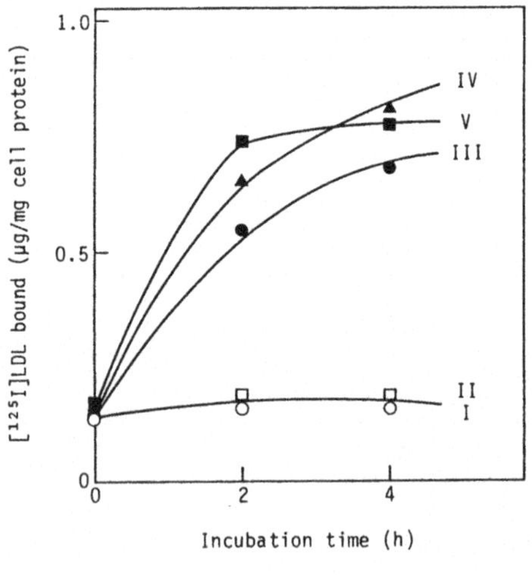

Fig. 8. Binding of [^{125}I]LDL pretreated with linoleic acid hydroperoxide to cultured smooth muscle cells from rabbit aorta. Treatment of [^{125}I]LDL was performed by incubation of it with definite concentrations of linoleic acid hydroperoxide at 25°C for 3 h, followed by gel filtration on a Sephadex G-25 column. Cells were incubated for the indicated times at either 4°C (open symbols) or 37°C (closed symbols) in 1.5 ml of Eagle's MEM containing 7.5 mg of bovine serum albumin and 15 μg of untreated [^{125}I]LDL (I,III) or that pretreated with 0.5 nmol/ml (IV) or 1.0 nmol/ml (II,V) of the hydroperoxide.

its internalization and degradation, leads us to consider that cholesterol should tend to accumulate in the cells. To check this point, we carried out morphological examination on cultured smooth muscle cells (Yagi et al., 1987). When the cells were incubated with either linoleic acid hydroperoxide or LDL, no significant accumulation of lipids was found in the cells. However, when the cells were pretreated with 3 nmol/ml of linoleic acid hydroperoxide at 37°C for 3 h and incubated with LDL, remarkable deposits of lipids were observed. In other words, the cells became lipid-laden.

EFFECT OF LIPID PEROXIDES ON UPTAKE OF LOW DENSITY LIPOPROTEIN BY MACROPHAGES

As another origin of lipid-laden cells, macrophages have been regarded as a possible candidate. Accordingly, we examined the effect of lipid peroxides on the possible formation of lipid-laden cells from macrophages (Yagi et al., 1987). Macrophages were obtained by culturing monocytes

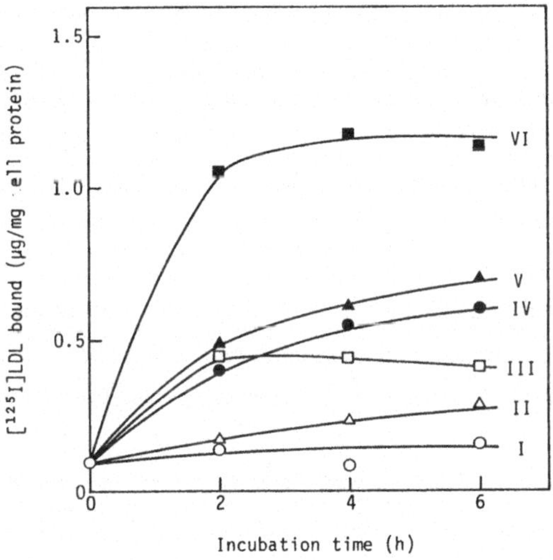

Fig. 9. Binding of $[^{125}I]$LDL to linoleic acid hydroperoxide-pretreated smooth muscle cells cultured from rabbit aorta. Treatment of the cells was performed by incubation of them with definite concentrations of linoleic acid hydroperoxide at 37°C for 3 h, followed by washing of the cells three times with Eagle's MEM. Untreated cells (I,IV) or those pretreated with 0.5 nmol/ml (II,V) or 3 nmol/ml (III,VI) of the hydroperoxide were incubated in 1.5 ml of Eagle's MEM containing 7.5 mg of bovine serum albumin and 15 µg of $[^{125}I]$LDL at either 4°C (open symbols) or 37°C (closed symbols) for the indicated times.

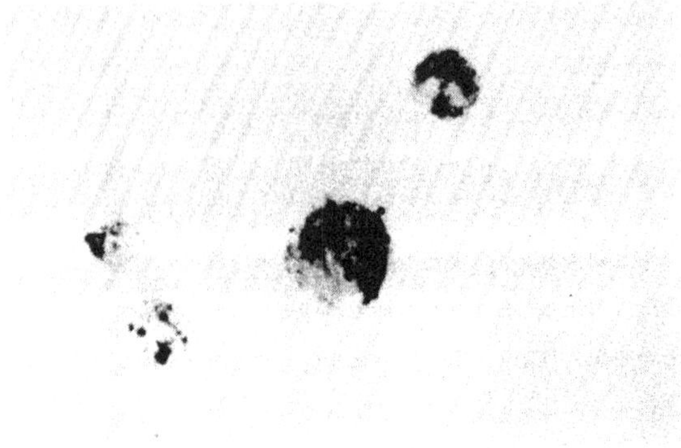

Fig. 10. Formation of lipid-laden cells from rabbit peripheral macrophages. Macrophages were derived from peripheral blood monocytes. LDL was preincubated with 5 nmol/ml of linoleic acid hydroperoxide at 25°C for 3 h. Macrophages were incubated for 6 days at 37°C in an atmosphere of 95% air and 5% CO_2 with hydroperoxide-pretreated LDL (12 mg in terms of cholesterol/ml). After fixation in 10% formalin, the cells were stained with Oil red O.

separated from rabbit blood, and similar experiments as those with smooth muscle cells were carried out. Light microscopic observation revealed that incubation of the cells with either linoleic acid hydroperoxide or LDL produced no significant deposition of lipids in the cells. However, when LDL was preincubated with linoleic acid hydroperoxide, enormous deposits of lipids were found in the cells, as shown in Fig. 10. Relating to this fact, it was found that susceptibility of macrophages to lipid peroxides is lower than that of the endothelial cells; and, therefore, macrophages are active when the endothelial cells are injured (unpublished results). Thus, macrophages recognize LDL as a foreign body, provided the LDL is modified by lipid peroxides, and scavenge it. Thereby, the macrophages become lipid-laden.

Since lipid-laden cells derived from macrophages as well as from smooth muscle cells would contribute to the formation of the atheromatous plaque, lipid peroxides associated with or incorporated into these cells would remain, or even propagate the formation of additional lipid peroxides, in the plaque. Lipid peroxides that injured the endothelial cells would behave in a similar way. Accordingly, the original finding of lipid peroxides in the atheromatous plaque by Glavind _et al_. (1952) and the demonstration of hydroperoxy derivatives of cholesterol linoleate in such plaques by Harland _et al_. (1971) become understandable.

REFERENCES

Baumgartner, H.R. and Studer, A., 1977. Platelet factors and the proliferation of vascular smooth muscle cells. In: G. Schettler, Y. Goto, Y. Hata and G. Klose (Editors), Atherosclerosis. Springer-Verlag, Heidelberg, Vol. IV, pp. 605-609.

Brown, M.S., Ho, Y.K. and Goldstein, J.L., 1976. The low-density lipoprotein pathway in human fibroblasts: relation between cell-surface-receptor binding and endocytosis of low-density lipoprotein. Ann. N. Y. Acad. Sci., 275: 244-257.

Bunting, S., Gryglewski, R.J., Moncada, S. and Vane, J.R., 1976. Arterial walls generate from prostaglandin endoperoxides a substance (prostaglandin X) which relaxes strips of mesenteric and coeliac arteries and inhibits platelet aggregation. Prostaglandins, 12: 897-913.

Cutler, M.G. and Schneider, R., 1974. Linoleate oxidation products and cardiovascular lesions. Atherosclerosis, 20: 383-394.

Glavind, J., Hartmann, S., Clemmesen, J., Jessen, K.E. and Dam, H., 1952. Studies on the role of lipoperoxides in human pathology II. The presence of peroxidized lipids in the atherosclerotic aorta. Acta Pathol., 30: 1-6.

Goldstein, J.L. and Brown, M.S., 1977. The low-density lipoprotein pathway and its relation to atherosclerosis. Ann. Rev. Biochem., 46: 897-930.

Goldstein, J.L., Ho, Y.K., Basu, S.K. and Brown, M.S., 1979. Binding site on macrophages that mediates uptake and degradation of acetylated low-density lipoprotein, producing massive cholesterol deposition. Proc. Natl. Acad. Sci. USA, 76: 333-337.

Gryglewski, R.J., Bunting, S., Moncada, S., Flower, R.J. and Vane, J.R., 1976. Arterial walls are protected against deposition of platelet thrombi by a substance (prostaglandin X) which they make from prostaglandin endoperoxides. Prostaglandins, 12: 685-713.

Harland, W.A., Gilbert, J.D., Steel, G. and Brooks, C.J.W., 1971. Lipids of human atheroma. Part 5. The occurrence of a new group of polar sterol esters in various stages of human atherosclerosis. Atherosclerosis, 13: 239-246.

Kagami, M., Iwashiro, Y., Kawamoto, M., Takaoka, S., Kato, T., Kasahara, N., Atarashi, J., Terashi, A., Nagatsumi, A., Miyazaki, T., Katsuragi, R. and Sakai, H., 1978. Relationship between lipid peroxide and tocopherol in sera of patients with acute cerebral vascular disorders. J. Lipid Peroxide Res., 2: 115-118.

Kawamoto, M., Kagami, M. and Terashi, A., 1986. Serum lipid peroxide level in apoplexia. J. Clin. Biochem. Nutr., 1: 1-3.

Kibata, M., Shimizu, Y., Miyake, K., Shimono, M., Shoji, K., Miyahara, K., Fuchimoto, T. and Nasu. Y., 1977. Alpha-tocopherol and TBA reactive substance (TBARS) in serum of the stroke at acute stage. Igaku no Ayumi, 101: 591-592.

Marcus, A.J., Weksler, B.B. and Jaffe, E.A., 1978. Enzymatic conversion of prostaglandin endoperoxide H_2 and arachidonic acid to prostacyclin by cultured human endothelial cells. J. Biol. Chem., 253: 7138-7141.

Moncada, S., Gryglewski, R.J., Bunting, S. and Vane, J.R., 1976a. An enzyme isolated from arteries transforms prostaglandin endoperoxides to an unstable substance that inhibits platelet aggregation. Nature, 263: 663-665.

Moncada, S., Gryglewski, R.J., Bunting, S. and Vane, J.R., 1976b. A lipid peroxide inhibits the enzyme in blood vessel microsomes that generates from prostaglandin endoperoxides the substance (prostaglandin X) which prevents platelet aggregation. Prostaglandins, 12: 715-737.

Moore, S., Mustard, J., Packham, M.A. and Kinlough-Rathbone, R.L., 1977.

Thrombosis and endothelial injury in atherogenesis. In: G. Schettler, Y. Goto, Y. Hata and G. Klose (Editors). Atherosclerosis. Springer-Verlag, Heidelberg, Vol. IV, pp. 601-605.
Nakao, J., Ito, H., Ooyama, T., Chang, W.-C. and Murota, S., 1983. Calcium dependency of aortic smooth muscle cell migration induced by 12-L-hydroxy-5,8,10,14-eicosatetraenoic acid. Effect of A23187, nicardipine and trifluoperazine. Atherosclerosis, 46: 309-319.
Nishigaki, I., Hagihara, M., Maseki, M., Tomoda, Y., Nagayama, K., Nakashima, T. and Yagi, K., 1984. Effect of linoleic acid hydroperoxide on uptake of low density lipoprotein by cultured smooth muscle cells from rabbit aorta. Biochem. Int., 8: 501-506.
Ohkawa, H., Ohishi, N. and Yagi, K., 1979. Assay for lipid peroxides in animal tissues by thiobarbituric acid reaction. Anal. Biochem., 95: 351-358.
Ross, R. and Vogel, A., 1978. The platelet-derived growth factor. Cell, 14: 203-210.
Sasaguri, Y., Nakashima, T., Morimatsu, M. and Yagi, K., 1984. Injury to cultured endothelial cells from human umbilical vein by linoleic acid hydroperoxide. J. Appl. Biochem., 6: 144-150.
Sasaguri, Y., Morimatsu, M., Kinoshita, T., Nakashima, T., Inagaki, T. and Yagi, K., 1985a. Difference in susceptibility to injury by linoleic acid hydroperoxide between endothelial and smooth muscle cells of arteries. J. Appl. Biochem., 7: 70-78.
Sasaguri, Y., Morimatsu, M., Nakashima, T., Tokunaga, O. and Yagi, K., 1985b. Difference in the inhibitory effect of linoleic acid hydroperoxide on prostacyclin biosynthesis between cultured endothelial cells from human umbilical cord vein and cultured smooth muscle cells from rabbit aorta. Biochem. Int., 11: 517-521.
Sato, Y., Hotta, N., Sakamoto, N., Matsuoka, S., Ohishi, N. and Yagi, K., 1979. Lipid peroxide level in plasma of diabetic patients. Biochem. Med., 21: 104-107.
Seder, A.W., Silver, M.J., Kocsis, J.J. and Smith, J.B., 1978. Fatty acids and the initial events of endothelial damage seen by scanning and transmission electron microscopy. Atherosclerosis, 30: 273-284.
Szczeklik, A. and Gryglewski, R.J., 1980. Low density lipoproteins (LDL) are carriers for lipid peroxides and inhibit prostacylin (PGI_2) biosyntheis in arteries. Artery, 7: 488-495.
Tomita, I., Sano, M., Serizawa, S., Ohta, K. and Katou, M., 1979. Fluctuation of lipid peroxides and related enzyme activities at time of stroke in stroke-prone spontaneously hypertensive rats. Stroke, 10: 323-326.
Yagi, K., 1976. A simple fluorometric assay for lipoperoxide in blood plasma. Biochem. Med., 15: 212-216.
Yagi, K., Ohkawa, H., Ohishi, N., Yamashita, M. and Nakashima, T., 1981. Lesion of aortic intima caused by intravenous administration of linoleic acid hydroperoxide. J. Appl. Biochem., 3: 58-65.
Yagi, K., Inagaki, T., Sasaguri, Y., Nakano, R. and Nakashima, T., 1987. Formation of lipid-laden cells from cultured arterial smooth muscle cells and macrophages of rabbits. J. Clin. Biochem. Nutr., in press.
Yoshikawa, T., Yamaguchi, K., Kondo, M., Mizukawa, N., Ohta, T. and Hirakawa, K., 1982. Thiobarbituric acid reactive substances and vitamin E in serum and cerebrospinal fluid from patients with cerebral apoplexy. Arch. Gerontol. Geriatr., 1: 209-218.
Valentovic, M.A., Gairola, C. and Lubawy, W.C., 1982. Lung, aorta, and platelet metabolism of ^{14}C-arachidonic acid in vitamin E deficient rats. Prostaglandins, 24: 215-224.

GPSR Compliance

The European Union's (EU) General Product Safety Regulation (GPSR) is a set of rules that requires consumer products to be safe and our obligations to ensure this.

If you have any concerns about our products, you can contact us on ProductSafety@springernature.com

In case Publisher is established outside the EU, the EU authorized representative is:

Springer Nature Customer Service Center GmbH
Europaplatz 3
69115 Heidelberg, Germany